Heart Disease
Second Edition

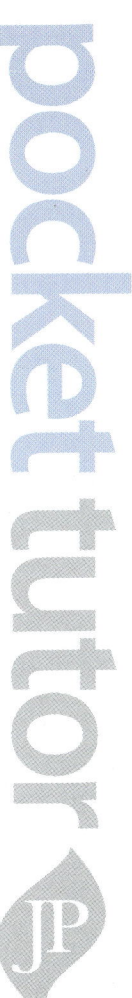

Heart Disease
Second Edition

Ravish Katira MBBS(Hons.) MD(Medicine) DM(Cardiology) FRCP(London)

Professor
Institute of Health Sciences
University of Greater Manchester
Bolton
Consultant Cardiologist
Merseyside & West Lancashire NHS Teaching Hospitals
Whiston Hospital
Merseyside, UK

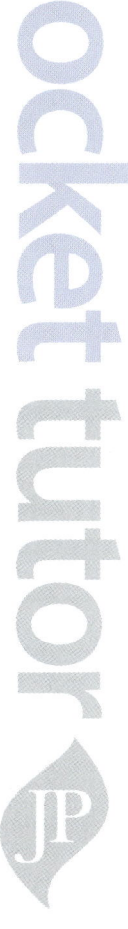

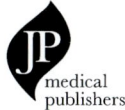

© 2026 JP Medical Ltd.

First Edition 2016

Published by JP Medical Ltd,
83 Victoria Street, London,
SW1H 0HW, UK
Tel: +44 (0)20 3170 8910
Email: info@jpmedpub.com
Web: www.jpmedpub.com

EU GPSR Authorised Representative
Logos Europe, 9 rue Nicolas Poussin
17000, La Rochelle, France
Phone: +33 (0) 6 67 93 73 78
E-mail: Contact@logoseurope.eu

The rights of Ravish Katira to be identified as the authors of this work have been asserted by them in accordance with the Copyright, Designs and Patents Act 1988.

All rights reserved. No part of this publication may be reproduced, stored or transmitted in any form or by any means, electronic, mechanical, photocopying, recording or otherwise, except as permitted by the UK Copyright, Designs and Patents Act 1988, without the prior permission in writing of the publishers. Permissions may be sought directly from JP Medical Ltd at the address printed above.

All brand names and product names used in this book are trade names, service marks, trademarks or registered trademarks of their respective owners. The publisher is not associated with any product or vendor mentioned in this book.

Medical knowledge and practice change constantly. This book is designed to provide accurate, authoritative information about the subject matter in question. However readers are advised to check the most current information available on procedures included and check information from the manufacturer of each product to be administered, to verify the recommended dose, formula, method and duration of administration, adverse effects and contraindications. It is the responsibility of the practitioner to take all appropriate safety precautions. Neither the publisher nor the authors assume any liability for any injury and/or damage to persons or property arising from or related to use of material in this book.

This book is sold on the understanding that the publisher is not engaged in providing professional medical services. If such advice or services are required, the services of a competent medical professional should be sought.

ISBN: 978-1-78779-194-7

British Library Cataloguing in Publication Data
A catalogue record for this book is available from the British Library

Library of Congress Cataloging in Publication Data
A catalog record for this book is available from the Library of Congress

Project Manager:	Bhavana Sharma
Editorial Assistant:	Keshav Kumar Baghel
Cover Design:	Seema Dogra

Preface

Coronary heart disease is the most common cause of death in the world. Many of the factors which place people at risk of coronary heart disease, such as physical inactivity, obesity, smoking and a diet high in fat and salt, are avoidable. A challenge for clinicians is that coronary heart disease develops silently over many years before manifesting as chest pain, heart attack, arrhythmia, heart failure or even sudden cardiac death.

Conditions such as hypertension, diabetes mellitus and hypercholesterolaemia can be considered as silent killers because these also predispose to atherosclerosis, the underlying cause of coronary heart disease, and are associated with few, if any, symptoms.

"Pocket Tutor Heart Disease" reinforces important principles and improves understanding of the basic science and clinical management of coronary heart disease, from atherosclerosis to the complications of acute myocardial infarction. We hope that this deeper understanding enables all healthcare professionals to improve coronary heart disease prevention and care for their patients more effectively when the disease manifests clinically. Lastly, a word on terminology: this book is called *"Pocket Tutor Heart Disease"* in the interests of brevity. The focus is upon coronary heart disease, its signs, symptoms, risk factors, presentations, and complications. That is the scope of this book.

Ravish Katira
June, 2025

Contents

Preface v
Acknowledgements ix

Chapter 1 First principles
1.1 Cardiovascular anatomy 2
1.2 Development of the cardiovascular system 22
1.3 Cardiovascular physiology 27

Chapter 2 Clinical essentials
2.1 History taking 90
2.2 Cardiovascular examination 103
2.3 Investigations 124
2.4 Cardiovascular risk assessment 145
2.5 Conservative management 146
2.6 Medication 149
2.7 Surgical management 164

Chapter 3 Atherosclerosis
3.1 Clinical scenario 169
3.2 Atherosclerosis 171

Chapter 4 Hypertension
4.1 Clinical scenario 183
4.2 Essential hypertension 185
4.3 Secondary hypertension 198
4.4 Hypertensive emergencies 202

Chapter 5 Hyperlipidaemia
5.1 Clinical scenario 205
5.2 Hyperlipidaemia 208
5.3 Familial hypercholesterolaemia 219

Chapter 6 Coronary heart disease
6.1 Clinical scenario 223
6.2 Angina 227

6.3	Acute coronary syndromes	235
6.4	Complications of myocardial infarction	244

Chapter 7 Arrhythmias

7.1	Clinical scenario	249
7.2	Mechanisms of arrhythmia	252
7.3	Bradyarrhythmias	258
7.4	Tachyarrhythmias	266
7.5	Atrial fibrillation	278

Chapter 8 Heart failure

8.1	Clinical scenario	285
8.2	Chronic heart failure	289
8.3	Acute heart failure	304

Chapter 9 Prevention of cardiovascular disease

9.1	Preventive measures	309
9.2	Secondary prevention/cardiac rehabilitation	318

Index   *321*

Acknowledgements

Figures 1.28, 1.30, 1.31, 1.35, 1.39, 1.40 and 1.41 are reproduced from: Mann J, Marples D. Eureka Physiology. London: JP Medical, 2015.

Figures 1.42, 1.43, 1.44, 1.45, 1.46, 1.47, 1.48, 1.49, 1.50 and 1.51 are reproduced from: Davison A, Milan A, Phillips S, Ranganath L. Eureka: Biochemistry & Metabolism. London: JP Medical, 2015.

Figure 2.2 is reproduced from: Craythorne E, Daly ML. Pocket Tutor Dermatology. London: JP Medical, 2015.

Figure 2.12 is reproduced from: Parker S. Eureka: General Surgery & Urology. London: JP Medical, 2015.

Figure 2.13 is copyright of Sam Scott-Hunter and reproduced from: Tunstall R, Shah N. Pocket Tutor Surface Anatomy. London: JP Medical, 2012.

Figure 2.14 is reproduced from: Borooah S, Wright M, Dhillon B. Pocket Tutor Ophthalmology. London: JP Medical, 2012.

Figure 2.19 is reproduced from: James S, Nelson K. Pocket Tutor ECG Interpretation. London: JP Medical, 2011.

First principles

chapter 1

The heart beats from the 3rd week of embryonic life until the moment of death – more than 3 billion times in a lifetime. Only the size of a fist and weighing 300 g, the heart pumps > 7,000 L of blood per day through nearly 100,000 km of blood vessels. The main purpose of the cardiovascular system (**Figure 1.1**) is to transport substances around the body, including:

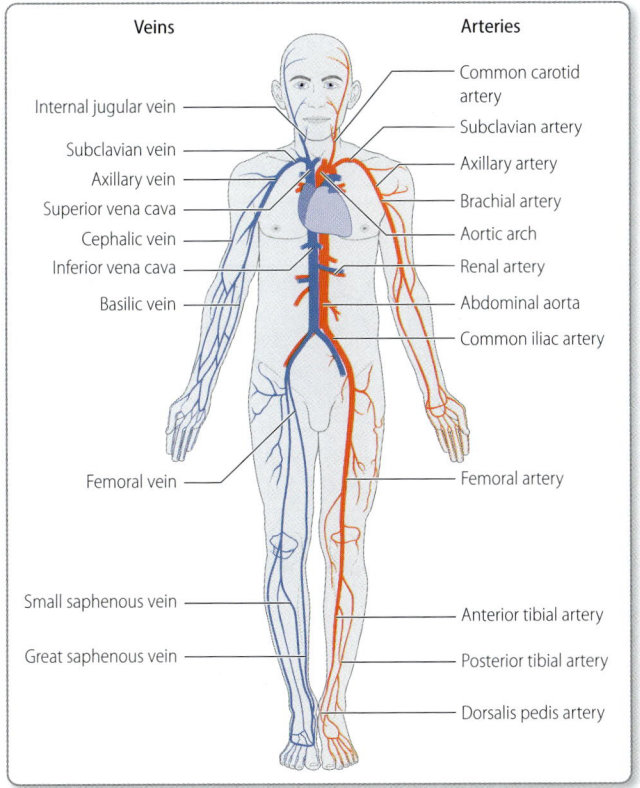

Figure 1.1 The cardiovascular system.

- Oxygen (O_2) and nutrients (e.g. glucose and amino acids) to tissues
- Waste products [e.g. carbon dioxide (CO_2), urea and lactate] from tissues
- Fluids and electrolytes
- Hormones to target organs
- White blood cells
- Clotting factors and platelets
- Heat, to aid thermoregulation

1.1 Cardiovascular anatomy

Heart

The heart is composed of muscle arranged around a framework of fibrous tissue and is the size of a fist. The two atria collect blood and fill the two ventricles, which pump blood into the pulmonary and systemic circulations (**Figure 1.2**). Its four valves prevent blood flow in the wrong direction.

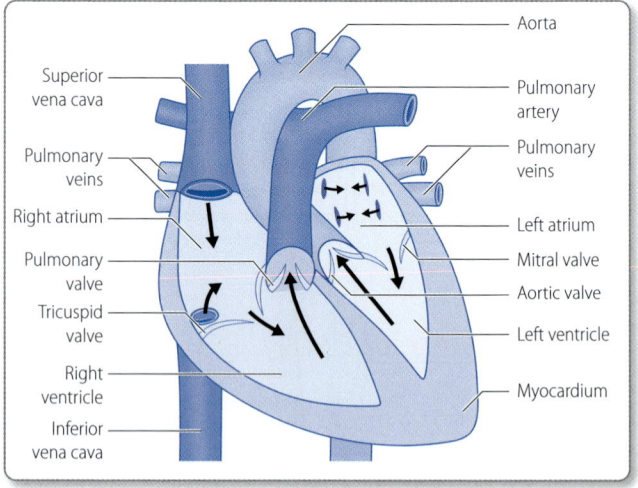

Figure 1.2 The heart.

Cardiomyocytes are the main cells of the heart. The interstitium between them contains collagen, elastin, fibrous connective tissue, blood and lymphatic vessels.

Surface anatomy and relations

The heart is in the middle mediastinum with its apex pointing inferolaterally (**Figures 1.3** and **1.4**). It is posterior to the

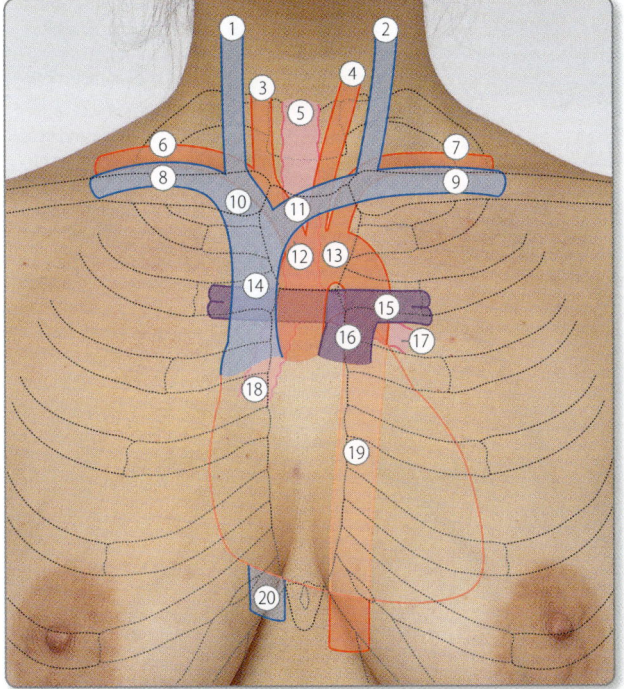

Figure 1.3 Surface anatomy of the heart and great vessels. ①, right internal jugular vein; ②, left internal jugular vein; ③, right common carotid artery; ④, left common carotid artery; ⑤, trachea; ⑥, right subclavian artery; ⑦, left subclavian artery; ⑧, right subclavian vein; ⑨, left subclavian vein; ⑩, right brachiocephalic vein; ⑪, left brachiocephalic vein; ⑫, brachiocephalic trunk; ⑬, arch of aorta; ⑭, superior vena cava; ⑮, left pulmonary artery; ⑯, pulmonary trunk; ⑰, left main bronchus; ⑱, right main bronchus; ⑲, descending aorta; and ⑳, inferior vena cava.

First principles

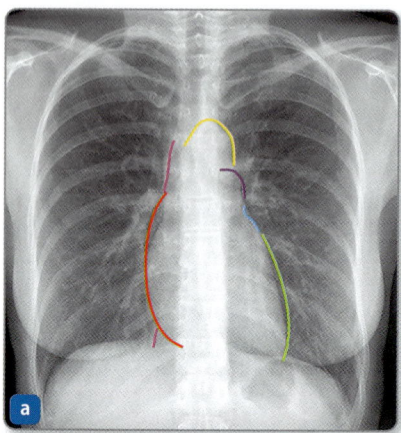

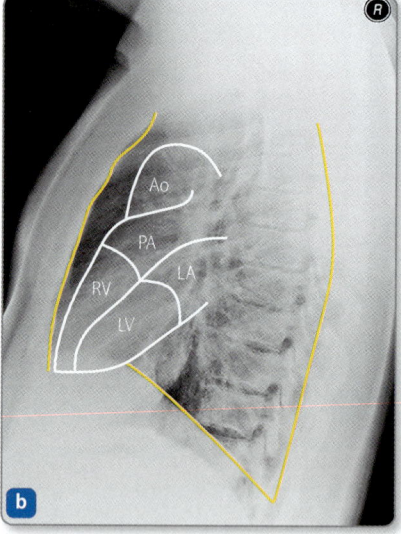

Figure 1.4 Radiographs showing the borders of the heart and great vessels. (a) Frontal view. The right heart border (red) is formed mainly by the right atrium. The left heart border is formed mainly by the left ventricle (LV, green) and the left atrium (LA, blue). The inferior surface (against the diaphragm) represents the right ventricle (RV).

Note: The vena cava (pink) is above and below the border of the right heart, and the aortic arch (yellow) and pulmonary trunk (purple) are above the left atrium. (b) Lateral view. The anterior, posterior and inferior relations of the heart (orange) are formed by the sternum or left lung pleura, thoracic spine and diaphragm, respectively. Ao, aorta; PA, pulmonary artery.

sternum, costal cartilages and left lung pleura and superior to the left diaphragm. Structures adjacent to the posterior heart are the thoracic vertebrae, oesophagus and descending aorta (**Table 1.1**).

Cardiac surface	Main structure	Extracardiac relation
Anterior (sternocostal)	Right ventricle	Sternum
		Costal cartilages
		Left lung pleura
Posterior (base)	Left atrium	Thoracic vertebrae
		Oesophagus
		Descending aorta
Inferior	Left ventricle	Left haemidiaphragm
Apex	Left ventricle	Sternum
		Costal cartilages
		Left lung pleura

Table 1.1 The structures and borders of the four cardiac surfaces.

Chambers and valves

The heart has four muscular chambers, each connected to a great vessel. The four valves lie between the ventricles and atria and the ventricles and the great arteries (**Figure 1.5**).

Left atrium

The mitral orifice and valve separate the left atrium and ventricle. The atrium receives its blood supply from the left circumflex coronary artery. The left atrial appendage or left auricle is a muscular outpouching continuous with the left atrium. The left and right atria are separated by the interatrial septum.

Mitral valve

The mitral valve prevents blood regurgitating back into the left atrium during systole. It has two leaflets (i.e. it is bicuspid):
1. The anterior leaflet attaches to the anterior aspect of the mitral orifice
2. The posterior leaflet attaches to the posterior orifice

The free edges of the leaflets are attached to the chordae tendineae, which attach to the left ventricular papillary muscles. This subvalvular apparatus prevents valve prolapse during systole.

6   First principles

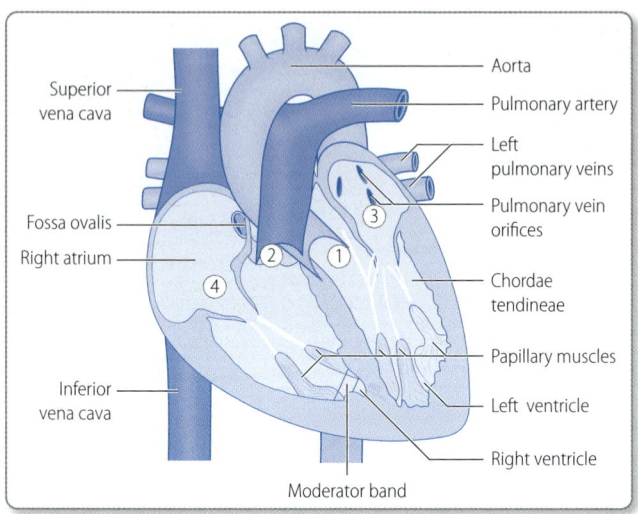

Figure 1.5 Anatomy of the heart valves. ① Aortic valve. ② Pulmonary valve. ③ Mitral valve. ④ Tricuspid valve.

Clinical insight

Ventricular dilatation or ischaemic damage to the papillary muscles can disrupt the subvalvular apparatus, allowing regurgitation to occur.

Guiding principle

The force countering systemic circulation (i.e. resistance) is five times higher than that of the pulmonary circulation. Consequently, the walls of the left ventricle are three times thicker (6–12 mm) than the right ventricle.

Left ventricle

The left ventricle is an elongated inverted cone that is circular in cross-section (**Figure 1.6**). Its internal surface is heavily trabeculated by muscle fibers (**Figure 1.7**).

The mitral valve chordae tendineae attach to an anterior and posterior papillary muscle.

Blood enters the left ventricle through the mitral valve and exits via the aortic valve. The outflow tract is posterior to the right outflow tract, which 'wraps' around the aorta. Blood supply is from the left anterior descending (LAD) artery and its diagonal branches.

Cardiovascular anatomy

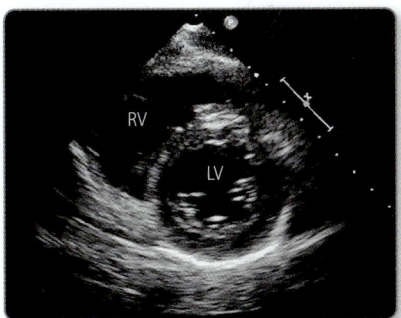

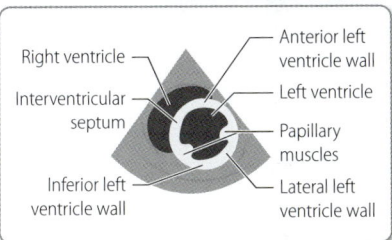

Figure 1.6 Transthoracic echocardiogram showing the circular left ventricle (LV). The lower pressure of right ventricle (RV) accommodates the higher pressure of LV.

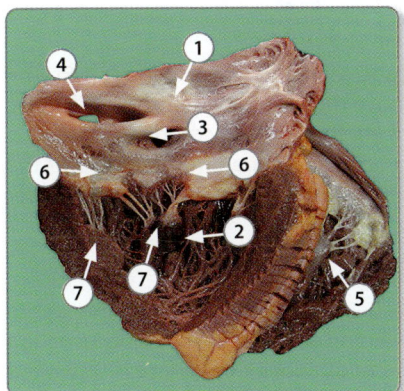

Figure 1.7 An exploded view of the left atrium (LA) (1), left ventricle (LV) (2) and mitral valve (3). The left atrial appendage orifice (4) and a pulmonary vein (5) are visible in the LA. Trabeculations of the LV are more coarse than those of the right ventricle (6). The mitral valve leaflets (3) are tethered to the papillary muscles (7) by the chordae tendineae. Courtesy of Dr K Suvarna.

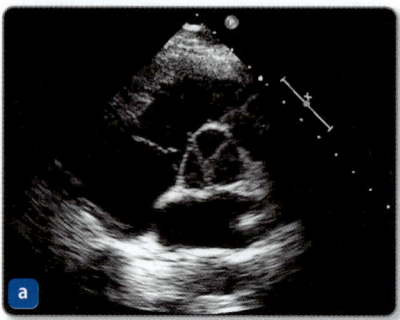
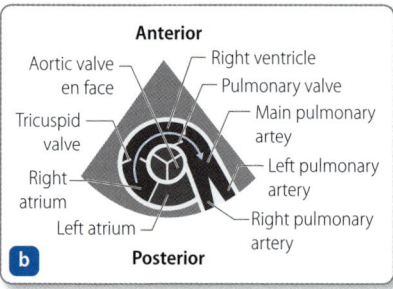

Figure 1.8 A transthoracic echocardiogram showing the aortic valve in cross-section.

Aortic valve and aortic root

The aortic valve has three semilunar cusps (**Figure 1.8**). The aortic root is directly above the valve, and has three dilations, or sinuses, two of which are the origin of coronary arteries.

The ascending aorta continues superiorly and towards the right before bending leftwards and posteriorly, arching over the left lung hilum.

Right atrium

The right atrium receives deoxygenated blood from the superior and inferior venae cavae and coronary venous blood through the coronary sinus. The smooth posterior surface is separated from the trabeculated anterior surface by the crescent-shaped crista terminalis muscle.

The trabeculated right atrial appendage – the auricle – projects from the superoanterior segment of the atrium.

Tricuspid valve

The tricuspid valve has anterior, posterior and septal leaflets. Their free edges are attached to the ventricular walls by the chordae tendineae and papillary muscles, which are smaller than the left subvalvular apparatus.

Right ventricle

The right ventricle, like the left, is an elongated inverted cone shape, but operates at a much lower pressure. As a result, the left ventricle and interventricular septum bulge into the right ventricular cavity (**Figure 1.6**).

The moderator band is a ridge of muscle that extends from the septum to the anterior wall at the base of the papillary muscle. It is part of the electrical conduction pathway that ensures the right-sided papillary muscles contract before the ventricle does, to ensure the tricuspid valve is braced for systole.

Pulmonary valve

The pulmonary valve is a tricuspid and semilunar valve at the apex of the right ventricular outflow tract.

Blood supply and drainage

Coronary heart disease (CHD) is a disease of the coronary arteries, and clinical understanding requires a thorough knowledge of the heart's blood supply.

Arterial supply

The left coronary artery (LCA) usually originates from the left coronary sinus, and the right coronary artery (RCA) emanates from the right coronary sinus.

The arteries run along the epicardial surface of the heart until they branch into smaller arteries, which penetrate and supply the myocardium. They are effectively end arteries, with only minimal anastomoses between them.

> **Clinical insight**
>
> Myocardium has a relative lack of collateral arterial connections; arterial occlusion quickly results in ischaemia and infarction.

Left coronary artery

The LCA passes behind the pulmonary artery and along the atrioventricular (AV) groove, where it divides into the left anterior descending and circumflex arteries (**Figure 1.9**).

The LAD artery roughly follows the line of the anterior septum down to the apex. It provides diagonal branches to the left ventricle laterally, and septal branches inferiorly to the interventricular septum.

The circumflex artery winds around the left lateral surface of the heart in the AV groove towards the inferior surface. Distally, it anastomoses with

> **Clinical insight**
>
> Coronary heart disease (CHD) kills more people worldwide than any other disease. It occurs when an atherosclerotic plaque disrupts and occludes the coronary arterial lumen.

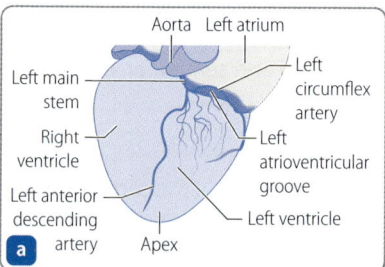

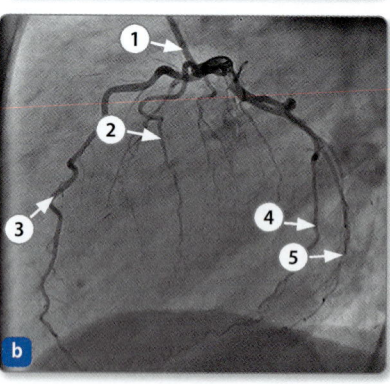

Figure 1.9 The left coronary artery. (a) Relations with other cardiac structures. (b) Left-sided angiogram of the left coronary artery. A coronary catheter is sitting in the aortic root, where it injects X-ray contrast material into the left main stem. ①, coronary catheter; ②, diagonal artery; ③, left anterior descending artery; ④, obtuse marginal artery; and ⑤, circumflex artery.

right-sided vessels on the inferior surface of the heart. Along its length, it supplies obtuse marginal branches that supply the high lateral wall of the left ventricle.

Right coronary artery

The RCA usually supplies the sinoatrial (SA) node, right ventricle, AV node and inferior surface of the left ventricle (**Figure 1.10**). It travels in the right AV groove to the inferior surface of the heart. From here, it usually supplies the posterior descending artery

> **Clinical insight**
>
> Occlusion of the left anterior descending (LAD) artery often results in left ventricular failure or death; occlusion of the right coronary artery (RCA) can result in arrhythmias, heart block, right ventricular failure or inferior left ventricular wall dysfunction.

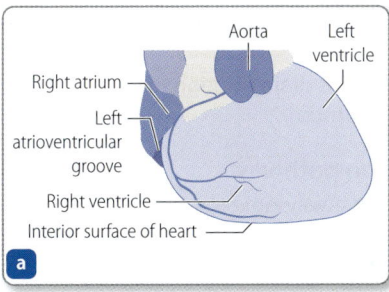

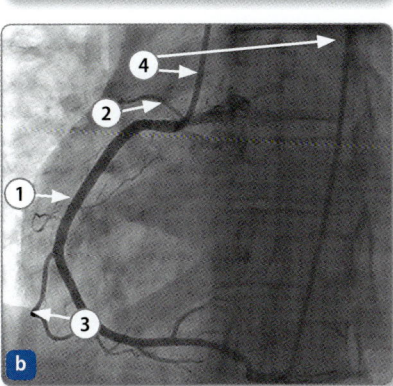

Figure 1.10 The right coronary artery. (a) Relations with other cardiac structures. (b) Angiogram taken from in front of the patient. The right coronary artery ① winds around the right atrioventricular (AV) groove, from which it branches to the sinoatrial (SA) node ② and right ventricle ③ before travelling down the inferior surface of the heart. A catheter ④ is visible in the descending aorta and in the aortic root at the right coronary ostium.

lying along the line of the inferior interventricular septum. Proximally, the RCA supplies a branch to the SA node. It also provides a branch to the right ventricle in its midsection.

Arterial dominance
Arterial dominance is determined by the artery that supplies the AV node (and usually the posterior descending artery):
- 75% are right-dominant (RCA)
- 15% are left-dominant (LCA)
- 10% are codominant.

Venous return
The great cardiac vein drains the anterior, posterior and lateral myocardial walls. It runs alongside the LAD artery and then in the left AV groove and empties into the right atrium through the coronary sinus. The middle cardiac vein begins at the apex, accompanies the posterior descending artery and drains into the coronary sinus.

Many right ventricular veins drain through the small cardiac vein directly into the right atrium.

The cardiac conduction pathway
The cardiac conduction pathway governs the route of myocardial depolarisation and therefore pattern of its contraction (**Figure 1.11**). It is formed by:

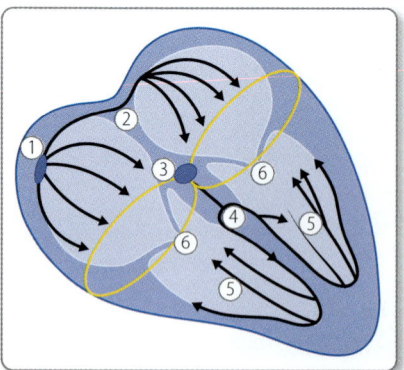

Figure 1.11 The conduction pathways of the heart. The sinoatrial (SA) node ①, Bachmann's bundle ②, atrioventricular node ③, bundle of His ④, which divides into left and right bundle branches. Purkinje fibres ⑤ rapidly conduct to the ventricles. Fibroannular rings ⑥ (shown in yellow) insulate the ventricles from the atria.

- The SA node – spontaneously depolarising pacemaker cells in the superior posterior right atrium
- Atrial cardiomyocytes that propagate depolarisation
- The AV node – normally the only electrical connection between the atria and the ventricles
- The bundle of His and Purkinje fibres – specialised conduction fibres in the ventricular septum and ventricles, respectively
- Ventricular cardiomyocyte propagation

Other than at the AV node, insulating fibrous tissue prevents conduction between the atria and ventricles. The node causes a pause in conduction, ensuring that ventricular filling is complete before contraction begins.

The bundle of His

The bundle of His descends in the ventricular septum and branches towards the right and left ventricles. The left bundle further divides into an anterior and a posterior branch, which subsequently form Purkinje fibres. These innervate the myocardium so that ventricular contraction starts at the apex and spreads to the base. This allows the efficient ejection of blood and ensures that the papillary muscles contract in time to prevent tricuspid or mitral valve regurgitation.

The pericardium

The pericardium is a double-membrane sac covering the heart and proximal segments of the great vessels. The outer tough fibrous pericardium protects the heart. The serous pericardium has two layers with a cavity in between:

- Parietal pericardium – a layer of mesothelial cells continuous with the fibrous pericardium
- The pericardial cavity containing a lubricating fluid to reduce friction
- Visceral pericardium that lines the epicardium

It also contains lymphatic tissue with a role in immune function.

The phrenic nerve innervates the fibrous and parietal layers, whereas the visceral layer is innervated by the autonomic nervous system (ANS).

Vessels

Ventricular contraction forces blood through the arteries under high pressure. As arteries branch, the number of blood vessels increases but their individual calibre decreases. Vast networks of capillaries perfuse tissues, in which substances are exchanged between blood and cells. Veins return blood to the heart under low pressure.

All vessels are cylindrical tubes of connective tissue and endothelial cells, and large vessels also have muscular, nervous, lymphoid and even vascular tissue.

Structure

All blood vessels, except capillaries, have three layers (**Figure 1.12**).

Tunica intima

This innermost layer is a single layer of endothelial cells, supported by a thin layer of connective tissue – lamina propria – and longitudinal elastic fibres, the internal elastic lamina. The luminal surface of the endothelial cells is in contact with blood in the lumen.

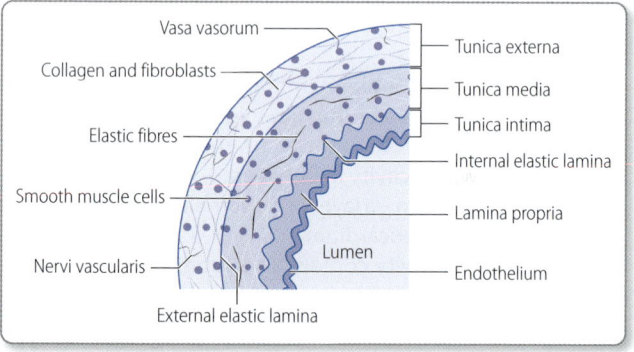

Figure 1.12 General structure of the walls of blood vessels. Vaso vasorum are the blood vessels to blood vessels; nervi vascularis are the nerves innervating vessels.

Tunica media

The middle layer consists of smooth muscle cells and elastic fibres in a circumferential arrangement. The smooth muscle is innervated by the sympathetic nervous system to control tone, i.e. vessel diameter. The external elastic lamina provides additional support.

Tunica externa

This outermost layer is mainly collagenous connective tissue and is fused with surrounding connective tissue to anchor vessels in place.

Types

The structure of each vessel type reflects its function (**Table 1.2**).

Vessel(s)	Main function	Description
Aorta and other elastic arteries	Compliance: distensibility and elasticity convert pulsatile to continuous flow	Thick media layer, rich in elastic fibres, collagen and smooth muscle
Muscular artery	Distribution of blood to the arterioles	Thick media layer, rich in smooth muscle
Arteriole	Generate peripheral resistance and control blood flow	Layers of smooth muscle
		Richly innervated by the autonomic nervous system
Capillary	Exchange of gases, nutrients and waste products	Single layer of endothelial cells
Venule	Collection of capillary blood	Thin and poorly developed tunica media
Vein	Acts as capacitance vessel (blood reservoir)	Thin media layer with scant elastic and smooth muscle fibres
		Compliant and contains valves
Vena cava	Returns blood to the right atrium	Very large vein in which flow is influenced by action of respiratory and cardiac pumps

Table 1.2 Structure and function of major vessels.

Elastic arteries

These are the major proximal arteries: the aorta and the brachiocephalic, carotid, subclavian, iliac and pulmonary arteries. Their tunica media contain many elastic fibres, which convert the intermittent, pulsatile blood flow from heart contraction into the continuous flow allowing constant tissue perfusion. They absorb energy during systole and discharge it in diastole.

Muscular arteries

Muscular – or distributing arteries – distribute blood to the resistance arterioles. They have multiple layers of smooth muscle in their tunica media, and include the radial, mesenteric and femoral arteries.

> **Clinical insight**
>
> Arteries become less elastic and more resistant as they age, causing an increase in systemic blood pressure from around 110 mmHg (average) at the age of 20 years to around 150 mmHg at 80 years.

Arterioles

Arterioles are known as resistance vessels because they regulate systemic vascular resistance (**Figure 1.13**). They contain one or two layers of smooth muscle that are autoregulating and affected by neuroendocrine control.

Arteriolar muscular tone is the primary controller of perfusion as these vessels supply capillary beds.

Capillaries

Capillaries consist of a single endothelial cell layer. They are 5–20 µm in diameter and about 1 mm long. However, they have a very large combined cross-sectional area, which results in a slow transit time. Known as 'exchange vessels', they are the site of gas, nutrient and waste product exchange between blood and tissues.

The microcirculation

The microcirculation is the functional unit of small vessels perfusing an organ or tissue (**Figure 1.14**). It consists of the:
- Terminal arterioles

Cardiovascular anatomy 17

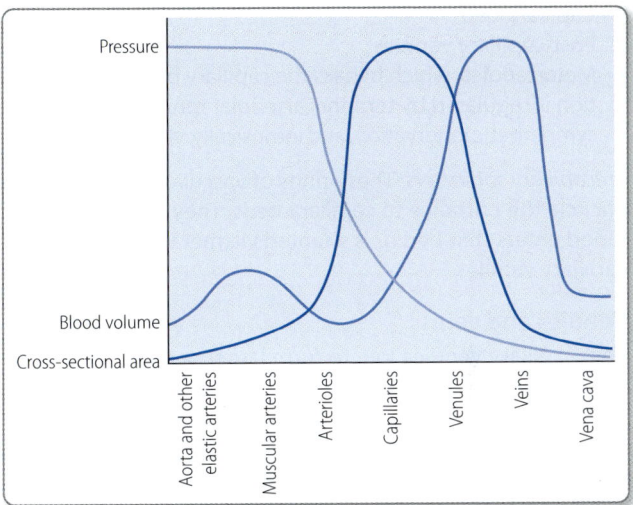

Figure 1.13 Pressure, blood volume and surface area at each level of circulation. The largest pressure drop occurs at the resistance vessels (arterioles), capillaries have the largest surface area and veins (capacitance vessels) hold the most volume.

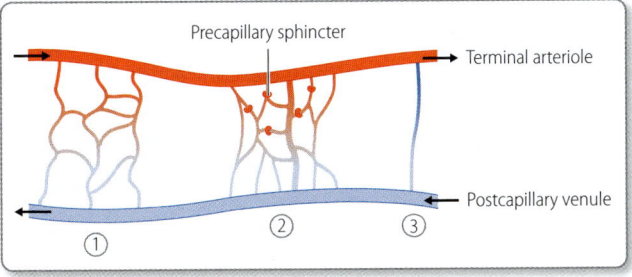

Figure 1.14 The microcirculation. ①, The simple branched microcirculation architecture present in most tissues. ②, Central metarteriole, a thoroughfare channel with branching capillaries. ③, Direct atrioventricular anastomosis found in cutaneous tissues.

- Capillary bed
- Post-capillary venules
- Metarterioles, which bypass the capillary bed. Microcirculation is regulated by terminal arteriolar tone, extrinsically by sympathetic innervation, and intrinsically, via autoregulation.

Precapillary sphincters: These rings of vascular smooth muscle encircle the entrance to capillary beds. They control whether blood enters that bed or is shunted via metarterioles to post-capillary venules.

Venules and veins

Post-capillary venules join to form larger venules, which join to form veins.

Venules and veins have a much thinner tunica media and less smooth muscle than arteries and arterioles. They are thin, compliant and lack elastic recoil. Consequently, they accommodate large increases in blood volume with minimal increase in pressure. The large combined cross-sectional area means resistance is low, so their low pressures are sufficient to return blood to the heart.

The large capacity of veins acts as a reservoir of blood and is regulated by the ANS. Sympathetic activation, e.g. results in venous constriction, increasing venous return (and central venous pressure, CVP). Venous return is aided by the skeletal muscle pump, where skeletal muscular contraction forces blood towards the heart and venous valves prevent backflow.

Key regional vascular anatomy

Carotid arteries

The right common carotid artery is a branch of the brachiocephalic artery. The left emerges directly from the aortic arch. The common carotid arteries bifurcate at the level of the C3–C4 vertebrae into the internal and external carotid arteries (**Figure 1.15**).

The internal carotid artery: The internal carotid artery enters the skull through the carotid canal, passes through the cavernous

Cardiovascular anatomy 19

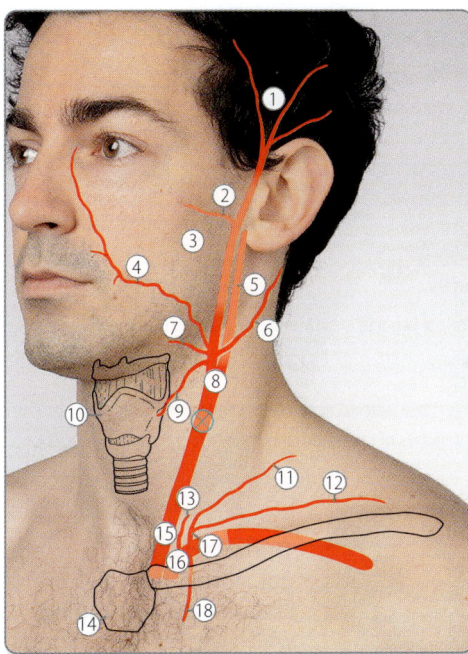

Figure 1.15 Arteries of the neck and face. ①, Superficial temporal artery; ②, maxillary artery; ③, masseter muscle; ④, facial artery; ⑤, internal carotid artery; ⑥, occipital artery; ⑦, lingual artery; ⑧, carotid bifurcation; ⑨, superior thyroid artery; ⑩, thyroid cartilage (vertebral level C5); ⑪, scalenus anterior; ⑫, transverse cervical artery; ⑬, suprascapular artery; ⑭, vertebral artery; ⑮, common carotid artery; ⑯, thyrocervical trunk; ⑰, subclavian artery; ⑱, internal thoracic artery. The best position to palpate the carotid artery is lateral to the larynx at the level of the thyroid cartilage ⊗.

sinus and supplies the ophthalmic artery. Its terminal branches are the middle and anterior cerebral arteries.

The external carotid artery: The external carotid artery supplies parts of the thyroid, larynx, tongue and superficial neck, face and head (**Table 1.3**).

Carotid sinus: The carotid sinus is a dilatation in the carotid artery, just below the bifurcation of the common carotid artery. It contains baro- and chemoreceptors involved in the regulation of blood pressure and ventilation.

Branch	Supplies
Superior thyroid artery	Larynx: Thyroid gland
Ascending pharyngeal artery	Skull base
Lingual artery	Tongue: Mouth floor
Facial artery	Superficial face
Occipital artery	Back of the head: Sternomastoid muscles
Posterior auricular artery	Scalp and ear
Maxillary artery (terminal branch)	Meninges, maxilla and mandible
Superficial temporal artery (terminal branch)	Scalp

Table 1.3 The main branches of the external carotid artery, inferior to superior.

Clinical insight

The carotid sinus is prone to atherosclerosis due to non-laminar blood flow. Atheroma can thromboembolise to cause a stroke. Risk is assessed via ultrasound.

Clinical insight

Thromboembolic disease of arteries supplying the gut can lead to bowel ischaemia and infarction which requires emergency surgery.

The gut

The arterial supply to the gut is from branches of the abdominal aorta (**Table 1.4**), which enters the abdomen behind the diaphragm at the level of the T12 vertebra.

It then descends, to the left of the midline, and divides at L4 into the common iliac arteries.

Renal vessels: The renal arteries arise as lateral branches from the aorta at the level of the L1 vertebra (**Figure 1.16**). They are large in caliber – 0.5–1 cm – reflecting the high level of kidney perfusion, about a quarter of total cardiac output (CO). They divide into segmental, lobar, interlobar and arcuate arteries before becoming the afferent arterioles supplying the glomeruli.

Cardiovascular anatomy 21

Branches	Supplies
Segmental arteries	Vertebrae
Coeliac and mesenteric arteries	Gastrointestinal tract
Renal arteries	Kidneys
Adrenal arteries	Adrenal glands
Gonadal arteries	Gonads

Table 1.4 Branches of the abdominal aorta.

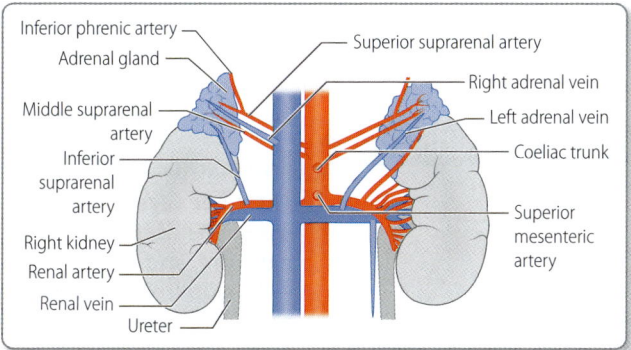

Figure 1.16 The arteries and veins of the kidneys and adrenal glands. The major vessels are the inferior vena cava and the abdominal aorta.

The renal veins mirror the arteries along their course.

Adrenal vessels: The adrenal glands also have a rich blood supply via their superior, middle and inferior suprarenal arteries. These usually arise from the inferior phrenic artery, aorta, and renal arteries, respectively. The right adrenal vein drains into the inferior vena cava, whereas the left drains into the left renal vein.

Clinical insight

Atherosclerosis or congenital diseases such as fibromuscular dysplasia can narrow the renal arteries. Such stenosis is a cause of resistant hypertension, kidney failure and atrophy.

1.2 Development of the cardiovascular system

The heart and vessels form by vasculogenesis, *de novo* vessel formation from endothelial precursors called angioblasts in the embryo. This stem cell budding is guided by genetic signals that orientate the direction and extent of growth. Further growth of small vessels occurs via angiogenesis, where vascular cells arise from already formed endothelial cells.

Development of the heart

The heart is the first organ to function and starts beating 3 weeks after fertilisation. It initially forms a single tube that then folds, loops and is divided by septae to form the four chambers and major vessels.

> **Guiding principle**
>
> In embryology:
> - Superior = cranial
> - Inferior = caudal
> - Anterior = ventral
> - Posterior = dorsal

Endocardial tubes

The three layers of cardiac tissue – endocardium, myocardium and epicardium – develop from cardiogenic mesoderm at the cranial end of the embryo:

- **Day 18:** Bilateral clusters of angioblasts form paired endocardial (heart) tubes
- **Embryonic folding** aligns these tubes in the midline on the ventral surface
- **Day 21:** The two tubes fuse to form a single-chambered heart with five segments that develop into chambers (**Figure 1.17** and **Table 1.5**). Myocyte rhythmic activity begins before tube fusion
- By week 4, contraction starts pumping blood in a caudal to cranial direction

Looping

On days 23–28, the growing tube folds and loops to the right (**Figure 1.17b**) to produce:

Development of the cardiovascular system 23

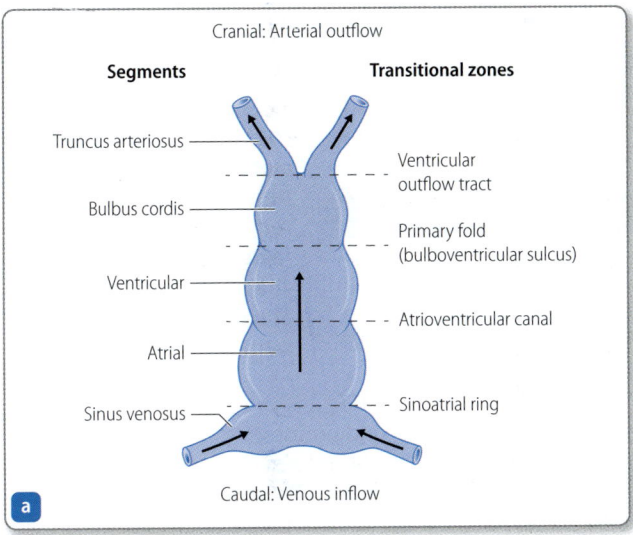

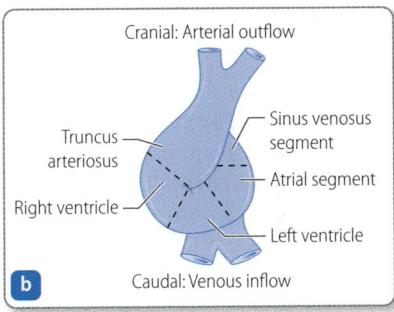

Figure 1.17 The heart tube. (a) Day 21: The heart tube has five distinct segments and four transitional zones. (b) Day 23–28: The tube folds and loops to resemble the mature heart.

Segment	Eventual structure
Truncus arteriosus	Aortic and pulmonary outflow tracts
Bulbus cordis	Right ventricle
Ventricular	Left and right ventricles
Atrial	Left and right atria
Sinus venosus	Coronary sinus and right atrium

Table 1.5 Structures originating from the five segments of the primitive heart tube.

- **Caudal segments:** Sinus venosus and primitive atria
- **Cranial segments:** Primitive ventricle and truncus arteriosus (the outflow tracts)

Once aligned, the atrial and ventricular segments begin to expand, differentiate and trabeculate. Externally, the heart starts to resemble the mature structure but internally remains a relatively simple folded, looped tube until the chambers and outflow tracts are divided by septation, the formation of tissue septa.

> **Guiding principle**
>
> The precision of heart tube looping is critical for the correct formation of chambers, vessels, and valves.

Atrioventricular septation

From *day 26*, cells surrounding the AV canal start to infiltrate the cardiac jelly, the gelatinous substance in-between the myocardium and endocardium. These form endocardial cushions – tissue that grows horizontally to form the valves and vertically, the septa.

Ventricular septation

Ventricular septation begins on *day 25*. From the apex of the cardiac loop, between the left ventricle and the bulbus cordis (the primary heart loop), the muscular interventricular septum starts to develop towards the endocardial cushions. The truncoconal septum extends inferiorly into the ventricular cavity to form the membranous portion of the interventricular septum.

Ventricular septation is completed in *week 7* when the primary muscular septum, the truncoconal septum and the AV endocardial cushions fuse. This joins the ventricular and outflow tract septae, which connect the left and right ventricles to the aortic and pulmonary outflow tracts, respectively.

Atrial septation

Atrial septation starts around *day 30*, when the septum primum descends from the roof of the atrium towards the endocardial cushions. In the fetus, blood shunts through the orifice primum.

Once this is obliterated by the fusion of the septum primum and the endocardial cushions, the second ostium develops.

The septum secundum then develops directly to the right of the septum primum. Septae have posteroinferior windows that together form the foramen ovale. This flap valve allows right-to-left blood flow (**Figure 1.18**) and closes when systemic blood pressure increases after birth.

Dorsally, the left horn of the sinus venosus forms the coronary sinus, which empties into the right atrium. The right horn becomes incorporated into the structure of the right atrium.

The primordial pulmonary vein merges with the left atrium in week 5. By *week 8*, all four pulmonary veins are absorbed.

Outflow tract septation

The truncus arteriosus is a common outflow tract. From week 5, along its length endocardial ridges form in a spiral arrangement. When these meet in the middle and fuse, they form a septum that separates the aortic outflow

> **Clinical insight**
>
> Failure of septation results in septal defects between the cardiac chambers, a common congenital heart disease.

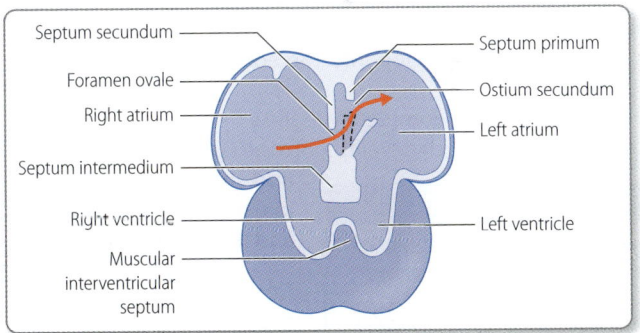

Figure 1.18 Fetal heart circulation. The interatrial septa and the foramen ovale flap valve (black dashed line). The rigid septum secundum grows alongside the septum primum. Fast flowing blood from the ductus venosus is directed across the atrial septae through the foramen ovale flap valve (red arrow). The valve closes after birth due to increased left atrial pressure.

tract from the pulmonary outflow tract). The same process is responsible for development of the aortic and pulmonary semilunar valves and is completed by the end of *week 8*.

The conduction tissue

Conduction tissue cells develop from the transitional zones of the heart tube. Regular contraction begins on *day 22*, before conduction tissues are formed. By the *7th week*, cells in the primitive atrium start to differentiate into the specialised pacemaker cells of the SA node, and cells of the sinus venosus into the AV node.

Development of vessels

Most vessels form by budding vasculogenesis from angioblasts. This initially forms a network of capillaries, with larger vessels formed as key pathways are enlarged. Further capillaries form via angiogenesis.

Arterial development

Arteries develop from the six, more ventral, paired aortic arches, along with the metabolic needs of the developing fetus (**Figure 1.19**):
- The first three arches develop into the arteries of the head and neck
- The 4th pair develop into the aortic arch and subclavian artery
- The 5th arches completely regress
- The 6th right arch develops into the right pulmonary artery, and the left arch develops into the left pulmonary artery and the ductus arteriosus.

> **Clinical insight**
>
> In the future, improved understanding of coronary artery embryology may allow the use of regenerated tissue to bypass sections blocked (i.e. stenosed) by atherosclerosis. Current materials used in coronary artery bypass grafts or stenting are prone to restenosis.

Coronary arteries

The coronary arteries originate from ventricular endocardial cells, at the right and left aortic sinuses of Valsalva.

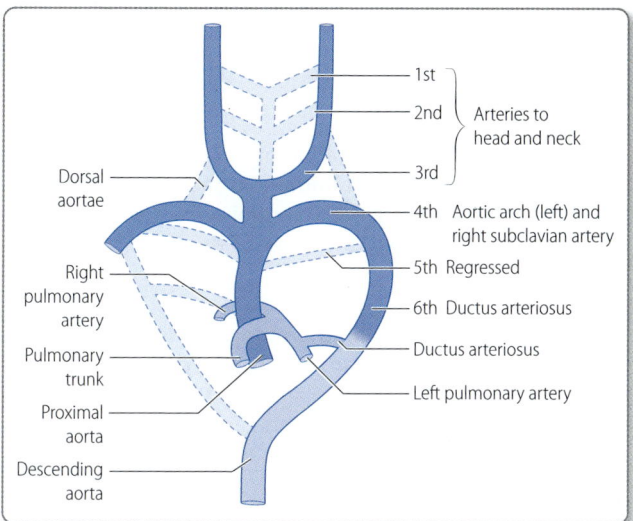

Figure 1.19 The aortic arches and dorsal aortae. The six arches develop and (some) regress at different times. Pair 1 regress but remnants form the adult maxillary and stapedial arteries. The 3rd pair form the carotid arteries. Pair 4 form the arch of the aorta (left) and the right subclavian artery. The 5th pair regress. Pair 6 contribute to the pulmonary arteries with the left also forming the ductus arteriosus. The dorsal aorta fuse in the midline forming the descending aorta.

Venous development: Veins mainly form from three bilateral veins in weeks 4–8:
- The cardinal system drains the head and body
- The umbilical system supplies O_2– and nutrient-rich blood from the placenta
- The vitelline system initially drains the yolk sac but develops into the hepatic, portal and superior mesenteric veins.

1.3 Cardiovascular physiology

Key physiological and biochemical processes to understand in CHD are:
- Electrophysiology
- The autonomic control of the heart

- The cardiac cycle
- Blood flow
- Blood pressure
- Haemostasis
- Lipid and cholesterol metabolism

Vascular inflammation and immunology, particularly endothelial cell involvement, are also central in the development of atheroma, but are beyond the scope of this book.

Electrophysiology

The cardiac cycle starts with the spontaneous initiation of an action potential – the cardiac impulse – by pacemaker cells of the SA node. This wave of depolarisation then conducts along specialised conduction tissues and cardiomyocytes, causing them to contract.

Cardiomyocytes

Cardiomyocytes are branched, tubular cells with a central nucleus (**Figure 1.20**). They connect end to end at intercalated

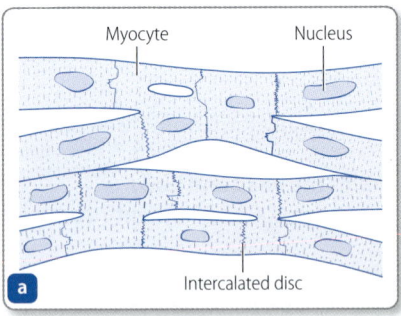

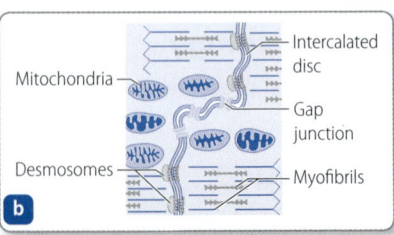

Figure 1.20 Cardiac muscle. (a) Cardiomyocytes are branched, nucleated, elongated, tubular cells joined at intercalated discs. (b) Close up of an intercalated disc: Desmosomes anchor cells, and gap junctions allow ions to pass freely between cells.

discs. The discs contain desmosomes that anchor cells together, and gap junctions, which allow action potentials to conduct freely between cells.

Resting membrane potential

Myocardial membranes have an electric charge – a resting potential of –90 mV, which allows them to conduct the cardiac impulse. This reflects unbalanced ion concentrations and selective membrane permeability maintained by membrane ion channels.

The main ions involved are the cations K^+, Na^+ and Ca^{2+} (**Table 1.6**).

Stage 1

Membrane-bound ion pumps actively pump K^+, Na^+ and Ca^{2+} out of the cell to make a small contribution to the resting membrane potential (RMP) (**Figure 1.21**):
- Na^+/K^+-ATPase pumps three Na^+ ions out of the cell and two K^+ ions into the cell
- Ca^{2+}-ATPase pumps Ca^{2+} out of the cell and into the sarcoplasmic reticulum
- The Na^+–Ca^{2+} exchanger exchanges three Na^+ ions for one Ca^{2+} ion

Stage 2

The membrane is permeable to K^+ but not other ions. K^+, therefore, passively diffuses out of the cell, down its concentration gradient, increasing the intracellular negative charge.

Cation	Intracellular concentration (mmol/L)	Extracellular concentration (mmol/L)
K^+	150	4
Ca^{2+}	10^{-4}	2
Na^+	15	145

Table 1.6 Intracellular and extracellular concentrations of important cations.

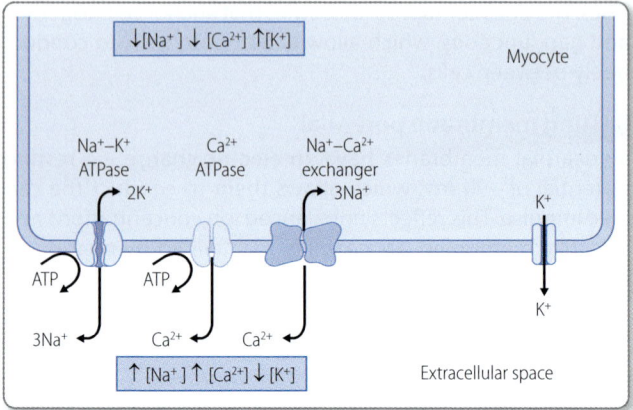

Figure 1.21 The resting membrane potential across the cardiomyocyte membrane. The three ion pumps (left) consume ATP to generate steep ionic concentration gradients. The membrane is permeable to K⁺ but less permeable to other ions. Therefore, K⁺ diffuses passively down its concentration gradient (right), leaving less positive charge (i.e. a net negative charge) on the inside of the cardiomyocyte.

> **Guiding principle**
>
> A myocyte with a resting membrane potential is polarised, i.e. there is a significant electrochemical gradient across the cell membrane. Depolarisation triggers myocardial contraction.

Stage 3

K⁺ efflux continues until equilibrium is reached between its concentration gradient and its electrochemical gradient. This equilibrium potential (E) is determined by ionic charge and the concentration gradient. For K⁺, E_K is around −96 mV.

Stage 4

The membrane potential (E_m) is equal to the sum of the equilibrium potentials of all the ions, proportional to their ability to cross the membrane (conductance, g):

$$E_m = (g_K \times E_K) + (g_{Ca} \times E_{Ca}) + (g_{Na} \times E_{Na})$$

This is predominately determined by E_K, as K⁺ has the highest conductance. Hence, overall RMP is close to E_K.

Gated ion channels

The cycles of depolarisation and repolarisation are controlled by membrane ion channels (**Table 1.7**). Ion channels are 'gated' in that they are activated (open) or inactivated (closed) by local factors such as voltage, ligand binding or receptor activation (**Table 1.8**).

Channel	Current	Function
Fast Na+ channel	I_{Na}	Rapid influx of Na+
Slow Na+ channel	I_b	Slow influx of Na+
'Funny' Na+ channel	I_f	Generates AP in pacemaker cells
Slow L-type Ca2+ channel	I_{Ca-L}	Prolongs AP in non-pacemaker cells
		Initiates AP in pacemaker cells
Transient T-type Ca2+ channel	I_{Ca-T}	Helps to initiate AP
Inwardly rectifying K+ channel	I_{ir}	Maintains resting membrane potential
Transient outward K+ channel	I_{to}	Contributes to phase 1 of AP
Delayed rectifier K+ channel	I_{Kr}	Contributes to repolarisation
AP, action potential.		

Table 1.7 Types of cardiomyocyte ion channel.

Gating mechanism	Stimulus	Example
Voltage-gated channels	Electrical potential	Generation of action potentials
Ligand-gated channels	Ligand binding	Hormones and neurotransmitters
Receptor-coupled channels	Physical stimulus	Myocardial stretch

Table 1.8 Different gating mechanisms of ion channels.

Clinical insight

Many antiarrhythmic drugs target Na^+, K^+ or Ca^{2+} channels. Flecainide and propafenone, for example, block fast Na^+ channels and delay phase 0.

Guiding principle

The action potential is 100 times longer in cardiomyocytes than skeletal myocytes (300 ms versus 3 ms). This allows time for the heart chambers to refill before contraction.

Movement of charged particles and ions generates an electrical current. Most of the current of depolarisation is from Na^+ influx (i.e. I_{Na}), which occurs until Na^+ channels are deactivated.

Cardiomyocyte depolarisation

The cardiomyocyte action potential has five phases (0–4) controlled by ion channel activation and inactivation (**Figure 1.22**). Phase 4 corresponds to diastole and phases 1 and 2 to systole.

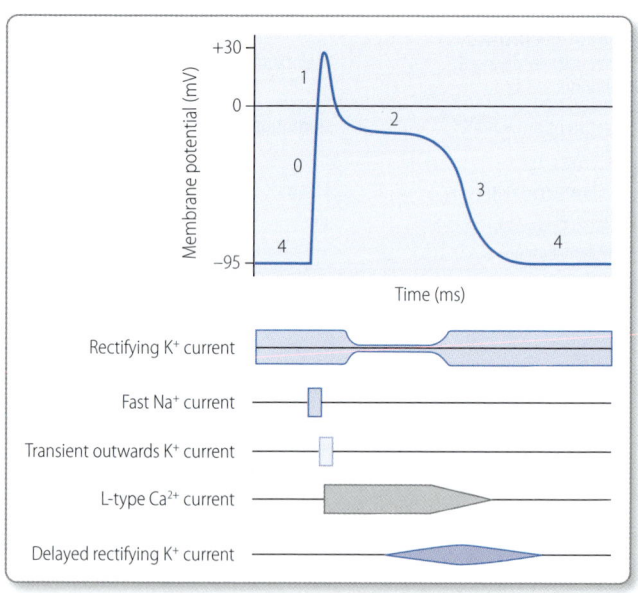

Figure 1.22 The cardiac action potential and the activation and inactivation of gated ion channels. The phases are 0, depolarisation; 1, transient partial repolarisation; 2, plateau; 3, repolarisation; and 4, resting.

Phase 4: Resting

The membrane is permeable to K^+ and relatively impermeable to other ions. Cardiomyocytes are held at RMP, and polarised between −90 and −95 mV.

Phase 4 ends when a depolarising electrical stimulus is conducted to the myocyte from a neighbouring cell. If it increases the membrane potential to −60 mV, an action potential (phase 0) is triggered.

Phase 0: Depolarisation

The threshold potential activates voltage-gated fast Na^+ channels and Na^+ ions rush into the cell, down a steep concentration gradient. INa rapidly increases the membrane potential to around +30 mV, when fast Na^+ channels abruptly inactivate.

Phase 1: Transient partial repolarisation

Voltage-gated, transient outward K^+ channels activate to allow a brief efflux of K^+ (Ito). This causes a brief partial repolarisation.

Phase 2: Plateau

Voltage-gated L-type Ca^{2+} channels activate and inactivate slowly, which prolongs inwards Ca^{2+} current (ICa); this sustains the action potential for around 250 ms and triggers myocyte contraction.

Towards the end of phase 2, Na^+–Ca^{2+} exchangers allow slow entry of Na^+, extending the plateau phase.

Ca^{2+} and Na^+ influx is opposed by outwards rectifying K^+ currents.

Phase 3: Repolarisation

As the L-type Ca^{2+} channels inactivate, delayed rectifying K^+ channels open. The now unopposed K^+ efflux causes rapid repolarisation.

Refractory periods

The absolute refractory period is the time during phases 1 and 2 in which another action potential cannot be initiated. It is due to inactivation of fast

> **Clinical insight**
>
> Calcium channel blockers (e.g. verapamil and diltiazem) block L-type Ca^{2+} channels to shorten phase 2. They are negative inotropes, i.e. they reduce cardiac contractility.

> **Clinical insight**
>
> Drugs that block K⁺ channels (e.g. amiodarone) prolong phase 3 and the refractory period. They are useful in alleviating the symptoms of certain re-entry tachycardias.

Na⁺ channels, which are not reactivated until phase 3. The relative refractory period is the time during their reactivation, when depolarisation can occur but depends on the magnitude of the stimulus and the number of reactivated channels (**Figure 1.23**).

Pacemaker depolarisation: Pacemaker cells are cardiomyocytes that can spontaneously depolarise, found in the SA and AV nodes and conducting tissues. This *automaticity* – regular, spontaneous firing – is due to:
- A less negative resting potential ($E_m = -60$ mV)
- Leaky Na⁺ channels.

A relatively high Na⁺ permeability means they slowly depolarise until a threshold at –20 mV. This opens voltage-gated Ca²⁺

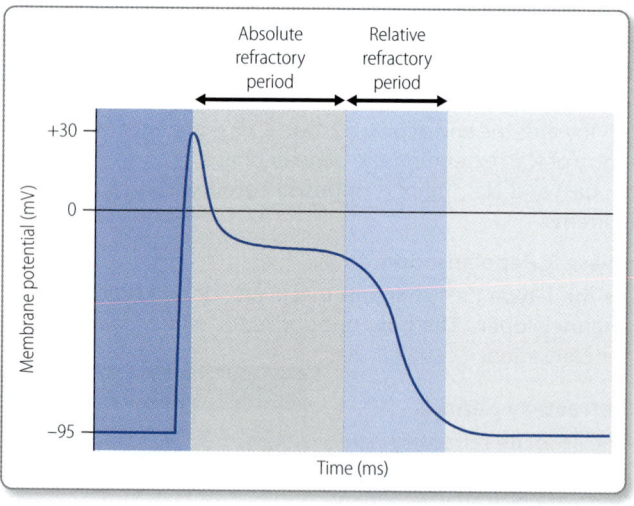

Figure 1.23 The absolute and relative refractory periods of an action potential in a cardiomyocyte.

Cardiovascular physiology

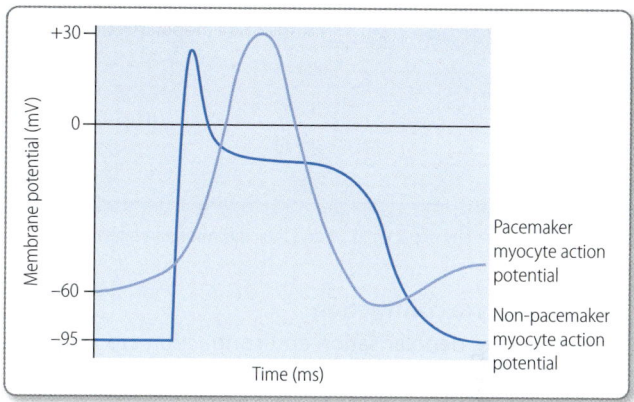

Figure 1.24 The action potentials of a pacemaker and a non-pacemaker cardiomyocyte. In a pacemaker cell, the resting potential (phase 4) is less negative and constantly drifts towards the firing threshold.

and slow Na⁺ channels, causing cation influx and an action potential spike (**Figure 1.24**).

Pacemaker potentials The rate of inwards Na⁺ and Ca²⁺ currents (INᵃ and ICᵃ) during phase 4 determines the rate of action potential generation and therefore heart rate.

Pacemaker hierarchy Multiple pacemaker sites provide a 'back up', though the fastest pacemaker functioning – the SA node in health – always assumes overall control. The more distal the pacemaker (relative to the SAN), the slower its intrinsic rate (**Table 1.9**).

Conduction pathway

The AV fibrous skeleton prevents the wave of depolarisation spreading into the ventricles. The AV node is normally the only electrical connection from the atria to the ventricles. The node slows conduction, allowing complete atrial emptying into the ventricles. Depolarisation then spreads rapidly down the septum via specialised Purkinje fibres in the bundle of His (**Figure 1.11**).

Pacemaker site	Intrinsic rate (depolarisations/min)
Sinoatrial node	100
Atrioventricular node	40–60
Bundle of His	30–40
Ventricles	≤30

Table 1.9 The hierarchy of pacemakers and their intrinsic heart rates.

Cardiomyocyte contraction

Cardiomyocyte depolarisation and contraction are linked via excitation–contraction coupling.

Myofibrils Myocytes contain elongated myofibrils composed of functional units called sarcomeres (**Figures 1.25** and **1.26**). Each sarcomere is bounded at each end by a Z line and contains contractile filaments made of the proteins actin and myosin. Peripherally, actin thin filaments attach to the Z line. Centrally, myosin thick filaments interdigitate (i.e. overlap) with the actin filaments.

Sarcolemma

The cell membrane – the sarcolemma – invaginates deeply into the myocyte around the Z lines to form T tubules. These are closely associated with sarcoplasmic reticulum, which contains intracellular stores of Ca^{2+}. This enables the rapid coupling of membrane (i.e. T tubule) depolarisation with the release of Ca^{2+} from the sarcoplasmic reticulum to stimulate myofibril contraction.

Myofibril contraction

Thin filaments consist of actin, tropomyosin and troponin complexes (**Figure 1.27**).
- Troponin T attaches each troponin complex to the tropomyosin
- Troponin I inhibits the binding of myosin heads to actin
- Troponin C binds to Ca^{2+}

The binding of Ca^{2+} to troponin C exposes the myosin-binding site, allowing actin–myosin cross-bridges to form.

Cardiovascular physiology 37

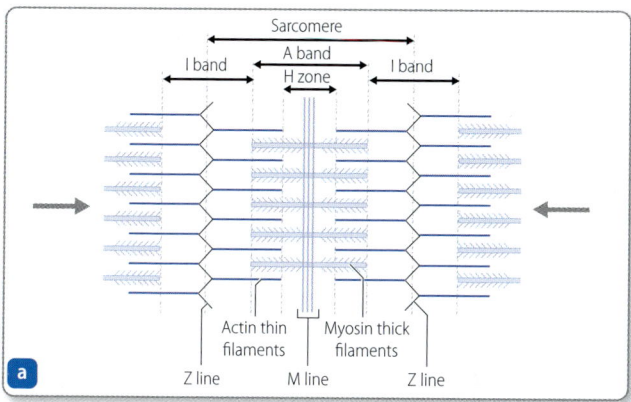

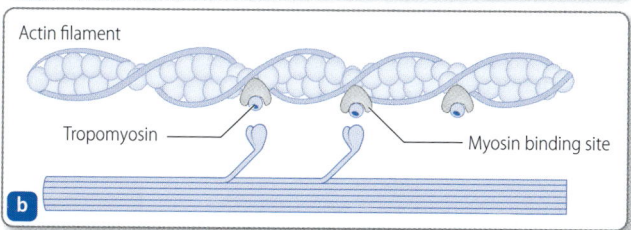

Figure 1.25 The sarcomere. (a) The sarcomere is bound by the Z lines – formed by the arbed ends of thin actin filaments. The filaments project centrally, where they interdigitate with thick myosin filaments. This gives the striated appearance of cardiomyocytes, defined by the M line, the H zone and the A and I bands. Actin–myosin interaction.

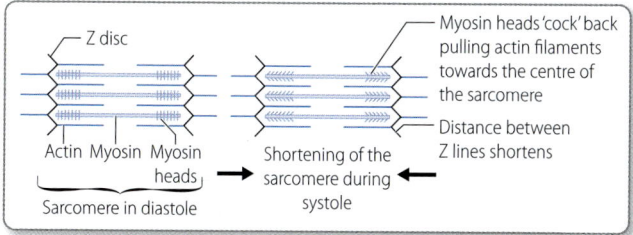

Figure 1.26 Sarcomeres and the sliding filament mechanism of myocardial contraction. Within the sarcomere, the central thick myosin filaments are surrounded by the thin actin filaments. Contraction of the many myocardial sarcomeres underlies contraction, and causes the H band to disappear, the A band to increase and the I band to shorten.

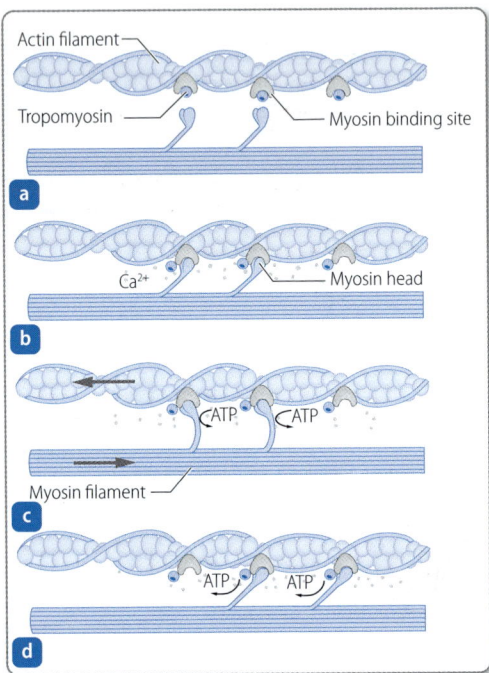

Figure 1.27 Mechanism of myocardial contraction. (a) Myosin-binding sites on actin filaments are blocked by tropomyosin. Ca^{2+} released after depolarisation binds to troponin. (b) Troponin changes conformation, exposing the binding site. Myosin heads bind actin. (c) Power stroke occurs as myosin heads pull filaments and shorten the sarcomere. (d) Myosin heads reset and can rebind. ATP, adenosine triphosphate.

Clinical insight

The regulatory troponin complex is found in cardiac and skeletal muscle, but not (vascular) smooth muscle. Subunits T and I are only found in cardiomyocytes whereas C is also found in skeletal muscle. Troponin T and I blood levels are indicators of myocyte damage associated with myocardial infarction.

The sliding filament model of contraction: The myosin 'power stroke' pulls the filaments so that they slide in opposite directions; this sliding shortens the sarcomere and, in turn, contracts the myocardium. Cycles of myosin-head binding to actin, contracting, disconnecting, and then reattaching – a 'ratcheting' effect – progressively shorten the sarcomere as long as intracellular Ca^{2+} remains high. Both contraction and relaxation are energy dependent (ATP consuming). In the heart, this is a continual cycle hence the large concentration of mitochondria and glycogen stores.

Inotropism

Inotropism is the ability of an agent to affect muscle contractility; positive inotropes enhance contractility and negative inotropes reduce contractility.

Autonomic control of the heart

The cardiovascular centre is a collection of nuclei in the medulla oblongata and is the branch of the ANS responsible for cardiovascular homeostasis and control. It receives sensory input from peripheral chemo- and baroreceptors, and higher control from the thalamus, hypothalamus and cerebral cortex (**Figure 1.28**). Through its modulated output it regulates:
- Heart rate
- Cardiomyocyte contractility
- Global blood flow
- Blood pressure.

The sympathetic nervous system

Sympathetic signals are transmitted from pre-ganglionic neurons in the lateral thoracic and lumbar spinal cord (levels T1–L2). These synapse with post-ganglionic neurons within the right and left paravertebral ganglia (the sympathetic chains).

Sympathetic nerves innervate the atrial and ventricular myocardium, SA node, AV node and conduction tissues. They release noradrenaline (norepinephrine), which – along with adrenaline (epinephrine) in the bloodstream – activates β1 adrenoreceptors in the heart.

Effects

Activation increases intracellular cyclic AMP (cAMP) and protein kinase A activation, causing changes in ion channel gating (**Table 1.10**), and thereby increases:
- Heart rate, i.e. chronotropicity
- Contractility, i.e. inotropicity

40 First principles

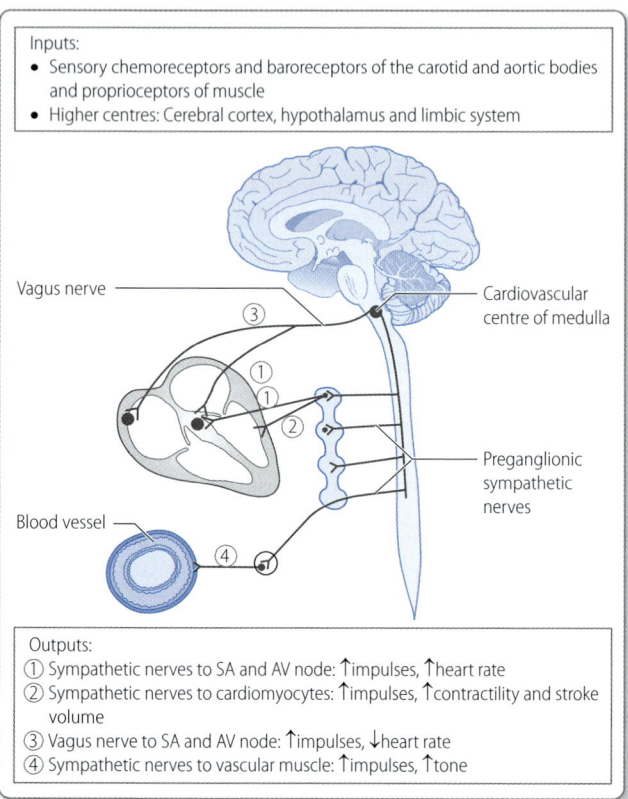

Inputs:
- Sensory chemoreceptors and baroreceptors of the carotid and aortic bodies and proprioceptors of muscle
- Higher centres: Cerebral cortex, hypothalamus and limbic system

Outputs:
① Sympathetic nerves to SA and AV node: ↑impulses, ↑heart rate
② Sympathetic nerves to cardiomyocytes: ↑impulses, ↑contractility and stroke volume
③ Vagus nerve to SA and AV node: ↑impulses, ↓heart rate
④ Sympathetic nerves to vascular muscle: ↑impulses, ↑tone

Figure 1.28 The cardiovascular centre of the medulla is responsible for the global control of heart rate, contractility and stroke volume, as well as vascular tone, the core determinant of blood pressure.

- Myocardial relaxation, i.e. lusitropicity
- Conduction through the AV node, i.e. dromotropicity

The parasympathetic nervous system

Efferent parasympathetic innervation of the heart is through the right and left vagus nerves (cranial nerve X), which originate in the nucleus ambiguous of the medulla oblongata.

Channel	Change	Effect
Na⁺ and Ca²⁺ channels	Activates	Increases phase 4 pacemaker currents and therefore heart rate
L-type Ca²⁺ channels	Augments	Increases Ca²⁺ influx, and therefore contractility (i.e. positive inotropicity)
Ca²⁺ pumps	Augments	More rapid Ca²⁺ clearance, which accelerates myocardial relaxation
Delayed rectifying K⁺ channels	Augments	Shortens action potential duration

Table 1.10 Noradrenaline (norepinephrine) induced changes in membrane ion transport.

Pre- and post-ganglionic neurons synapse very close to the heart. Post-ganglionic neurons primarily innervate the atrial myocardium, SA node and AV node.

Vagal activation releases acetylcholine, which binds to muscarinic M_2 receptors, antagonising cAMP production and protein kinase A activation. Vagal activation also results in K⁺ channel activation and hyperpolarisation of the myocyte membrane.

Clinical insight

Atropine blocks muscarinic acetylcholine receptors to reduce parasympathetic activation.

Guiding principle

At rest, parasympathetic (i.e. vagal) tone dominates the control of heart rate.

During activity, vagal tone is reduced, and during exercise, sympathetic activity dominates.

The parasympathetic nervous system reduces heart rate by reducing pacemaker potentials.

The cardiac cycle

The cardiac cycle is the series of the events occurring every heart beat (**Figure 1.29** and **Table 1.11**).

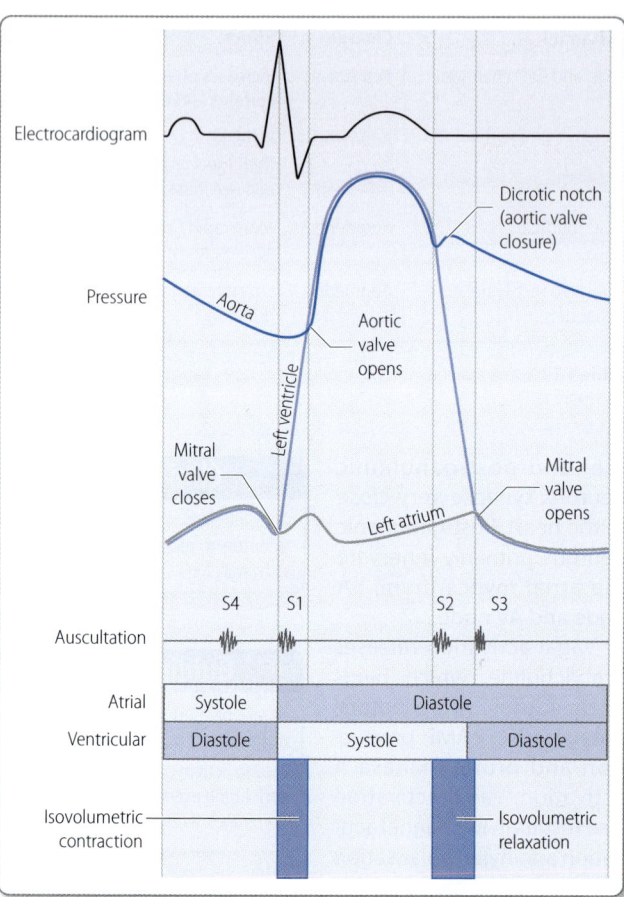

Figure 1.29 The cardiac cycle can be interpreted by electrocardiography, blood pressure dynamics and heart sounds.

Atrial systole

Atrial contraction (systole) is the active phase of ventricular filling that follows passive filling. At rest, it contributes 10–20% of total end-diastolic volume. This contribution decreases as the heart rate increases.

Heart sound	Mechanism	Timing	Circumstance
1st (S1)	Atrioventricular valve closure	Immediately before the carotid pulse	Normal
2nd (S2)	Semilunar valve closure	Immediately after the carotid pulse	Normal
3rd (S3)	Rapid early (passive) ventricular filling	Shortly after S2	Can be normal in young fit people but is also a sign of increased end-diastolic pressure, which occurs in heart failure
4th (S4)	Atrial systole against stiffened ventricle	Shortly before S1	Indicates stiffened (hypertrophied) ventricular walls

Table 1.11 The physiological basis of the heart sounds.

A small pressure wave – the *a* wave – is detectable in the veins during this phase, as the atria are continuous with the great veins which do not have valves.

Atrial systole indirectly contributes to CO as ventricular stroke volume is proportional to end-diastolic volume.

Ventricular systole
During ventricular systole:
- Ventricles contract
- Atrioventricular valves close (heart sound S1)
- Semilunar valves open
- Blood is ejected.

As the AV valves bulge into the atria, they produce a *c* pressure wave in the venous pulse when they close.

Ventricular pressure increases
The semilunar valves remain closed until the ventricular pressure exceeds the aortic and pulmonary artery pressures. This phase is called isovolumetric contraction because the ventricular pressure increases without any change in ventricular volume.

> **Clinical insight**
>
> On electrocardiography (ECG):
> - *p* wave = Atrial depolarisation
> - QRS complex = Ventricular systole
> - T wave = Ventricular repolarisation
>
> Atrial repolarisation is 'hidden' in the QRS.

Ventricular ejection

Once the semilunar valves open, the pressure gradient across the valves is minimal and blood is powerfully ejected into the aorta and pulmonary arteries.

Atrial diastolic filling occurs during ventricular systole with a corresponding increase in atrial pressure (the *v* wave).

Ventricular diastole

During ventricular diastole:
- Ventricles relax
- Semilunar valves close
- AV valves open

Ventricular systole continues until arterial pressures are slightly greater than ventricular. This allows a very brief reversal of flow that closes the semilunar valves (S2).

Ventricular relaxation

Ventricular pressure continues to decrease after the semilunar valves close. Ventricular volume is unchanged until the AV valves open, hence this phase is isovolumetric relaxation time. Ventricular relaxation is not passive, and active recoil of the ventricles helps to suck in blood during the next phase.

Atrioventricular valves open

The AV valves open as soon as atrial pressure exceeds ventricular, just after the point of peak atrial filling and pressure (the *v* pressure wave). Atrial pressure decreases rapidly. Ventricular filling is rapid at first and then slows as the pressure gradient declines.

Finally, atrial systole starts the next cycle.

Blood flow

At rest, total blood flow – cardiac output (CO) – is about 5 L/min. This can increase to 30 L/min during strenuous exercise. Both the total and local flow of blood are closely regulated to match global and local metabolic need.

Global control – the cardiovascular centre

The cardiovascular centre controls the rate and force of heart contraction and global vascular tone (see **Figure 1.28**).

> **Clinical insight**
>
> A lack of blood flow leads to tissue ischaemia, O_2 and nutrient starvation. A sustained or severe lack of perfusion causes infarction, tissue death.
>
> Excessive blood flow can damage vessels and lead to oedema – fluid leak into the extracellular compartment.

Cardiac output

$$CO = \text{heart rate (HR)} \times \text{stroke volume (SV)}$$

Therefore, the cardiovascular centre controls total blood flow by adjusting heart rate or stroke volume.

Stroke volume

Stroke volume is the volume of blood ejected with each heartbeat:

SV = End-diastolic volume (EDV) – End-systolic volume (ESV)

It is influenced by preload, myocardial contractility and afterload.

The ejection fraction (EF) is the percentage of blood ejected from the ventricle with each heartbeat. It is normally 50–70% but is reduced in heart failure.

$$\text{Ejection fraction (\%)} = \frac{SV}{EDV} \times 100$$

Cardiac preload: Preload is end-diastolic ventricular pressure. An increase in preload increases end-diastolic and stroke volume. The myocardium is at its most stretched at the end of diastole, which has two effects:
1. More active actin–myosin cross-bridges form
2. The affinity between Ca^{2+} and troponin C increases

This is the basis for the Frank–Starling law: 'The mechanical energy discharged during ventricular systole is a function of initial fibre length', i.e. more myocardial stretch leads to a more forceful contraction (**Figure 1.30**). This is how:

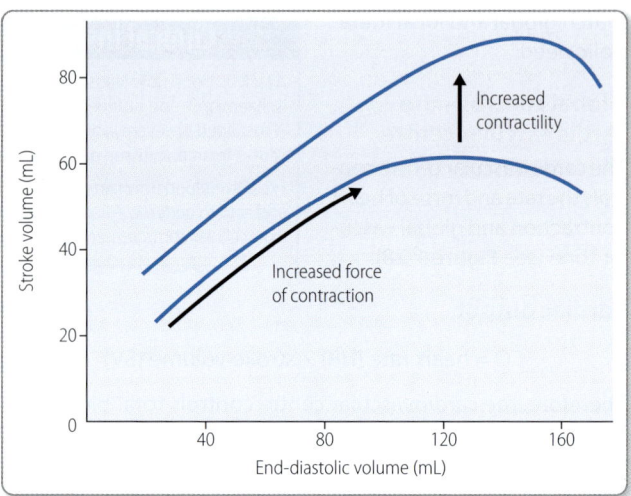

Figure 1.30 The Frank–Starling curve. An increase in end-diastolic volume results in a greater stroke volume. In the physiological range, the curve is steep as ventricles are particularly sensitive to changes in end-diastolic volume. Beyond the physiological range, the curve plateaus; further increases in end-diastolic volume do not increase stroke volume. The effect of raised contractility (often referred to as increased sympathetic tone) is demonstrated in the upper curve.

- Left and right circulations equalise
- Exercise increases venous return and therefore CO
- Reduced venous return (e.g. haemorrhage) decreases CO.

Venous muscular tone can also affect venous return:

- An increase – e.g. sympathetic activation – increases venous return
- A decrease in tone decreases venous return.

Contractility: Contractility is the force of myocardial contraction, independent of preload. Inotropes affect contractility (**Table 1.12**) and are also the name of a class of drugs with positive inotropic effects (e.g. digoxin).

A positive inotropic agent – such as sympathetic activation or increased myocardial stretch – increases cardiomyocyte contraction, usually by increasing Ca^{2+} influx, which causes more actin–myosin cross-bridges to form.

Positive inotropes	Negative inotropes
Increase contractility	Decrease contractility
<ul><li>Sympathetic nervous activation</li><li>Hormones, e.g. adrenaline (epinephrine) and thyroxine</li><li>Serum ions (Ca^{2+})</li><li>β_1 agonists (e.g. dobutamine, isoprenaline and adrenaline)</li><li>Phosphodiesterase inhibitors (e.g. milrinone)</li></ul>	<ul><li>General ill health (e.g. myocardial ischaemia, acidosis and hypoxia)</li><li>β_1 antagonists (β-blockers)</li><li>Calcium-channel blockers</li></ul>

Table 1.12 Positive and negative inotropes.

Sympathetic activation increases contractility and heart rate via β1-adrenoceptors. An increase in contractility shifts the Frank–Starling curve upwards.

Parasympathetic activation reduces rate but has no effect on contractility due to minimal parasympathetic innervation of myocardium.

Afterload: Afterload is the ventricular tension required to eject blood against aortic or pulmonary artery pressures. An increase in afterload increases end-systolic volume and reduces stroke volume.

Tension is a factor of volume and pressure and is therefore increased in conditions of ventricular dilatation. It is also increased by arterial hypertension and aortic stenosis.

Heart rate

As heart rate affects cardiac output and therefore blood pressure, the mechanisms controlling it and blood pressure are integrated. Sympathetic activation increases heart rate and contractility, as increasing the rate alone would decrease diastolic filling time and therefore end-diastolic volume (preload).

> **Guiding principle**
>
> An increase in central venous pressure increases cardiac output by:
> - Frank–Starling's law – increased cardiomyocyte stretch causes increased contraction
> - Bainbridge's reflex – right atrial stretch receptors increase sympathetic activation to the heart

Peripheral signals to the cardiovascular centre include pressure and chemical sensors in the carotid and aortic bodies:
- Baroreceptor activation (by being stretched) results in vagal activation and bradycardia
- Chemoreceptor stimulation, for example, via low O_2 or glucose or raised CO_2, also leads to bradycardia, though the effect is less direct.

Hormones such as thyroxine and its metabolites increase heart rate. Extreme cold causes a reduction in heart rate, and higher body temperatures result in an increase in heart rate.

Total peripheral resistance

Total blood flow is also affected by total peripheral resistance (TPR), which is the sum force opposing blood flow, determined by the diameter of resistance vessels. This is dependent on vascular tone, the degree of smooth muscle contraction, and therefore constriction, of a vessel. Therefore, global blood flow is also affected by changes in vascular tone. This is affected by innervations from the ANS and global hormones.

Vascular tone is also locally controlled by hormones and autoregulation – an intrinsic response of vascular muscle to maintain tone.

Vascular smooth muscle

Vascular smooth muscle contraction – like all muscle – involves Ca^{2+} release and the sliding filament model. However, vascular contraction is slower and sustained compared to cardiac or skeletal muscle. It always has some degree of 'tone'. Unlike cardiac muscle, it lacks the troponin complex, and cells are not arranged into a striated pattern.

Contraction occurs in response to electrical, mechanical or chemical stimulation:
- Membrane depolarisation
- Stretch
- Receptor binding

Stimulation causes Ca^{2+} influx from the extracellular space and Ca^{2+} release from sarcoplasm:
- Ca^{2+} binds to the protein calmodulin

- Ca^{2+}-calmodulin complex activates myosin light chain kinase (MLCK)
- Myosin light chain kinase phosphorylates myosin light chains
- Actin–myosin cross bridges form and contraction occurs

Cycles of sliding filament contraction progressively shorten the myofibrils as long as intracellular Ca^{2+} remains high. Ca^{2+}ATPase and Na^+ Ca^{2+} exchanger membrane proteins actively remove Ca^{2+}.

Vascular tone

Vascular tone is proportional to the intracellular Ca^{2+} concentration. This is influenced globally by autonomic control and hormones and locally by chemicals and intrinsic autoregulation.

Extrinsic control of vascular tone. This is affected by external factors:
- Vasoactive chemicals in the blood
- Autonomic nervous system activity (which releases vasoactive chemicals)
- Variations in membrane receptors for afferent nerves or hormones

Vasoactive chemicals: Vasoactive compounds work via four main mechanisms: Three different G-protein linked signal transduction pathways (Gq, Gs and Gi), and nitric oxide (**Table 1.13**). Nitric oxide is one of the few gas signalling molecules.

Pathway	Examples	Mechanism	Effects
Gq-protein coupled	Catecholamines (adrenaline, noradrenaline–epinephrine, norepinephrine) angiotensin II, thromboxane A_2, endothelin I, and vasopressin	Gq-protein linked receptor activates phospholipase C and diacylglycerol, causing Ca^{2+} release and myosin light chain phosphorylation	Vasoconstriction, membrane depolarisation, Ca^{2+} sensitisation

Table 1.13 Mechanisms of vasoactive compounds. *Continues overleaf*

Pathway	Examples	Mechanism	Effects
Adenylate cyclase (Gs- and Gi-coupled)	Catecholamines (via β_2 adrenoreceptors), adenosine, acetylcholine, and prostacyclin	Gs-protein linked receptor activates adenylate cyclase to convert ATP into cAMP, which inhibits MLCK, reducing contractility	Vasodilation
	Catecholamines (via α_2 adrenoreceptors)	Gi-protein linked receptor inhibits adenylate cyclase, reducing cAMP, increasing MLCK activity	Vasoconstriction
Nitric oxide	NO	Activates guanylate cyclase to convert GTP into cGMP, which inhibits Ca^{2+} influx, inositol triphosphate synthesis, membrane depolarisation and increases myosin light chain dephosphorylation	Vasodilation
Sympathetic nerves: catecholamine release	α_1 receptor	Gq-protein linked receptor	Vasoconstriction
	α_2 receptor	Gi-protein linked	Vasoconstriction
	β_2 receptor	Gs-protein linked receptor	Vasodilation (primary action)
Parasympathetic nerves: acetylcholine release	Muscarinic M_3 receptors	Gq-protein linked receptor	Vasoconstriction (primary action and secondary effect)
	Muscarinic M_3 receptors	NO release (secondary action, principal effect)	Vasodilation (genitals, salivary glands and bladder)

ATP, adenosine triphosphate; cAMP, cyclic adenosine monophosphate; cGMP, cyclic guanosine monophosphate; GTP, guanosine triphosphate; MLCK, myosin light chain kinase; NO, nitric oxide.

Table 1.13 *Continued*

It is synthesised by endothelial cells – stimulated, e.g., by acetylcholine released by parasympathetic efferent neurons. It diffuses through vascular myocyte membranes to cause vasodilation.

Autonomic nervous system activity: Generally, sympathetic adrenergic activation (via α receptors) vasoconstricts systemic vessels to increase TPR and, therefore, blood pressure, and cholinergic activation (via muscarinic receptors) stimulates sweating and dilates skin arteries. Most blood vessels have very little parasympathetic innervation. At rest, vagal tone dominates in the heart, whereas sympathetic tone dominates in vascular smooth muscle.

Intrinsic control of vascular tone: Autoregulation is the intrinsic response of arteriolar smooth muscle to changes in perfusion or blood constituents to moderate local blood flow. Different networks can have different responses due to receptor variation. For example, hypoxia in the pulmonary circulation causes vasoconstriction to match ventilation and perfusion; elsewhere, it induces vasodilatation to correct the abnormality.

The myogenic response: Increased blood flow/pressure activates stretch receptors, causing reflex vasoconstriction and a decrease in local flow. This myogenic response maintains constant flow despite fluctuating mean arterial blood pressure (**Figure 1.31**).

Metabolic adaptation: Increased cellular metabolism produces metabolites that are vasodilators, thereby matching blood

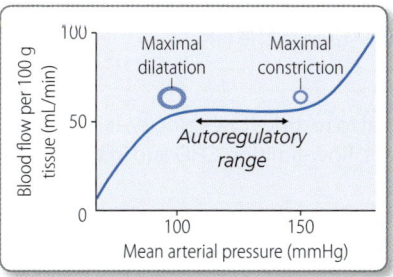

Figure 1.31 Myogenic autoregulation. Within the autoregulatory range a rise in pressure in the arterioles perfusing a tissue will cause reflex constriction, which increases resistance and maintains constant blood flow through the tissue.

flow to metabolic demand. They include K^+ ions, adenosine and CO_2.

Coronary blood flow

Myocardium has a high metabolic rate, reflected in its large numbers of mitochondria, and receives a high blood flow via an extensive capillary network. It is the most efficient organ at extracting O_2 from blood – about 70% that enters its circulation. Therefore, it relies on metabolic adaptation to match blood flow and O_2 supply. Its resting blood flow of 200–250 mL/min can increase to 1 L/min during exercise.

Contrary to other organs, coronary blood flow is impeded during systole and enhanced during diastole, particularly on the most muscular left side. The transmural pressure generated by systole compresses subendocardial arterioles so that myocardium is not perfused. Some systolic perfusion does occur in the outermost (i.e. subepicardial) myocardium, where transmural pressure is lower.

> **Clinical insight**
>
> The heart is unique in its efficiency in extracting O_2 from blood, which it does at a nearly constant maximum rate.
>
> Increasing blood flow is the only way to meet increased O_2 demand.

Left coronary artery flow

The highest LCA flow occurs during diastole (**Figure 1.32**). The lowest is during the isovolumetric phases of systole, when ventricular pressure is high but coronary flow is low.

Right coronary artery flow

Right ventricular myocardial perfusion is more consistent as wall tension is much lower than in the left.

Coronary flow reserve

This is the ratio of maximal to resting flow velocity. It is reduced in patients with significant, flow-limiting CHD and in those with microvascular disease.

Velocity is measured with an intracoronary Doppler wire during coronary angiography. Maximal velocity is induced

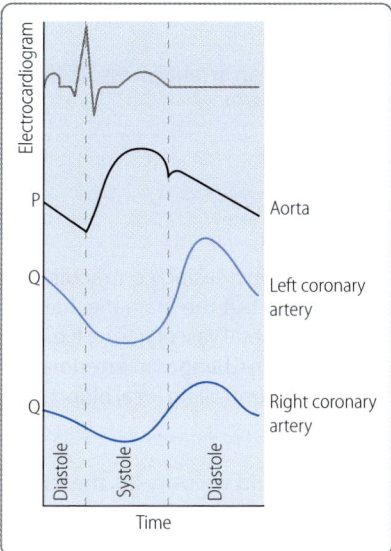

Figure 1.32 Coronary blood blow (schematic representation). Aortic pressure (P) peaks in systole; left coronary artery (LCA) flow (Q) peaks in diastole, due to high systolic resistance caused by compression of vessels in the ventricular wall. This effect is less in the right coronary artery (RCA) as right ventricular pressures are lower.

pharmacologically, usually with adenosine. The ratio is calculated as the hyperemic flow velocity divided by baseline velocity.

Haemodynamics

Haemodynamics is the study of physical laws governing blood flow.

Pressure, flow and resistance

The heart is an intermittent pump, generating pressure (P) to drive blood flow (Q) through the circulation against the force of resistance (R):

This can be rearranged:

$$\Delta P = QR$$

$$Q = \frac{\Delta P}{R}$$

i.e. an increase in driving pressure, or a reduction in resistance to flow both increase blood flow.

Applying this to the circulatory system:
- Flow (Q) is cardiac output (CO)
- The change in pressure (ΔP) is mean arterial pressure (MAP) minus central venous pressure (CVP)
- Resistance (R) is TPR

Hence:

$$CO = \frac{MAP-CVP}{TPR}$$

Cardiac output can be increased by increasing contractility (to generate higher MAP) or heart rate, but the main mechanism of regulation is via changes in peripheral vascular tone (i.e. TPR) as explained by Poiseuille's equation. Changes in arteriolar diameter are the main mechanism of controlling local blood flow.

Poiseuille's equation

This law relates to the influence of fluid viscosity (η), the length of tube (L) and its radius (r) on resistance:

$$R = \frac{8\eta L}{\pi r^4}$$

Substituting in the previous resistance equation gives:

$$Q = \frac{\Delta P}{L} \cdot \frac{\pi r^4}{8\eta}$$

As blood viscosity and vessel length are relative constants, this simplifies to:

$$Q \propto \Delta P \cdot r^4$$

In effect, this means:
- Most peripheral resistance is due to arterioles, because of the small diameter
- Blood flow increases linearly with blood pressure and to the fourth power of vessel radius
- Therefore, very small changes in vessel radius profoundly affect resistance, e.g. doubling the radius increases flow 16-fold

Poiseuille's equation also defines how an increase in blood viscosity increases resistance and blood pressure.

Flow velocity

Flow velocity is the velocity of blood in centimeters per second in a vessel or group of vessels. Unlike the overall volumetric flow (measured in mL/min), flow velocity varies in different circulatory networks. It is inversely proportional to the cross-sectional area of the network (**Table 1.14**). The combined cross-sectional area of capillaries is very large. Consequently, slow capillary flow (<0.1 cm/s) allows time for exchange of nutrients, gases and waste between blood and cells.

> **Clinical insight**
>
> Anaemia – a reduction in erythrocytes – decreases blood viscosity and therefore blood pressure. Polycythaemia has the opposite effect.

Laminar and turbulent flow

Blood flow is normally laminar, i.e. concentric layers of fluid move parallel to the axis of the vessel (**Figure 1.33**). Vessel wall friction creates a gradient of velocity, with slower flow closer to the wall.

Turbulent, or disturbed, flow may occur if:
- Velocity increases as it goes through narrower spaces
- Viscosity reduces
- Vessel diameter increases

Turbulent flow requires more pressure to achieve a given flow rate and is less efficient.

Vessels	Cross-sectional area (cm^2)	Flow velocity (cm/s)
Aorta	4	40
Capillaries	5,000	<0.1
IVC and SVC	14	15
IVC, inferior vena cava; SVC, superior vena cava.		

Table 1.14 Cross-sectional area and flow velocity in the aorta, capillaries and vena cavae.

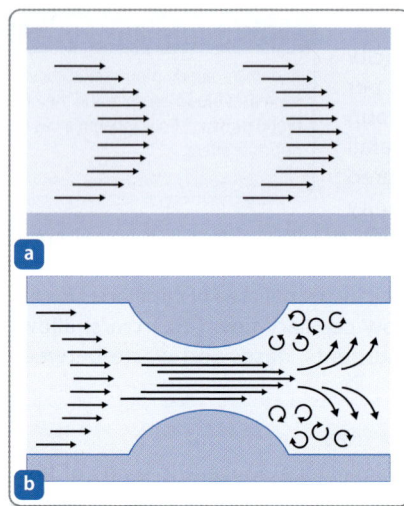

Figure 1.33 Flow through blood vessels. (a) Laminar flow. Friction between the vessel wall and flowing blood causes a parabolic velocity profile with the highest flow velocity centrally and the slowest at the periphery. (b) Turbulent flow: acceleration through narrowed segment causes flow separation and vortex formation in the post-stenotic region.

> **Guiding principle**
>
> 1 mmHg = 133.3 pascals (Pa)

Blood pressure

Blood pressure is the force that blood exerts on vascular walls. It is measured in millimeters of mercury (mmHg), i.e. the number of millimeters by which it can raise a column of mercury in a manometer. In this section, blood pressure refers to systemic blood pressure, routinely measured with a sphygmomanometer at the brachial artery.

Blood pressure is expressed as the systolic value over the diastolic value, e.g. 120/80 mmHg. MAP is the average blood pressure over the period of the cardiac cycle (**Figure 1.34**).

Maximum blood pressure is reached during systole, and the minimum occurs in diastole. Although the heart is an intermittent pump, blood pressure is maintained during diastole by elastic recoil of the large arteries (**Figure 1.35**). Blood pressure declines the most distal a vessel is from the left ventricle, as flow energy is lost via friction and resistance decreases.

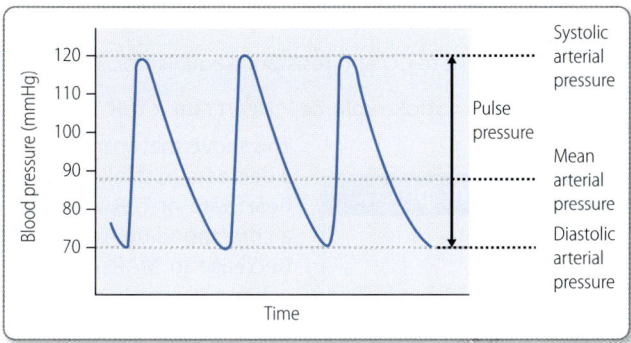

Figure 1.34 Systolic, diastolic and mean arterial blood pressure. The pulse pressure is the difference between the systolic pressure and the diastolic pressure.

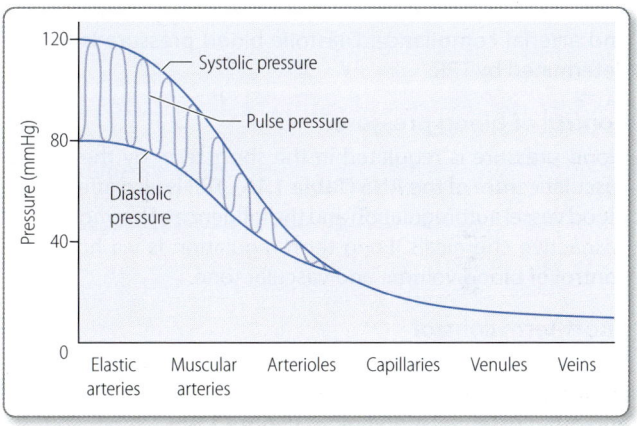

Figure 1.35 The first vessels in the arterial tree, the elastic and muscular arteries, transmit blood pressure with minimal loss. Through the arterioles there is a large fall in blood pressure and the pulse pressure falls until it is eventually lost.

Determinants of blood pressure

Blood pressure is the sum of the arterial and venous pressures. However, CVP is usually discounted as it is close to zero (normally 2–5 mmHg). Recall the following relationship:

$$\text{Pressure } (P) = \text{Flow } (Q) \times \text{Resistance } (R)$$

Flow is equivalent to CO and resistance equals TPR. Therefore:

$$\text{MAP} = \text{Stroke volume} \times \text{Heart rate} \times \text{TPR}$$

> **Guiding principle**
>
> Mean arterial blood pressure can be approximated by:
> MAP = 1/3 systolic BP + 2/3 diastolic BP

This shows that an increase or a decrease in stroke volume, heart rate or TPR will cause a corresponding increase or decrease in MAP. As stroke volume is closely related to blood volume, the major determinants of MAP are:

- Total peripheral resistance
- Cardiac output (stroke volume × heart rate)
- Blood volume

Systolic blood pressure is mainly determined by stroke volume and arterial compliance. Diastolic blood pressure is mainly determined by TPR.

Control of blood pressure

Blood pressure is regulated in the short term by the cardiovascular centre of the ANS (**Table 1.15**). TPR is also affected by blood vessel autoregulation and the influence of hormones and vasoactive chemicals. Long-term regulation is via hormonal control of blood volume and vascular tone.

Short-term control

The medullary cardiovascular centre co-ordinates fast homeostatic mechanisms to ensure tissues have sufficient O_2, glucose and other essential metabolites (**Figure 1.36**).

Baroreceptors Stretch receptors of the aortic arch and carotid sinus send signals to the cardiovascular centre via cranial nerves IX and X. An increase in the rate of baroreceptor action potential firing stimulates the PNS, and inhibits the SNS, to decrease blood pressure. A decrease in pressure has the opposite effect. This baroreflex system

> **Clinical insight**
>
> In essential hypertension, the baroreflex threshold is reset to a higher point.

Cardiovascular physiology

Factor	Sympathetic activation	Parasympathetic activation
Heart rate	↑ (increasing CO)	↓
Contractility	↑ (increasing SV and CO)	–
Arterial vascular tone	↑ (increasing TPR)	↓
Venous tone	↑ (increasing CVP and CO)	↓
Hormone release	Adrenaline (epinephrine) from adrenal glands and renin from the kidneys	–
Blood pressure	↑	↓

ANS, autonomic nervous system; CO, cardiac output; CVP, central venous pressure; SV, stroke volume; TPR, total peripheral resistance.

Table 1.15 The ANS is central to global blood pressure control.

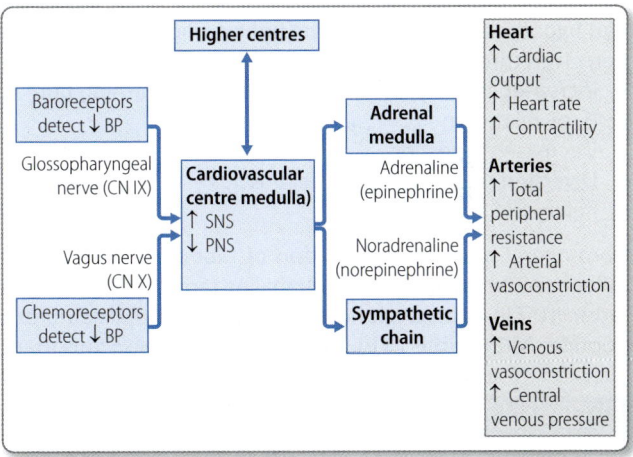

Figure 1.36 Short-term mechanisms of blood pressure control. A decrease in blood pressure is detected by baroreceptors and chemoreceptors. The cardiovascular centre coordinates the response through activation of the sympathetic nervous system (SNS) and inhibition of the parasympathetic nervous system (PNS) to cause a compensatory increase in blood pressure.

is rapid and modifiable (e.g. to accommodate exercise) but does not affect long-term control.

Chemoreceptors: Chemoreceptors of the aortic arch and carotid bodies are sensitive to changes in blood O_2, CO_2 and pH. Their signals also travel in the IX and X cranial nerves to the medulla. They have a greater effect on the respiratory than the cardiovascular centre.

Chemoreceptors are activated by decreased O_2 and pH and increased CO_2, and cause an increase in vascular tone and *decrease* in heart rate. The bradycardic effect is concurrently overridden by sympathetic stimulation due to lung stretch receptor activation, so that the overall effect is an increase in heart rate, vascular tone and blood pressure.

Muscle receptors: Muscle chemo- and stretch receptors activate the SNS during activity.

Influence of higher brain regions: Higher brain regions can influence blood pressure homeostasis. For example, the amygdala and hypothalamus stimulate the fight-or-flight response to a perceived threat:
- Increased blood pressure, heart rate and breathing rate
- Pupil dilatation
- Decreased digestion
- Diversion of blood to skeletal muscles
- Release of stored energy

Hormones: Short-term regulation of blood pressure is also influenced by the hormones adrenaline (epinephrine), angiotensin II (AT II), antidiuretic hormone (ADH) and atrial natriuretic peptide (ANP) (**Table 1.16**). The latter three are also important in long-term blood pressure regulation.

> **Clinical insight**
>
> Chronic stress can increase risk of coronary heart disease (CHD), via increases in blood pressure, triglycerides (TG) and cholesterol leading to atherosclerosis.

Long-term control

Long-term blood pressure regulation is largely via control of blood volume. This is modified by systems of Na^+

Hormone	Source	Stimulant	Action
Adrenaline (epinephrine)	Adrenal medulla	SNS	Nonselective adrenoreceptor agonist – similar to noradrenaline (norepinephrine) action
Angiotensin II	Liver	Hypotension	Vasoconstriction, renal water and salt retention
Antidiuretic hormone	Hypothalamus/ Posterior pituitary gland		
Atrial natriuretic peptide	Atrial myocardium	Atrial stretch	Vasodilation, and augments renal salt and water clearance

SNS, sympathetic nervous system.

Table 1.16 Hormones influencing blood pressure.

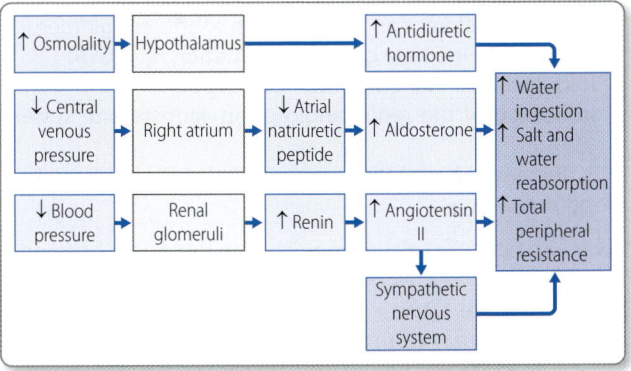

Figure 1.37 Long-term blood pressure regulation through control of blood volume. The overall effect is a reflex increase in blood pressure by increasing both blood volume and total peripheral resistance.

and water reabsorption and excretion in the renal tubules (**Figure 1.37**).

Antidiuretic hormone: Osmoreceptors in the hypothalamus sense fluctuations in serum osmolality, i.e. in how concentrated

plasma is with electrolytes (particularly Na+). An increase in osmolality results in ADH secretion via the posterior pituitary. ADH causes:
- Peripheral vasoconstriction
- Thirst
- Increased aquaporin expression in cells of the distal renal tubule and collecting dust, resulting in increased water reabsorption.

> **Clinical insight**
>
> A low salt diet is advised for hypertensive patients as Na+ is the main contributor to plasma osmolality, and increases blood volume.

This dilutes blood and increases TPR and blood volume and therefore blood pressure.

Atrial natriuretic peptide Atrial myocardial cells release ANP in response to stretch, i.e. increased blood volume or venous return. ANP causes:
- Peripheral vasodilation
- Dilation of afferent and constriction of efferent glomerular arterioles to increase glomerular filtration rate (GFR)
- Reduced renal Na+ and water reabsorption
- Inhibition of the renin–angiotensin–aldosterone system (RAAS).

This decreases both TPR and blood volume, and therefore blood pressure.

Renin–angiotensin–aldosterone system: RAAS is a hormonal cascade that increases TPR and blood volume to raise blood pressure (**Figure 1.38**).

Renin is an enzyme produced by granular cells of the renal juxtaglomerular apparatus (JGA). Release is stimulated by:
- Decrease in arterial blood pressure – detected by JGA
- Low Na+ detected in the ultrafiltrate – detected by macula densa of JGA
- Sympathetic nervous system stimulation to the JGA

Renin converts plasma angiotensinogen produced by liver cells into angiotensin (AT). AT is subsequently converted by angiotensin-converting enzyme (ACE) into AT II. AT II causes:
- Powerful vasoconstriction

Cardiovascular physiology

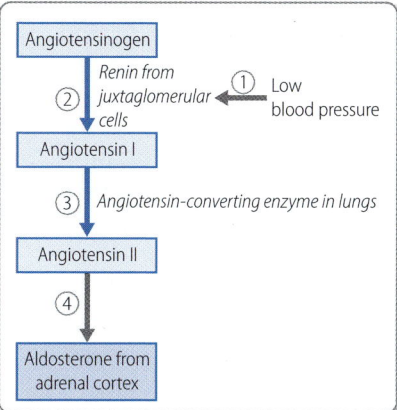

Figure 1.38 The renin–angiotensin–aldosterone cascade. (**1**), Renin is released from the response to low blood pressure; (**2**), renin cleaves angiotensinogen into angiotensin I; (**3**), angiotensin I is converted angiotensin-converting into angiotensin II by enzyme; (**4**), angiotensin II stimulates aldosterone release from the adrenal cortex.

- Increase in renal Na^+ and water reabsorption
- Sympathetic nervous system stimulation
- Aldosterone release
- Antidiuretic hormone release.

> **Clinical insight**
>
> Angiotensin converting enzyme (ACE) inhibitors and angiotensin II receptor blockers (ARBs) are two antihypertensive drugs that block renin–angiotensin–aldosterone system (RAAS) activation.

Aldosterone is a mineralocorticoid hormone that, like ADH, increases renal Na^+ and water reabsorption at the distal convoluted tubule (DCT) and collecting ducts.

Haemostasis

Blood is a water-based fluid that distributes metabolic nutrients, gases and waste products as well as blood cells and many proteins (**Table 1.17**).

Haemostasis is a sequence of events that prevents blood loss from damaged vessels and is the start of wound healing. It has three stages:
1. Vasoconstriction
2. Platelet aggregation forming a 'platelet plug'
3. The coagulation cascade forming a fibrin clot

Blood composition			Example	Function
55% plasma	92% water		-	Solvent
	8% dissolved substances	Nutrients	Glucose	Energy metabolism
		Respiratory gases	O_2 and CO_2	Cellular respiration
		Proteins	Albumin	Transport of substances, maintain intravascular oncotic pressure
			Clotting factors	Blood clotting
			Immunoglobulins	Adaptive immune response
		Lipids		Cell membranes, energy, and hormones
		Electrolytes	$Na^+, K^+, Ca^{2+},$ and Cl^-	Membrane potentials and transport
			H^+ and HCO_3^-	Body fluid acidity
44% red blood cells (erythrocytes)				O_2 transport
1% white blood cells (leucocytes)				Immune

Table 1.17 Blood constituents and their functions.

The result is a thrombus; a collection of platelets, dead (predominately red) cells and a matrix of the protein fibrin. Platelet aggregation is quicker but weaker than the fibrin deposition of the cascade and is of greater importance in high-flow, arterial vessels – forming paler, platelet-rich white clots. Fibrin deposition occurs more in low-flow venous vessels, resulting in fibrin and erythrocyte-rich red clots.

Vasoconstriction

Injury to a blood vessel results in vasoconstriction to limit blood loss. Constriction is triggered by:
- A direct vascular smooth muscle cell response
- Endothelial cell release of vasoconstrictive mediators
- Local pain reflexes

> **Clinical insight**
>
> Thromboembolism is when a piece of a thrombus breaks off and embolises (i.e. travels) downstream to partially or completely occlude a vessel. Deep vein venous thromboembolism is the most common and can result in pulmonary embolism.

Platelet aggregation

Platelets are anuclear fragments of megakaryocytes produced in the bone marrow. They are continually produced and last for 10–12 days. Platelets contain vesicles (granules):
- *α-granules:* Clotting factors, inflammatory mediators and growth factors
- *Dense granules:* ATP, adenosine diphosphate (ADP), serotonin (a potent vasoconstrictor) and Ca^{2+}
- Lysosomes

A number of platelet agonists trigger specific pathways of platelet activation, resulting in activation of the GPIIb/IIIa complex. Platelet aggregation is initiated by exposure to subendothelial components in the extracellular matrix (ECM). von Willebrand factor (vWF), a circulating protein, binds to both ECM collagen and to platelet surface glycoprotein GpIb (**Figure 1.39**). This results in translocation of glycoprotein complex IIb/IIIa (GpIIb/IIIa) to the platelet surface. Platelets aggregate by bonding via GpIIb/IIIa complexes.

Platelet activation

Platelets are activated to release their secretory vesicles (i.e. degranulate) by:
- Adenosine diphosphate
- Thrombin, an enzyme of the coagulation system
- Calcium

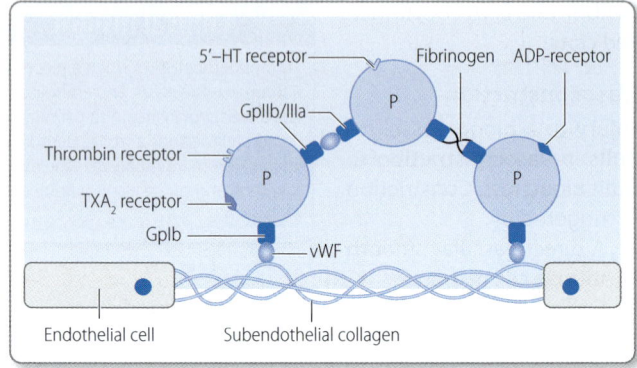

Figure 1.39 Platelets constitutively express GpIb on their surface, but once activated they express GpIIb/IIIa, which mediates strong bonds between them. ADP, adenosine diphosphate; Gp, glycoprotein; P, platelet; TXA_2, thromboxane; vWF, von Willebrand factor.

- Thromboxane A2, a lipid signalling molecule. Degranulation promotes aggregation, further platelet activation, the coagulation cascade and inflammation. Conversely, prostacyclin release by endothelial cells and leucocytes inhibits platelet aggregation and their release from the bone marrow.

The coagulation cascade

The coagulation cascade is a series of amplifying reactions of clotting factors resulting in fibrin clot formation. Clotting factors are soluble proenzymes (e.g. factor X or FX) present in circulation that are cleaved to become active enzymes (e.g. FXa).

The reactions of the coagulation system often take place on the surface of platelets and require Ca^{2+} as a co-factor. The cascade can be initiated by endothelial damage (the extrinsic pathway) or intrinsic to ongoing haemostasis (the intrinsic pathway).

> **Guiding principle**
>
> Clotting factors are synthesised by the liver and have a short half-life. FII, FVII, FIX and FX require vitamin K for their synthesis.

The extrinsic pathway

Endothelial damage exposes tissue factor (TF), which binds factor VII (FVII), activating factor VII to FVIIa–TF. This complex activates FX, which associates with its co-factor, FV, to form FXa–FVa (a small amount of active FV is present spontaneously). FXa–FVa converts prothrombin (FII) into thrombin (FIIa), which cleaves soluble, circulating fibrinogen – the soluble precursor of fibrin – into insoluble fibrin. Only a small clot is formed, but the intrinsic pathway is activated to form a full fibrin clot. Thrombin produced by the extrinsic pathway activates:

- Factor V
- Factor VIII (by cleavage from circulating FVII–vWF complexes)
- Factor XI
- Platelets

The extrinsic pathway is rapidly terminated by the extrinsic pathway inhibitor (EPI) that blocks activation of FX by FVIIa–TF.

The intrinsic pathway

This is triggered by thrombin generated by the extrinsic pathway or from platelet degranulation. FIXa–FVIIIa complexes activate FX, which is able to generate large amounts of thrombin and, therefore, a fibrin clot.

Thrombolysis

Thrombolysis (or fibrinolysis) is the process of cleaving insoluble fibrin into soluble degradation products, to remove clots (**Figure 1.40**). This limits thrombus size allows remodelling and breaks the thrombus down once the causative damage has been repaired.

Cleavage is mediated by plasmin, which circulates as inactive plasminogen and is activated by tissue plasminogen activator (tPA). Endothelial cells release tPA in response to the presence of thrombin.

Anti-coagulation systems

The body has several systems to prevent unnecessary activation of the coagulation cascade:

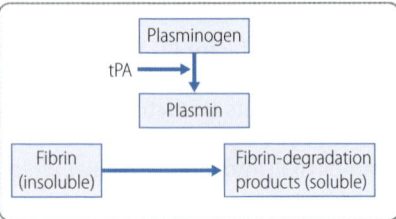

Figure 1.40 Mechanism of thrombolysis: plasmin breaks down insoluble fibrin into soluble degradation products. tPA, tissue plasminogen activator.

- Antithrombins (e.g. antithrombin III) inhibit thrombin and other active clotting factors, blocking progression of the cascade
- Heparin works by activating antithrombin III, making it rapidly effective
- *The protein C system:* In response to the presence of thrombin, thrombomodulin is expressed on the surface of intact endothelial cells. Circulating protein C and its co-factor protein S bind to thrombomodulin and break down FVa and FVIIIa.

Clinical insight

Synthetic (recombinant) tPA is used to promote thrombolysis and reopen blocked vessels in cases of ischaemic stroke and myocardial infarction.

Clinical insight

Warfarin is an anticoagulant that antagonises the effects of vitamin K, preventing the formation of clotting factors (II, VII, IX and X). Its onset is much slower (2–3 days) than heparin anticoagulation (<12 hours). Over-anticoagulation can cause spontaneous bleeding with serious clinical consequences.

Lipid metabolism

Lipid molecules contain carbon, hydrogen and oxygen, and principally consist of non-polar carbon–hydrogen (C–H) bonds. They are consumed in the diet and synthesised *de novo*. Lipids can be hydrolysed to yield fatty acids or complex alcohols, which are important energy fuels for cellular metabolism.

They are a diverse group of substances with diverse chemical structures and functions (**Table 1.18**).

Function	Examples	Structure
Principle component of biological membranes	Glycerophospholipids	Derivatives of phosphatidic acid
	Sphingolipids	Derivatives of the amino acid sphingosine
Hormones	Prostaglandins	Fatty acid (mostly arachidonic acid) derivatives
	Steroids	Cholesterol based
Energy storage	Acylglycerols	Glycerol backbone with fatty acid attached
Energy metabolite	Fatty acids	12–20 carbon hydrocarbons with COOH group. Saturated have no double bonds
Vitamins	Terpenes, e.g. vitamins A, E and K	Polymer of 5 carbon isoprene
Transport of lipophilic compounds	Lipoproteins	Protein-emulsified lipid assemblies

Table 1.18 Lipid functions. COOH, carboxylic acid.

Polarity

Lipids have a hydrophobic tail group which is non-polar. This makes them soluble in organic solvents and insoluble in water. Some lipids also contain other polar groups that make them amphiphilic (amphipathic), i.e. they have both polar, soluble, water-loving (hydrophilic) and non-polar, fat-loving (lipophilic) properties. Amphiphilic lipids have important biological functions, e.g. phospholipids constitute the lipid bilayer structure of cell membranes.

Lipolysis

Lipids are hydrolysed to fatty acids and glycerol in adipose and muscle tissues when energy is required.

> **Guiding principle**
>
> Carbon–carbon double bonds:
> - Saturated fatty acids – 0
> - Monounsaturated fatty acids – 1
> - Polyunsaturated fatty acids > 1

1. *Triglyceride (TG) hydrolysis:* Fasting, exercise or stress stimulates TG hydrolysis by lipase. Glycerol is then phosphorylated to glycerol 3-phosphate before being oxidised to dihydroxyacetone phosphate. Glyceraldehyde-3-phosphate can be converted to either pyruvate or glucose in the liver.
2. *Fatty acid co-linkage to coenzyme A (CoA):* Fatty acids are first activated in the cytosol when they are bound by a CoA. This is catalysed by acyl CoA synthetase and is irreversible.

   Step 1: Fatty acid + ATP → acyl adenylate + Pyrophosphate

   Step 2: Acyl adenylate + CoASH → acyl CoA + AMP

   A thioester bond is formed between the fatty acid carboxyl group and the sulfhydryl group of CoA.
3. *The carnitine shuttle:* Acyl CoA can only enter mitochondria via the carnitine shuttle. Carnitine is a nitrogenous cation that binds to acyl CoA to form acylcarnitine. This can cross the outer and inner mitochondrial membranes in exchange for unbound carnitine moving out of mitochondria. This is the rate-limiting step in fatty acid oxidation.

Regulation of lipolysis

Lipolysis is regulated through the control of lipase activity (**Figure 1.41**). Counter regulatory hormones stimulate lipase when energy reserves are low: adrenaline (epinephrine), noradrenaline (norepinephrine), growth hormone, cortisol and glucagon. Conversely, insulin inhibits lipase.

Fatty acid oxidation

Fatty acids are oxidised by β-oxidation in mitochondria and peroxisomes to generate acetyl CoA, nicotinamide adenine dinucleotide (NADH) and flavin adenine dinucleotide ($FADH_2$). Acetyl-CoA enters the citric acid cycle and the latter acts as oxidising co-factors in the electron transport chain. Each $FADH_2$ and NADH generates two and three molecules of ATP, respectively.

Before oxidation, unsaturated fatty acids must have their double bonds broken by isomerase and reductase enzymes.

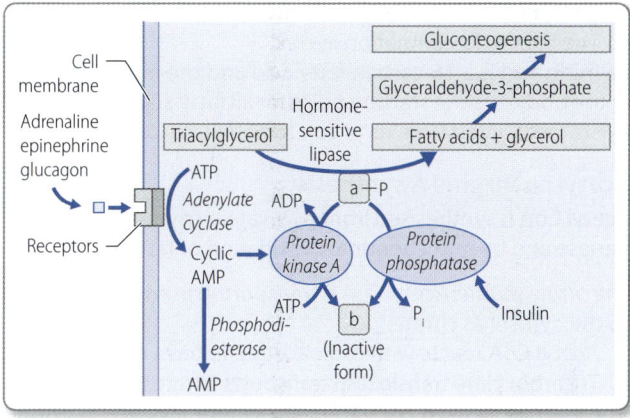

Figure 1.41 Regulation of lipase activity. ADP, adenosine diphosphate; AMP, adenosine monophosphate; ATP, adenosine triphosphate.

Glycerol

Glycerol is a 3-carbon polyol (sugar alcohol) with 3-hydroxyl groups and is the backbone of all TG lipids. Once converted to glyceraldehyde-3-phosphate, it can enter glycolysis or gluconeogenesis in the liver. Alternatively, it can be used as a substrate for triacylglycerol or phospholipid synthesis in the liver and adipose tissue.

> **Guiding principle**
>
> Peroxisomes are small organelles that break down very long chain and branched chain fatty acids, polyamines, amino acids and synthesise plasmalogens. Peroxisomal oxidation is stimulated by a fat-rich meal or some lipid-lowering drugs such as fibrates.

Lipogenesis

Fatty acids synthesis is the production of palmitic acid from acetyl CoA and malonyl CoA. It occurs in the liver, lactating mammary glands and adipose tissue if dietary intake is insufficient. There are four stages, the later three occurring in the cytosol:
1. Acetyl CoA synthesis and the citrate shuttle
2. Malonyl CoA synthesis

3. Formation of malonyl transferase
4. The fatty acid elongation cycle

Palmitic acid is a 16-carbon fatty acid and the most abundant in the body. It is the starting point for all fatty acids. It normally exists dissociated from its H⁺ ion as palmitate ion.

Acetyl coenzyme A synthesis

Acetyl CoA is synthesised from pyruvate by pyruvate dehydrogenase and by mitochondrial β-oxidation of fatty acids.

The citrate shuttle: Acetyl CoA is transported from mitochondria to the cytosol as citrate:
1. Acetyl CoA reacts with oxaloacetate to form citrate
2. Tricarboxylate translocase transports citrate to the cytosol
3. Citrate is cleaved back to oxaloacetate and acetyl CoA in the cytosol by an ATP-dependent enzyme called ATP-citrate lyase

This requires 14-nicotinamide adenine dinucleotide phosphate (NADPH) as reducing agents and produces 8 for every molecule of palmitate produced. The pentose phosphate pathway provides the deficit.

Malonyl coenzyme A synthesis

Some acetyl CoA is carboxylated to form malonyl CoA in an irreversible two-step reaction that requires bicarbonate, biotin and ATP. It is a commitment step in fatty acid synthesis, as malonyl CoA is only involved in fatty acid synthesis.

Both steps are catalysed by acetyl CoA carboxylase:
1. Acetyl CoA is converted to carboxybiotin; one ATP is used
2. The carboxyl group is transferred from the biotin to the acetyl CoA to form malonyl CoA

This is the key regulatory step for fatty acid synthesis. The 'extra' carbon of malonyl CoA is what allows lipogenesis to be thermodynamically possible.

Fatty acid synthase

Fatty acid synthase is a dimeric, 7-enzyme complex that synthesises palmitic acid from either acyl CoA or malonyl CoA. Each domain is responsible for different steps of synthesis (**Table 1.19**).

Domain	Enzymes/Proteins	Function
Condensing unit	Acetyl transferase	Substrate binding
	Malonyl transferase	
	β-ketoacyl ACP synthase	Decarboxylation – liberation of CO_2; condensation (merging) of acetyl and malonyl groups to form acetoacetyl-ACP
Reduction unit	ACP	Binds acetoacetyl group
	β-ketoacyl reductase	Reduces acetoacetyl-ACP to β-hydroxybutyryl-ACP
	β-hydroxybutyryl-ACP dehydratase	Dehydrates β-hydroxybutyryl-ACP to trans-Δ^2-butenoyl-ACP (with a double bond)
	Enoyl reductase	Reduces trans-Δ^2-butenoyl-ACP to remove double bond and form butyryl-ACP
Palmitate release unit	Thioesterase	Releases palmitic acid via hydrolysis
ACP, acetyl carrier protein.		

Table 1.19 The three domains of the fatty acid synthase complex and their functions.

Firstly, acetyl CoA or malonyl CoA attach to an oxygen atom of acetyl transferase or malonyl transferase, respectively. Acetyl groups are transferred to the condensing enzyme β-ketoacyl synthase. Malonyl groups are then transferred to the acyl carrier protein.

> **Guiding principle**
>
> Biotin is a water-soluble B vitamin (B7) and important for carboxylase catalysed reactions.

The two carbons of the malonyl group attached to the acyl carrier protein are elongated by a cycle of condensation and reduction reactions to form 16-carbon palmitoyl. Finally, this is hydrolysed to palmitate. The stoichiometry can be summarised as:

$$8 \text{ acetyl CoA} + 7 \text{ ATP} + 14 \text{ NADPH} + 6 \text{ H}^+$$
$$\downarrow$$
$$\text{Palmitate} + 14 \text{ NADP}^+ + 8 \text{ CoA} + 6 \text{ H}_2\text{O} + 7 \text{ ADP} + 7 \text{ P}_i$$

Further elongation

Longer fatty acids are synthesised by microsomes – vesicles of budded endoplasmic reticulum. Two carbon units are added to the carbonyl end of saturated and unsaturated fatty acids. Solubility rapidly decreases as chain length increases.

Unsaturation of fatty acids

Microsomal enzymes also add double bonds to unsaturated long chain acyl CoAs, such as converting stearoyl CoA to oleoyl CoA. An oxidase enzyme introduces a *cis*-Δ^9 double bond, and requires O_2 and NADH, and releases two molecules of water.

Regulation of fatty acid metabolism

Fatty acid metabolism is predominately regulated by hormones that affect acetyl CoA carboxylase activity (**Figure 1.42**):

- When energy is required, adrenaline (epinephrine) and glucagon inactivate it via phosphorylation by AMP protein kinase
- When energy is not required, insulin activates it via dephosphorylation by phosphatase 2A.

Acetyl CoA carboxylase is also activated by citrate and inhibited by AMP and palmitoyl CoA.

Lipogenesis is tightly co-ordinated with fatty acid breakdown, i.e. β-oxidation (**Table 1.20**).

> **Guiding principle**
>
> Double bonds in unsaturated fatty acids increase solubility and lower melting point. This underlies the fluidity of cell membranes.

> **Clinical insight**
>
> Fibric acid derivatives (fibrates) are used as drugs to lower triglyceride concentration. They:
> - Induce gene expression of lipolytic enzymes such as lipoprotein lipase
> - Decrease the expression of apolipoprotein C3, a protein that inhibits lipoprotein lipase
> - Promote a shift towards larger, more buoyant low-density lipoprotein (LDL) particles that are less susceptible to oxidation and have increased affinity for the LDL receptor

Prostaglandins

Arachidonate is a 20-carbon polyunsaturated fatty acid derived from linoleate. It is

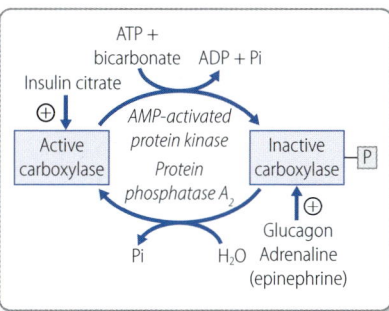

Figure 1.42 Regulation of acetyl coenzyme A carboxylase activity. +, activates; ADP, adenosine diphosphate; AMP, adenosine monophosphate; ATP, adenosine triphosphate; P, phosphate; Pi, inorganic phosphate.

Feature	Synthesis	Oxidation
Intracellular location	Cytoplasm	Mitochondria
Initial substrates	Acetyl CoA or malonyl CoA	Fatty acyl CoA
Thioester linkage of intermediates	Protein-SH (acyl carrier protein)	CoA
Coenzymes	NADPH	FAD^+ and NAD^+
Bicarbonate dependence	Yes	No
Energy state favouring process	High ATP	High ADP
Citrate activation	Yes	No
Acyl CoA inhibition	Yes	No
Highest activity	Fed	Fasting or starvation

ATP, adenosine triphosphate; CoA, coenzyme A; CoASH, acetyl coenzyme A; FAD^+, flavin adenine dinucleotide (oxidised form); NAD^+, nicotinamide adenine dinucleotide (oxidised form); NADPH, nicotinamide adenine dinucleotide phosphate (reduced form).

Table 1.20 Comparison of fatty acid synthesis and breakdown (β-oxidation).

the starting point for the basis of the prostaglandins: prostacyclins, thromboxanes and leukotrienes (**Figure 1.43**). These locally acting hormones have a short half-life but have vital functions, including:

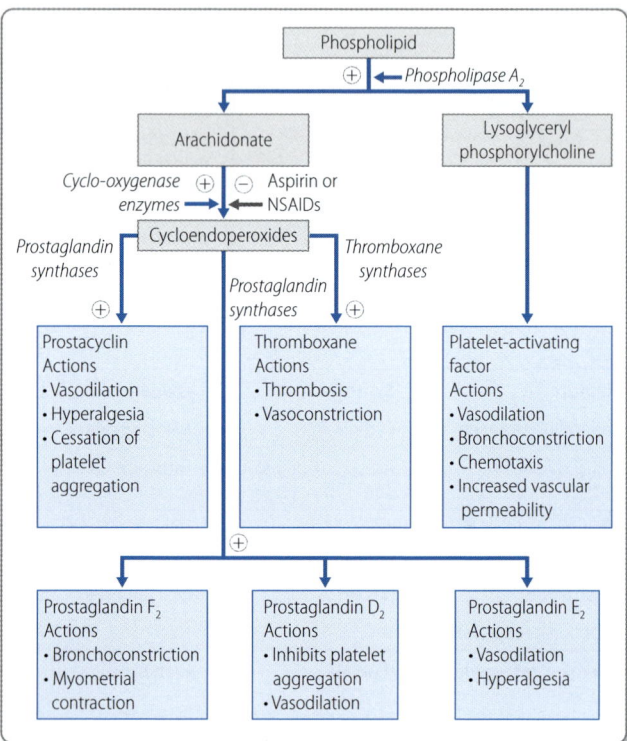

Figure 1.43 Prostaglandin biosynthesis and their actions. +, activates; −, inhibits; NSAID, non-steroidal anti-inflammatory drug.

- Stimulating the inflammatory response
- Regulating local blood flow
- Modulating ion transport across membranes
- Propagating synaptic transmission
- Sleep induction

Cholesterol metabolism

Cholesterol is a 27-carbon steroid alcohol (sterol) lipid (**Figure 1.44**). It is a key component of cell membranes, allowing their fluid movement, and is the precursor to vitamin

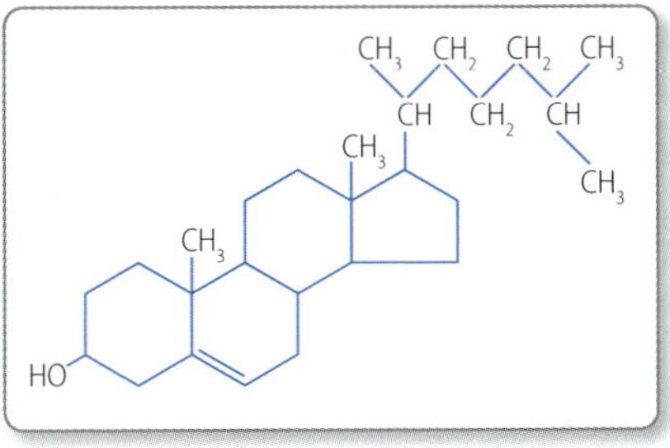

Figure 1.44 Cholesterol.

D, bile acids and steroid hormones, including testosterone and cortisol.

Cholesterol is consumed in the diet and synthesised de novo in the liver and intestine. On average, 800 mg of cholesterol is synthesised daily in a person on a low-cholesterol diet.

> **Clinical insight**
>
> Aspirin (acetylsalicylate) decreases inflammation by inhibiting the activity of prostaglandin synthase. It irreversibly inhibits the cyclo-oxygenase activity of this enzyme by acetylating the serine hydroxyl group. It is also an antithrombotic agent, because it blocks the production of prostaglandin A_2, a potent aggregator of blood platelets.

Cholesterol synthesis

Cholesterol biosynthesis begins with formation of isopentenyl pyrophosphate from acetyl CoA (**Figure 1.45**). The first step is the condensation of acetyl CoA with acetoacetyl CoA, forming 3-hydroxy-3-methylglutaryl CoA (HMG-CoA), a reaction catalysed by HMG-CoA synthase.

Formation of mevalonate: HMG-CoA, which is present in the cytosol and mitochondria of the liver, is reduced to mevalonate by HMG-CoA reductase. This reaction requires NADPH. This is the first irreversible, committed step of cholesterol synthesis. Mevalonate is then converted to isopentenyl pyrophosphate in a series of three ATP-dependent reactions.

> **Clinical insight**
>
> Statins lower blood cholesterol by inhibiting HMG-CoA reductase, the rate-limiting enzyme of cholesterol biosynthesis.

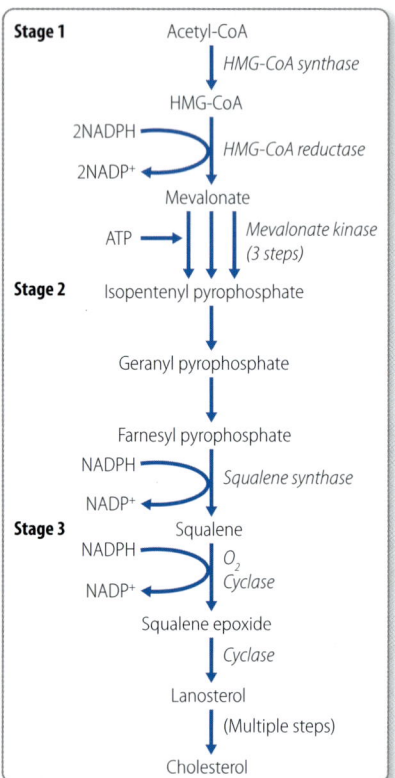

Figure 1.45 Biosynthesis of cholesterol. ATP, adenosine triphosphate; HMG-CoA, 3-hydroxy-3-methylglutaryl coenzyme A; NADPH, nicotinamide adenine dinucleotide phosphate.

Synthesis of squalene: The second stage of cholesterol synthesis is the synthesis of squalene, a 30-carbon hydrocarbon molecule, from five five-carbon molecules of isopentenyl pyrophosphate. This process starts with the isomerisation of isopentenyl pyrophosphate to form dimethylallyl pyrophosphate.

Formation of squalene epoxide: The third stage is the cyclisation of squalene to form squalene epoxide. This requires O_2 and NADPH. Squalene epoxide then undergoes cyclisation to lanosterol in a reaction catalysed by cyclase. Lanosterol is then converted

Cardiovascular physiology

to cholesterol, a 27-carbon molecule, by the removal of three methyl groups and the reduction of a double bond by NADPH.

Regulation of cholesterol synthesis: Cholesterol synthesis is regulated by mechanisms that sense the cellular level of cholesterol and modifies HMG-CoA reductase levels and activity:
- *Sterol regulatory element:* A transcription factor that inhibits enzyme gene expression in the presence of sterols
- *Non-sterol metabolites:* Derivatives of mevalonate inhibit enzyme gene expression
- *AMP-activated protein kinase:* Phosphorylates and decreases enzyme activity when ATP levels are low
- Enzyme degradation is also tightly regulated

Cholesterol absorption

Cholesterol esters in the gut are hydrolysed by cholesterol esterases, secreted by the pancreas and small intestine, to free cholesterol. Cholesterol must be emulsified to be absorbed: conjugated bile acids form micelles with free cholesterol, fatty acids, monoglycerides, and phospholipids.

Most cholesterol is absorbed in the middle jejunum and terminal ileum through the transmembrane transporter protein Niemann–Pick C1-like 1 protein. 30–60% of dietary cholesterol is absorbed daily. Once absorbed into the intestinal mucosa cell, it is packaged into large lipoproteins called 'chylomicrons'.

Cholesterol esterification: As free cholesterol is cytotoxic, it is esterified in the liver to cholesterol ester by acyl cholesterol acyl transferase. Cholesterol esters are stored in intracellular lipid drops and constitute 70% of plasma cholesterol.

Esterification requires energy-dependent activation of a fatty acid with CoA to

> **Clinical insight**
>
> Ezetimibe is a potent cholesterol-lowering drug that works by blocking cholesterol absorption mediated by the Niemann–Pick C1-like 1 protein.

> **Clinical insight**
>
> Familial hypercholesterolemia is an inherited condition causing high blood cholesterol concentrations. There are heterozygous and homozygous forms, affecting 1 in 500 and 1 in 1,000,000 of the UK population, respectively.

form an acyl CoA. The acyl CoA reacts with a hydroxyl group on cholesterol to form an ester.

Lipoprotein esterification: Esterification also occurs in the blood, in lipoproteins, the lipid transport vesicles. This is catalysed by lecithin-cholesterol acyl transferase and does not require CoA; instead, a fatty acid is transferred from lecithin. The enzyme is activated by apolipoprotein A-I, the major apolipoprotein in high-density lipoprotein (HDL). Cholesterol esters are in the hydrophobic core of the lipoprotein molecule (**Table 1.21**).

Lipid absorption and transport: Lipoproteins

Lipoproteins are spherical particles with non-polar neutral lipids in their core (i.e. TG and cholesterol esters) and more polar amphipathic lipids (i.e. phospholipids and cholesterol) on their surface (**Figure 1.46**). They also have apolipoproteins on their surface, which bind lipids, cell receptors and act as cofactors for enzymes of lipid metabolism (**Table 1.22**).

Types

Lipoproteins are classified by their physiochemical properties (**Tables 1.21** and **1.23**). Generally, larger lipoproteins contain more core lipids, TG and cholesterol esters, and less protein.

Class	Cholesterol (%)	Phospholipids (%)	Apolipoproteins (%)	Triglycerides (%)	Cholesterol ester (%)
CM	2	7	2	86	3
VLDL	7	18	8	55	12
IDL	9	19	19	23	29
LDL	8	22	22	6	42
HDL-2	5	33	40	5	17
HDL-3	4	25	55	3	13

CM, chylomicron; HDL, high-density lipoprotein; IDL, intermediate-density lipoprotein; LDL, low-density lipoprotein; VLDL, very-low-density lipoprotein.

Table 1.21 Chemical composition of lipoproteins.

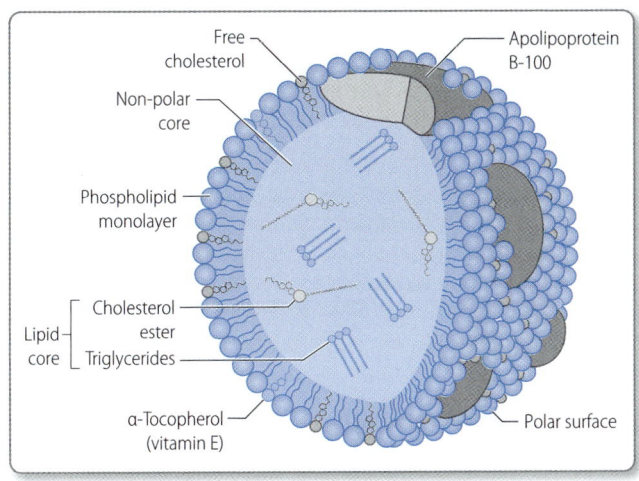

Figure 1.46 Lipoprotein structure.

Apolipoprotein	Function	Lipoprotein carrier
A-I	Co-factor for cholesteryl ester transfer protein	CM and HDL
A-II	Unknown	HDL
A-IV	• Activates lecithin cholesterol acyltransferase • Secretion of TG from liver binding protein to LDL receptor	CM and HDL
B-100	Secretion of TG from intestine	VLDL, IDL and LDL
B-48	Secretion of TG from liver binding protein to LDL receptor	CM
C-I	Activates lecithin cholesterol acyltransferase	CM, VLDL and HDL
C-II	Co-factor for lipoprotein lipase	CM, VLDL and HDL

Table 1.22 Functions of apolipoproteins. *Continues overleaf*

Apolipoprotein	Function	Lipoprotein carrier
C-III	Inhibits apo C-II Activates lipoprotein lipase	CM, VLDL and HDL
E	Facilitates uptake of CM and IDL remnants	CM, VLDL and HDL
(a)	Unknown	Lipoprotein (a)

CM, chylomicron; HDL, high-density lipoprotein; IDL, intermediate-density lipoprotein; LDL, low-density lipoprotein; TG, triglyceride; VLDL, very-low-density lipoprotein.

Table 1.22 *Continued*

Variable	Chylomicron	VLDL	IDL	LDL	HDL	Lp(a)
Density (g/mL)	<0.95	0.95–1.006	1.006–1.019	1.019–1.063	1.063–1.210	1.040–1.130
Electrophoretic mobility	Origin	Pre-beta	Slow pre-beta	Beta	Alpha	Pre-beta
Molecular weight (Da)	$0.4–30 \times 10^9$	$5–10 \times 10^6$	$3.9–4.8 \times 10^6$	2.75×10^6	$1.8–3.6 \times 10^5$	$2.9–3.7 \times 10^6$
Diameter (nm)	>70	26–70	22–24	19–23	4–10	26–30
Lipid: lipoprotein ratio	99:1	90:10	85:15	80:20	50:50	75:26–64:36
Major lipids	Exogenous TG	Endogenous TG	Endogenous TG, CEs	CEs	PLs	CEs and PLs
Major proteins	A-I	B-100	B-100	B-100	A-I	(a)
	B-48	C-I	E		A-II	B-100
	C-I	C-II				

Table 1.23 Properties of lipoproteins. *Continues opposite*

Variable	Chylomicron	VLDL	IDL	LDL	HDL	Lp (a)
	C-II	C-III				
	C-III	E				

CE, cholesterol ester; CM, chylomicrons; HDL, high-density lipoprotein; IDL, intermediate-density lipoprotein; LDL, low-density lipoprotein; Lp(a), lipoprotein(a); PL, phospholipid; TG, triglycerides; VLDL, very-low-density lipoprotein.

Table 1.23 *Continued*

Pathways

Lipoprotein metabolism has four main pathways with discrete functions in lipid transport.
1. The exogenous pathway
2. The endogenous pathway
3. Intracellular cholesterol transport
4. Reverse cholesterol transport.

The exogenous pathway The exogenous lipoprotein pathway transports lipids absorbed by the intestine to the liver and peripheral cells (**Figure 1.47**).
- Chylomicrons are assembled in the endoplasmic reticulum of endocytes by combining TG with apolipoprotein B-48
- They are secreted into the circulation, where they acquire additional lipoproteins (e.g. apolipoproteins E and CIIII) from HDL
- Apolipoprotein C-II activates lipoprotein lipase on the luminal surface of endothelial cells, which hydrolyses chylomicrons to free fatty acids
- The free fatty acids are either taken up by adipose tissue and stored as TG or taken up by muscle and used as an energy source

Remnant particles: Chylomicrons are progressively hydrolysed to chylomicron remnant particles. The surplus phospholipids and apolipoprotein A-I are transferred back to HDL. Remnant particles are taken up by the liver through via

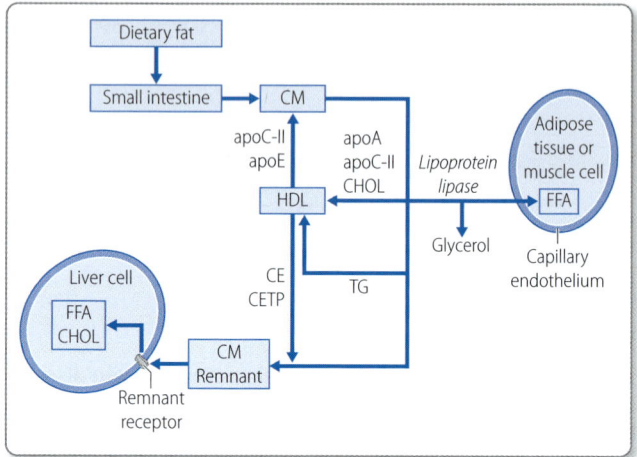

Figure 1.47 The exogenous lipoprotein pathway. apo, apolipoproteins; CE, cholesteryl ester; CETP, cholesteryl ester transfer protein; CHOL, cholesterol; CM, chylomicrons; FFA, free fatty acids; HDL, high-density lipoprotein; IDL, intermediate-density lipoprotein; TG, triglycerides; VLDL, very-low-density lipoprotein.

hepatic apolipoprotein E and B-48 receptors. The TG returned to the liver are used to power the biosynthetic activity of the liver, or they are repackaged with apolipoprotein B100 and secreted as very-low-density lipoprotein (VLDL) particles.

The endogenous pathway This pathway transfers TG synthesised by/transferred to the liver to peripheral cells for energy metabolism (**Figure 1.48**).

Lipoproteins in the endogenous pathway contain apolipoprotein B-100, particularly VLDLs, which also contain apolipoprotein E and apolipoprotein C. The apolipoprotein C-II on the surface of VLDLs activates lipoprotein lipase on the surface of endothelial cells, which hydrolyse TG to glycerol and fatty acids. The progressive hydrolysis of TG in the core of a VLDL particle transforms it into intermediate density lipoprotein and eventually LDL.

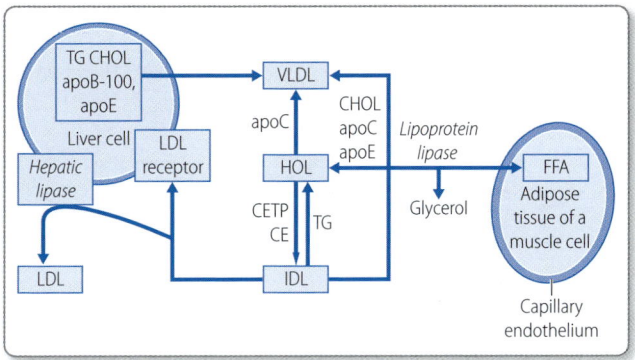

Figure 1.48 The endogenous lipoprotein pathway. apo, apolipoproteins; CE, cholesteryl ester; CETP, cholesteryl ester transfer protein; CHOL, cholesterol; CM, chylomicrons; FFA, free fatty acids; HDL, high-density lipoprotein; IDL, intermediate-density lipoprotein; LDL, low-density lipoprotein; TG, triglycerides; VLDL, very-low-density lipoprotein.

About half of the apolipoprotein B100 particles in the exogenous pathway are removed by hepatic remnant receptors before undergoing complete hydrolysis. The remaining portion is converted to LDL. The TG in LDL is further depleted by the cholesteryl-ester transfer protein, a plasma enzyme that removes TG from LDL in exchange for cholesterol esters from HDL. During the transformation from VLDL to LDL, excess surface phospholipid and lipoproteins (except apolipoprotein B-100) are transferred to HDL.

Most LDL is returned to the liver through the LDL apolipoprotein B-100 receptor. The cholesterol can then be:
- Incorporated into lipoproteins
- Used in bile salt syntheses
- Excreted in bile

Intracellular cholesterol transport The intracellular transport of cholesterol is tightly regulated (**Figure 1.49**), as cholesterol affects membrane properties and is cytotoxic in excess.

Cellular cholesterol is derived from cellular synthesis, or through lipoprotein uptake via the LDL receptor. Receptor

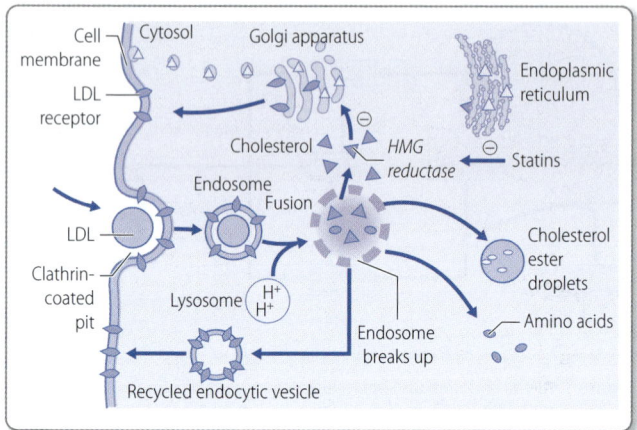

Figure 1.49 Overview of intracellular cholesterol transport. HMG-CoA, 3-hydroxy-3-methylglutaryl coenzyme A; LDL, low-density lipoprotein.

binding leads to lipoprotein endocytosis and lysosomal breakdown.

Apolipoproteins are degraded to small peptides and amino acids. Cholesterol esters are converted to free cholesterol by lysosomal acid lipase. Cholesterol is:
- Used for membrane biogenesis
- Stored in intracellular lipid drops after re-esterification
- Excreted in the reverse cholesterol transport pathway.

Regulation: Excess intracellular cholesterol has a negative feedback effect on its own biosynthesis via HMG-CoA reductase and LDL receptor down-regulation. It also induces the synthesis of proteins of the reverse cholesterol transport pathway.

Reverse cholesterol transport

This removes excess, potentially toxic, cellular cholesterol and transfers it to the liver for excretion (**Figure 1.50**). The main lipoprotein involved is HDL.

Cardiovascular physiology

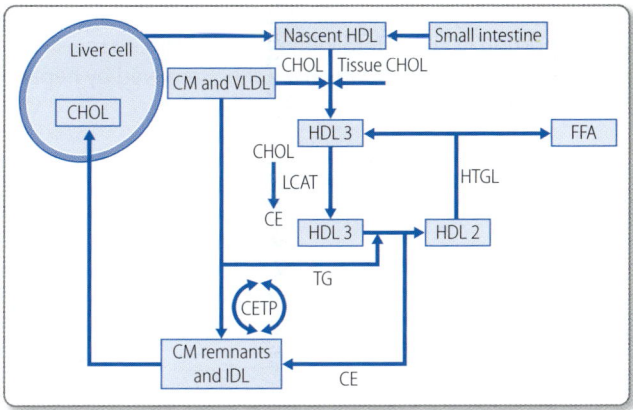

Figure 1.50 The reverse cholesterol transport lipoprotein pathway. CE, cholesteryl ester; CETP, cholesteryl ester transfer protein; CHOL, cholesterol; CM, chylomicrons; FFA, free fatty acids; HDL, high-density lipoprotein; HTGL, hepatic triglyceride lipase; IDL, intermediate-density lipoprotein; LCAT, lecithin-cholesterol acyltransferase; TG, triglycerides; VLDL, very-low-density lipoprotein.

Cholesterol is actively pumped out of cells by the ATP-binding cassette transporter 1 (ABCA1) on to apolipoprotein A-I, which binds to cells to form nascent HDL.

Lecithin cholesterol acyl transferase is important in reverse cholesterol transport, as esterification produces the most hydrophobic cholesterol esters that remain trapped in the HDL core, until they reach the liver.

> **Clinical insight**
>
> (LDL) (mmol/L) = (total cholesterol) − (HDL cholesterol) − [(triglyceride)/2.2]

> **Clinical insight**
>
> Increasing HDL (good) cholesterol has been proposed to reduce cardiovascular risk. HDL concentration is increased by exercise, taking nicotinic acid (vitamin B3), consuming alcohol in moderation, losing weight and stopping smoking.

The liver selectively removes some of the cholesterol esters to allow the lipid-depleted HDL to return to the circulation for further rounds of cholesterol removal.

The cholesteryl-ester transfer protein is also key, as it allows a large portion of cholesterol removed from HDL to transfer to LDL as cholesterol esters, which are then removed by hepatic LDL receptors.

Clinical essentials

chapter 2

The terms 'ischaemic heart disease, coronary artery disease, atherosclerotic heart disease and coronary heart disease (CHD)' are synonymous (in this book we use the latter). All are used to describe the condition whereby coronary arterial blood flow becomes restricted secondary to an accumulation of atherosclerotic plaque. The resulting ischaemia presents as angina, or as one of the acute coronary syndromes: unstable angina or myocardial infarction (MI) with or without ST elevation.

The clinical management of CHD centres on the recognition and treatment of signs and symptoms of atherosclerosis and cardiovascular risk factors including hypertension, hyperlipidaemia, and arrhythmia, as discussed in Chapters 3 to 7. Complications include arrhythmias and heart failure (see Chapters 7 and 8).

Guidelines for diagnosis and management are continually changing, because there is such a large amount of research and a wide spectrum of diseases, including sub-clinical presentations.

Management depends largely on the stage of disease. Many people are at a stage early enough that primary and secondary prevention can have a significant effect with changes in lifestyle, exercise and diet, supplemented with drugs to lower risk factors and treat angina symptoms.

Treatment is graded from conservative to pharmacologic, then finally to surgical interventions if all else fails. CHD can be treated by all approaches at once, with a hybrid invasive and bypass strategy and medications to reduce the risk of graft and stent thrombosis. Structural heart diseases, such as aortic stenosis, are managed conservatively until percutaneous or surgical intervention is indicated.

2.1 History taking

The patient's history should produce a shortlist of potential diagnoses.

Symptoms

The key cardiovascular symptoms are chest pain, dyspnoea, palpitations, ankle swelling and syncope.

Chest pain

Chest pain can be caused by benign, serious or life-threatening cardiac and non-cardiac conditions (**Table 2.1**).

Most cardiac chest pain (angina) is caused by myocardial ischaemia due to atherosclerosis. It is less commonly caused by non-ischaemic disease, including aortic dissection or pericarditis.

Character Angina is usually described by patients as a tight band around – or dull weight on, tightness of or discomfort in – the chest, making breathing difficult (**Figure 2.1**). It is usually brought on by exertion and relieved by rest. In contrast, non-cardiac chest pain is felt as a local sharpness (musculoskeletal pain), or diffuse burning [e.g. pain due to gastro-oesophageal reflux disease (GORD)]. Aortic dissection is usually experienced as a tearing or gripping pain.

Like any pain, chest pain should be carefully characterised (**Table 2.2**) to differentiate the cause (**Table 2.3**).

Cause of chest pain	Percentage of presentations (%)
Musculoskeletal	36–45
Gastrointestinal conditions	8–19
Stable angina	10–12
Psychogenic	7.5–11.5
Acute cardiac ischaemia	3
Pulmonary embolism	<1

Table 2.1 Causes of chest pain presentations in primary care.

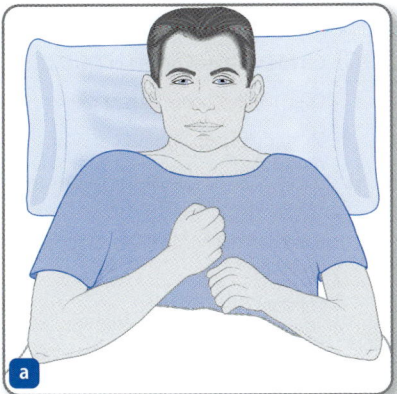
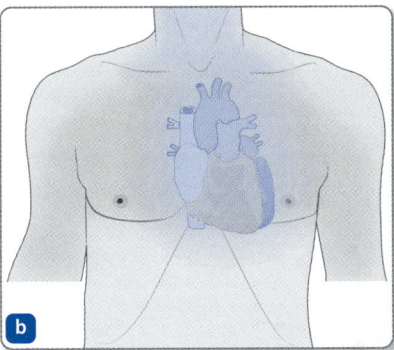

Figure 2.1 Angina. (a) In Levine's sign, patients use a clenched fist in the centre of their chest to describe the pain. Pointing with a single finger suggests a non-ischaemic cause. (b) Pain is typically across the centre of the chest and often radiates into the arms, neck and jaw.

Onset This can be:
- Sudden, spontaneous – aortic dissection, pneumothorax or massive pulmonary embolism (PE)
- Gradual, spontaneous – myocardial infarction
- Gradual, which increases during exertion – angina
- Gradual, decreasing on exertion – normally due to musculoskeletal problems.

Radiation Cardiac pain radiates to the neck, jaw or shoulders/arms (typically left) as these areas share spinal nerves T1–T4 with afferents from the heart. Aortic dissection radiates to the back.

Characteristic	Example
Site	Central, unilateral, diffuse or focal?
Onset	Over minutes, hours, days or weeks?
Character	Sharp, dull, stabbing, heavy or constricting?
Radiation	Neck, jaw, back or arm?
Associated symptoms	Nausea, vomiting, dizziness, dyspnoea or collapse?
Timing	Constant or intermittent?
Exacerbating and relieving factors	E.g. exertion or rest
Severity	Graded out of 10

Table 2.2 The SOCRATES mnemonic for characterising pain.

Aspect of chest pain	GORD	Angina	Pericarditis	Pneumonia or PE
Site	Epigastric/Retrosternal	Retrosternal, left pectoral region and the epigastrium	Central/Left pectoral	Anywhere
Character	Burning	Crushing/Aching	Sharp	Sharp
Radiation	Neck	Arms, neck and jaw	No	No
Associated symptoms	Water brash	Nausea, dyspnoea, and sweating	Fever	Shortness of breath, cough, and fever
Exacerbating factors	Food, lying down	Exertion, cold, and stress	Breathing and lying down	Breathing and coughing
Relieving factors	Milk and antacid	GTN and rest	NSAIDs and sitting forward	Holding breath

GERD, gastro-oesophageal reflux disease; GTN, glyceryl trinitrate; NSAIDs, non-steroidal anti-inflammatory drugs; PE, pulmonary embolism.

Table 2.3 Differentiating chest pain.

Pain that radiates to the left axilla is usually non-cardiac (e.g. anxiety, pleural or musculoskeletal disease).

> **Clinical insight**
>
> Chest pain that has been present constantly for years without complications is unlikely to be cardiac.

Associated symptoms Acute severe chest pain is associated with tachycardia, sweating, nausea and vomiting.

Coronary heart disease pain often presents with symptoms of heart failure, including shortness of breath and ankle swelling.

Exacerbating/Relieving factors Cardiac chest pain usually increases with myocardial oxygen demand; exercise, cold weather, consuming a large meal or stress. Chest pain that increases during rest or a specific movement is normally non-cardiac, such as anxiety or musculoskeletal causes.

Severity Rating pain on a scale of 0–10 helps to understand the patient's relative concept of their pain and to monitor changes.

Dyspnoea

Dyspnoea – shortness of breath – is the sensation of not being able to breathe enough. It often occurs with chest pain but has non-cardiac causes (**Table 2.4**).

Types of breathlessness include:
- Orthopnoea – breathlessness on lying supine; common in heart disease where alveolar fluid shifts with gravity to increase ventilation–perfusion mismatch when the patient lays supine
- Paroxysmal nocturnal dyspnoea – intermittent breathlessness which occurs during the night
- Tachypnoea – increased respiratory rate of >20 breaths/min

Onset Defining the onset of breathlessness helps to differentiate the cause and what action can be taken:
- 1 week after ceasing a diuretic indicates a medication review
- Sudden onset following a long-haul flight can suggest pulmonary embolus
- Intermittent breathlessness that coincides with palpitations suggests paroxysmal atrial fibrillation (AF)

Type of feature	Angina	Asthma/ COPD	Heart failure	Pulmonary embolism	Pneumonia
Associated symptoms	Chest pain	Wheeze and cough	Fatigue	Pain and cough	Fever and cough
Exacerbating factors	Exertion	Allergens and aspirin	Supine	None	None
Relieving factors	Rest	β-agonists	Diuretics	None	Oxygen
Risk factors	Hypertension and smoking	Occupation and smoking	Myocardial infarction	DVT and immobility	Malnutrition, immuno-suppression
Onset	Gradual	Acute	Gradual	Acute	Gradual

COPD, chronic obstructive pulmonary disease; DVT, deep vein thrombosis.

Table 2.4 Differentiating between causes of dyspnoea.

Associated symptoms Other symptoms experienced during dyspnoea may include pain, wheeze or cough (**Table 2.5**).

Exacerbating factors Most breathlessness is worse on exertion and better at rest; the inverse suggests a psychological cause.

Severity Monitoring the severity of dyspnoea helps to gauge quality of life, and guide and monitor treatment.

> **Clinical insight**
>
> Anxiety or allergens can exacerbate pre-existing breathlessness.

Palpitations

Palpitation is awareness of heartbeat and have a variety of sensations and causes (**Table 2.6**).

It is useful to ask the patient to tap the rhythm they feel and how long they feel it for (**Table 2.7**).

Most irregular rhythms are AF, and most regular rhythms are sinus tachycardia, atrial flutter or supra-ventricular tachycardias (SVT).

Associated symptoms Breathlessness, chest pain and pre-syncope suggest serious underlying cardiac pathology.

Dyspnoea symptom	Indicates	
Pain	On exertion indicates myocardial ischaemia	
Wheeze	Cardiac asthma – pulmonary edema due to left ventricular failure	
Cough	White/Frothy sputum	Pulmonary oedema
	Pink/Blood-stained sputum	Mitral valve disease with pulmonary capillary rupture
		Infiltrative lung malignancy
	Grey/Green/Brown and purulent sputum	Infection
	Dry/Non-productive/Tickly	Side effect of angiotensin-converting enzyme inhibitors
		Asthma

Table 2.5 Symptoms associated with dyspnoea and their causes.

Syncope

Syncope, or fainting, is a sudden and transient loss of consciousness with rapid recovery and no long-term consequences. It is caused by temporary global hypoperfusion of the brain due to hypotension. It can suggest serious cardiac pathology, pulmonary emboli, sepsis, or significant blood loss (**Table 2.8**).

Cardiac syncope This is suggested by:
- Onset within seconds
- Onset during exercise – this is a red flag for cardiac pathology
- Concurrent palpitations, chest pain, dyspnoea
- Symptoms while sat or supine

Ankle swelling

Ankle swelling is often due to oedema (**Table 2.9**). Gradual onset is often due to cardiac or systemic disease, whereas acute causes include insect bite, surgery, cellulitis, or deep vein thrombosis (DVT).

A history should confirm the location, speed of onset and any associated symptoms.

Arrhythmia	Character	Exacerbating factors	Relieving factors
Bradyarrhythmias	Tired and dizziness	CCB, β-blockers and HD	Atropine, PPM and stop drugs
Ventricular ectopics	Thump or missed beat	Electrolyte disturbance and caffeine excess	Correct electrolytes and reduce caffeine
Sinus tachycardia	Fast heartbeat	Pain, exercise, anxiety and fever	Treat underlying problem
Atrial fibrillation	Fluttering in chest, dizziness, dyspnoea and transient loss of consciousness	Infection, dehydration, alcohol excess, ischaemia, hyperthyroidism and caffeine	Treat underlying problem, anti-arrhythmic medication, DC cardioversion and ablate focus of the arrhythmia
Atrial flutter			
AVRT/AVNRT		Stress, caffeine and alcohol	
Ventricular tachycardia		Myocardial ischaemia and cardiomyopathy	

AVNRT, atrio-ventricular nodal re-entry tachycardia; AVRT, atrio-ventricular re-entry tachycardia; CCB, calcium-channel blockers; HD, heart disease; PPM, permanent pacemaker.

Table 2.6 Common causes of palpitations and their features.

Duration of palpitation	Cause
Seconds	Ectopic beats, i.e. not serious pathology
Minutes	Atrial fibrillation/flutter, SVT or sinus tachycardia
Hours	Atrial fibrillation/flutter or SVT lasts for several hours but normally self-terminate
Days	Normally anxiety/depression

SVT, supra-ventricular tachycardia.

Table 2.7 Duration of palpitations and their likely cause.

Cause	Speed of onset	Recovery	Initiating events	Associated symptoms
Carotid sinus hypersensitivity	Sudden	Rapid	Turning head, shaving and tight shirt collar	Dizziness
Hypoglycaemia	Gradual	Gradual	Exercise, hypoglycemics and missed meal	Sweating and tremulous
LV outflow obstruction	Sudden	Rapid	Exercise	Chest pain and palpitations
Orthostatic hypotension	Sudden	Rapid	Change in posture, anti-hypertensives	Tunnel vision and weakness
Postural orthodromic tachycardia syndrome	Sudden	Gradual	Increased heart rate on standing	CFS, IBS and JHS
Pseudo-seizure	Gradual	Rapid	Stress and trauma	Psychiatric illness
Pulmonary embolus	Sudden	Gradual	Immobility, travel, trauma and surgery	Chest pain and dyspnoea
Seizure	Sudden	Gradual	Fatigue, alcohol and flashing lights	Incontinence and mouth bite
Stokes–Adams attack	Sudden	Rapid	Prolonged asystole	None
Tachycardia	Sudden	Rapid	None	Chest pain and palpitations
Vasovagal syncope	Sudden	Rapid	Pain, emotion, coughing and micturition	Dizziness and weakness

CFS, chronic fatigue syndrome; IBS, irritable bowel syndrome; JHS, joint hypersensitivity syndrome; LV: left ventricle.

Table 2.8 Features of the different causes of syncope.

Cause	Pathophysiology	Onset	Associated symptoms	Symmetry
Cellulitis	Infection and inflammation	Sudden	Fever, pain and redness	Unilateral
Deep vein thrombosis	Blood clotting	Sudden	Pain, dyspnoea (pulmonary embolism)	Unilateral
Heart failure	Increased venous intra vascular hydrostatic pressure	Gradual	Dyspnoea (pulmonary oedema), fatigue and weight loss	Bilateral
Renal failure	Proteinuria leading to low oncotic pressure	Gradual	Dyspnoea (pulmonary oedema), anaemic fatigue and frothy urine	Bilateral
Liver failure	Low-serum albumin leading to low oncotic pressure	Gradual	Jaundice, abdominal swelling and easy bruising	Bilateral
Myxoedema/ Hypothyroidism	Accumulation of mucin leading to non-pitting oedema	Gradual	Weight gain, neck (thyroid) swelling and fatigue	Bilateral
Pregnancy	Increased hydrostatic and decreased oncotic pressure	Gradual		Bilateral
Travel	Prolonged immobility, decreased lymphatic and venous return	Sudden	None, but at risk of DVT/ pulmonary embolism	Bilateral

DVT, deep vein thrombosis.

Table 2.9 Causes of ankle oedema and their features.

Types

Pitting oedema – where a finger indentation remains for 5 seconds or more – occurs in heart failure, renal and liver disease. It worsens with gravity and improves on elevation.

Non-pitting oedema occurs with lymphatic blockage (lymphoedema) or hypothyroidism (myxoedema), and causes a firm swelling.

Taking a history

After introducing yourself to the patient, ask their permission to take the history, choose an area of privacy and ask if you can make notes as you proceed.

Presenting complaint

Begin with open questions, such as 'what brings you to hospital today?' Then move on to increasingly closed questions.

History of presenting complaint

This includes:
- When it started?
- Duration
- Frequency
- Exacerbating or relieving factors
- Associated symptoms

Pain should be systematically characterised (see **Table 2.2**).

Past medical history

Inquire about any prior illnesses, particularly CHD risk factors:
- Hypercholesterolaemia
- Diabetes
- Kidney disease
- Hypertension

Key differentials include chronic airways disease causing breathlessness or malignancy presenting with cachexia and oedema.

Drug history

This includes recent medications, dosage, route and frequency:
- Use full generic names
- Be clear on dosages
- Include over-the-counter and alternative medications. Common cardiotoxins include non-steroidal anti-inflammatory drugs (NSAIDs), anabolic steroids, radiotherapy and chemotherapeutic agents.

Allergy history

Allergies may include drugs, latex, peanuts, shellfish or other substances. Specify the drug, route, nature and severity of the reaction. Side effects should also be noted.

> **Guiding principle**
>
> Smokers should always be encouraged to stop and be provided with sufficient information and support to aid cessation.

Family medical history

Construct a family tree to document any heritable conditions (**Table 2.10**) in first-degree relatives, including MI or sudden cardiac death in those under 60 years.

Disorder	Inheritance	Complications
Arrhythmogenic right ventricular dysplasia	AD	SCD and arrhythmia
Amyloidosis	AD	Heart block and heart failure
Brugada's syndrome	AD	SCD and arrhythmia
Long QT	AD/R	SCD and arrhythmia
Hypertrophic cardiomyopathy	AD	SCD and arrhythmia
Dilated cardiomyopathy	AD/R	Heart failure and arrhythmia
Marfan's syndrome	AD	MVP and aortopathy
Atrial myxoma	AD	Stroke and syncope

AD, autosomal dominant; AD/R, autosomal dominant/recessive; HF, heart failure; MVP, mitral valve prolapse; SCD, sudden cardiac death.

Table 2.10 Inherited cardiac conditions.

Social history

Occupation Some occupations, e.g. owning a bar, are associated with cardiovascular risk factors. It is also important to be aware of how disease or a diagnosis may limit livelihood.

Smoking Smoking is the biggest risk factor for cardiovascular disease. One 'pack year' is 20 cigarettes a day for 1 year.

Alcohol Record weekly consumption in units. Moderate alcohol consumption appears beneficial for cardiovascular health, but regular and excessive consumption leads to dilated cardiomyopathy and/or rhythm disturbance such as AF.

Caffeine Excessive caffeine consumption can lead to sinus tachycardia or ectopic beats.

Recreational drugs Amphetamines are sympathomimetic and can cause palpitations and hypertension. Cocaine can lead to coronary artery spasm, thrombosis, myocarditis and sudden death.

Functional capacity Functional capacity should be regularly documented to monitor changes and influence decisions of treatment and prognosis. Ask about mobility, what type of home they live in and if they have any help.

Exercise Atherosclerosis is lifestyle disease; exercise helps lower blood pressure, increase energy and decrease depression.

> **Guiding principle**
> All patients should be encouraged to exercise a minimum of 30 minutes of moderate exercise five times a week.

Systems review

A systems review ensures that nothing relevant is missed (**Table 2.11**).

> **Guiding principle**
> Avoid interrupting patients: the diagnosis is usually given to you in the history.

Summary

Briefly summarise the history back to the patient to check the facts have been recorded correctly. Lastly, ask the patient if they have any questions, concerns or expectations.

System	Sign/Symptom	Cardiac and related causes
Respiratory	Cough	Infection, heart failure or angiotensin-converting enzyme inhibitors
	Wheeze	Cardiac asthma due to heart failure
	Haemoptysis	Pulmonary embolism, pulmonary oedema or mitral stenosis
	Stroke	Following aortic dissection or atrial fibrillation
Endocrine	Changes in mood, weight or energy	Thyroid disease
	Sweating, weakness and headaches	Adrenal disease
Musculoskeletal	Myalgia	Statins, unaccustomed exercise or tissue ischaemia
Neurological	Dizziness	Postural hypotension
	Syncope	Cardiac diseases, e.g. aortic stenosis and medications, e.g. anti-hypertensive agents
	Headache	Cardiac medication, e.g. nitrates
	Stroke	Aortic dissection and atrial fibrillation
Gastrointestinal	Weight loss	Cardiac cachexia – a poor prognostic indicator
	Gastric reflux	Cardiac drugs causing chest pain
	Diarrhoea	Arrhythmia due to loss of potassium
	Nausea and vomiting	Complication of MI
Genitourinary	Impotence	Underlying vascular disease
	Haematuria	Glomerulonephritis or endocarditis
	Proteinuria	Peripheral oedema due to renal disease
	Frequency	Prostatic disease or diuretic use

MI, myocardial infarction.

Table 2.11 Systems review: Key clinical features associated with cardiac disease.

2.2 Cardiovascular examination

Clinical examination requires a systematic routine (**Table 2.12**).

System or category	Examination	Signs
General inspection	Appearance	Systemically well or unwell, underweight (cachexia), overweight or obese
	Environment	Clues suggesting disease
	Face	Central cyanosis (blue discolouration)
	Neck	Visible jugular venous pulse (fluid overload)
	Chest	Breathlessness at rest
Hands	Nails	Nail abnormalities
	Fingers	Peripheral cyanosis (bluish discolouration)
Arterial pulse	Palpation	Heart rate and rhythm
Respiration	Inspection	• Respiratory rate • Breathing pattern
Head and neck	Inspection	• Central cyanosis (blue discolouration of the lips or tongue) • Xanthelasma • Jugular venous pulse
Chest	Inspection	• Surgical scars, pacemakers or chest wall deformities
	Palpation	• Apex beat • Heaves • Thrills
	Auscultation	• Heart sounds • Murmurs • Pericardial rub • Lung signs: Wheeze, crepitations and dullness

Table 2.12 A systematic approach to cardiovascular examination. *Continues overleaf*

System or category	Examination	Signs
Lower limb	Inspection	• Xanthomata • Ankle oedema
	Palpation	• Ankle oedema • Peripheral pulses
Abdomen	Inspection	Ascites
	Palpation	• Ascites • Abdominal aorta
	Auscultation	Renal arteries
Blood pressure		Hypertension
Fundi	Inspection	Hypertensive and diabetic retinopathy

Table 2.12 *Continued*

Starting the examination

To prepare:
- Wash your hands, introduce yourself and check the patient's identity
- Obtain verbal consent for 'a heart and chest examination, which will require removal of clothing from the waist upwards'
- Ensure modesty is preserved and, if appropriate, ask if the patient would like a chaperone
- Position the patient at 45°

General inspection

Carefully survey the patient and surroundings:
- Does the patient look well, i.e. pink, talkative, smiling, not in pain or distress?
- Are there any medications or other treatments present?

> **Clinical insight**
>
> The hands convey a great deal of information about a patient, e.g. signs of chronic disease, circulation, occupation, hobbies, smoking, hygiene, nervousness and strength.

Hands

Ask the patient to rest their hands on a pillow.

Finger clubbing

Digital clubbing is characterised by increased soft tissue and vasodilation (**Figure 2.2** and **Table 2.13**) and is a sign of chronic pulmonary, cardiac, liver or gastrointestinal disease that increases circulating growth factors.

Cardiac causes include:
- Benign cardiac tumours
- Cyanotic congenital heart disease
- Infective endocarditis

Signs of infective endocarditis

Infective endocarditis can present with finger signs (**Figure 2.3**).

Splinter haemorrhages are short, thin, and linear discolourations in the nail that are initially red then brown and finally black within a few days. Most are due to trauma, but they can be a sign of microemboli from vasculitis or infective endocarditis.

Osler nodes are tender, raised, purple papules in the finger pulps, due to immune complex deposition.

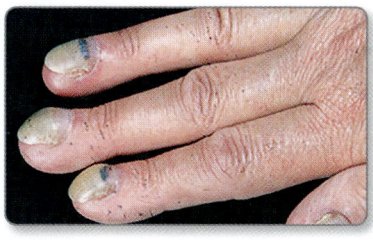

Figure 2.2 Finger clubbing.

Stage	Description
1	Increased sponginess of the nail bed
2	Loss of the nail angle (usually <165°)
3	Increased convexity of the nail bed
4	Thickening of finger (drumstick appearance)
5	Shiny aspect and striation of finger and nail

Table 2.13 The stages of clubbing.

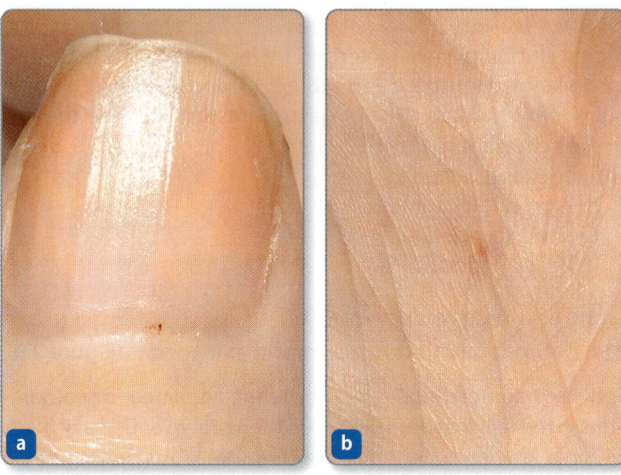

Figure 2.3 Signs of infective endocarditis. (a) A small splinter haemorrhage. (b) Janeway lesion.

Janeway lesions are non-tender, flat, purple, macules found in the palm of the hand due to septic emboli.

Palmar erythema

Reddening of the thenar and hypothenar eminences of the palm occurs with:
- **Pregnancy:** Palmar erythema arises in 30% of pregnant women due to increased oestrogen
- Polycythaemia, as a manifestation of the increased number of red blood cells
- Syphilis and vasculitis, i.e. inflammation

Peripheral cyanosis

Cyanosis is the blue discolouration associated with low oxygen. Peripheral cyanosis (**Figure 2.4**) occurs with:
- Reduced central circulation – central cyanosis (e.g. blue tongue)
- Cold
- Acute limb ischaemia
- Arterial vasospasm

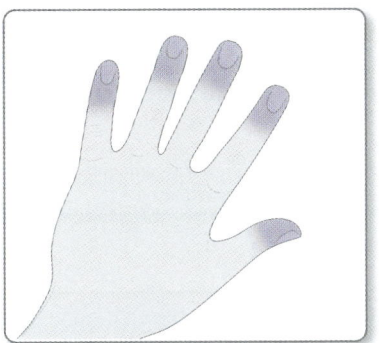

Figure 2.4 Peripheral cyanosis.

Capillary refill time

Press the fingernail for 5 seconds; it should return to 'normal' within 2 seconds. A delay suggests reduced peripheral perfusion, for example:
- Cardiogenic shock
- Heart failure
- Dehydration
- Acute limb ischaemia

Arterial pulse

The arterial pulse gives information on heart rate, rhythm, cardiac output, and heart valve and vascular function.

Radial pulse

The radial pulse is felt between the radial styloid and the palmaris longus and flexor digitorum superficialis tendons.

Heart rate Palpate for 1 minute using the index and middle finger and count the beats/min (bpm) (**Table 2.14**).

Pulse rhythm A pulse can be regularly irregular, where the period varies but has a pattern, or irregularly irregular, where there is no pattern (**Table 2.15**).

Collapsing (waterhammer) pulse Elevate the arm above the patient's head; a collapsing radial pulse of aortic regurgitation

Rate (bpm)	Term	Causes
<60	Bradycardia	Sleep, hypothermia, hypothyroidism, athletic training, arrhythmia, and medication
60–100	Normal	–
>100	Tachycardia	Pain, anxiety, fever, exercise, arrhythmia, shock, and hyperthyroidism

Table 2.14 Causes of slow and fast heart rates.

Rhythm	Description	Causes
Regularly regular	Consistent time between each pulse	Sinus rhythm, 1st or 3rd degree heart block
Regularly irregular	Period varies but has a pattern	Sinus arrhythmia, 2nd degree heart block
Irregularly irregular	No pattern	Atrial and ventricular ectopic beats, AF, atrial flutter with variable block, and MAT
AF, atrial fibrillation; MAT, multi-focal atrial tachycardia.		

Table 2.15 Causes of cardiac rhythms.

rapidly increases and collapses to feel like it is knocking against your fingertips.

Delayed pulses These include:

- Radio-radial delay, which suggests aortic dissection proximal to the left subclavian artery
- Radio-femoral delay, which suggests coarctation (i.e. narrowing) of the aortic arch distal to the subclavian arteries

Carotid pulse

Palpate the carotid pulse in the anterior cervical triangle, between the trachea and the sternocleidomastoid muscle, to assess pulse character and volume.

Pulse character Assess for changes in pulse waveform, including the slow rising, broad pulse of aortic stenosis and the collapsing, narrow pulse of aortic regurgitation (**Figure 2.5**).

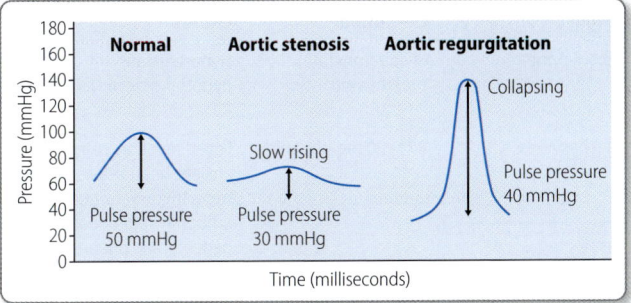

Figure 2.5 Pulse character and pulse pressure.

Pulse volume A low volume or 'thready' pulse can reflect a reduced stroke volume felt in shock, heart failure, anxiety, and anaemia or reduced vascular resistance associated with hyperthermia and hyperthyroidism.

> **Clinical insight**
>
> A patient cannot be anaemic and cyanotic at the same time. In fact, many cyanotic patients have compensatory polycythaemia, a raised red cell count.

Respiration

A normal respiratory rate is 12–20 breaths/min. To avoid distortion, observe the rate and breathing pattern while still palpating the radial pulse (**Table 2.16**).

Head and neck

Inspect the hair, skin, eyes and mouth (**Table 2.17**).

Jugular venous pulse Moving down to the neck, examine the pulse of the internal jugular vein as an indicator of central venous pressure (CVP) (**Figure 2.6**):
- Position the patient at an angle of 45°, with their head turned to the left
- Observe the supraclavicular fossa and anterior cervical triangle on the patient's right for the characteristic double waveform, distinct from the carotid pulse

Sign	Definition	Causes
Bradypnoea	Respiratory rate < 12 breaths/min	Hypertension, hypothyroidism, decreased ICP and sedatives
Tachypnoea	RR > 20 breaths/min	Fever/infection, pain, anxiety, heart failure, hyperthyroidism, pulmonary embolism, pulmonary oedema, and pneumothorax, ILD, COPD, asthma, and sympathomimetics
Dyspnoea	Shortness of breath	Heart failure, asthma and COPD
Rapid shallow breathing		Pleuritic chest pain, ILD, hyperventilation
Stridor	Inspiratory wheeze	Upper airway obstruction
Kussmaul's breathing	Rapid deep sighing; 'air hunger'	Acidosis (e.g. diabetic ketoacidosis)
Excess abdominal/accessory muscle movement on inspiration		COPD and respiratory distress
Cheyne–Stokes breathing	5–30 seconds of apnoea followed by increased and then decrease RR	Severe pulmonary oedema and brainstem lesions
Prolonged expiratory phase		Significant airway obstruction due to asthma or COPD, etc.

COPD, chronic obstructive pulmonary disease; ICP, intracranial pressure; ILD, interstitial lung disease; RR, respiratory rate.

Table 2.16 Signs of respiratory rate and breathing pattern and their causes.

- The JVP should be <3 cm vertically above the sternal angle. 3 cm is equivalent to 3 cm H_2O (2 mmHg).

Raised JVP The JVP is normally hidden behind the right clavicle. It is increased in:
- Biventricular/right heart failure

Cardiovascular examination 111

Area	Sign	Indication
Hair	Brown tar stains	Smoking
Skin	Malar erythema	Mitral stenosis, systemic lupus erythematosus
	Grey cheekbones	Amiodarone, an antiarrhythmic agent
Eyes	Xanthelasma – yellow fat deposits in the skin around the eyes (see **Figure 2.11**)	Hypercholesteraemia
	Corneal arcus – white ring of lipid deposits in the cornea	Hypercholesteraemia, old age
	Subconjunctival pallor (pale under eyelids)	Anaemia
Mouth	Dental caries (tooth decay)	Risk factor for bacterial endocarditis
	Central cyanosis	Deoxygenated haemoglobin > 5.0 g/dL (>50 g/L), chronic lung disease, myocardial infarction, congenital heart disease, or cardiogenic shock
	Pale mucous membranes	Anaemia

Table 2.17 Signs of the hair, skin, eyes and mouth.

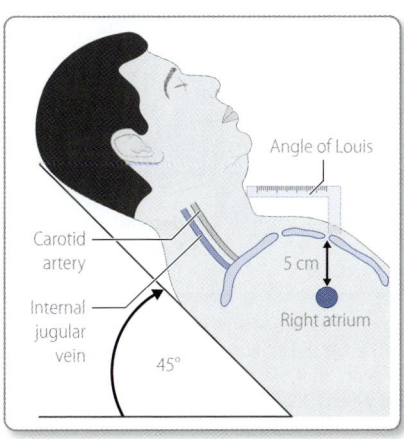

Figure 2.6 Observing the jugular venous pulse (JVP). The internal jugular vein courses from the ear lobe to between the sternal and clavicular head of sternocleidomastoid muscle at the clavicle. Note that the JVP is best observed with the patient's head turned to the left (not shown here).

- Right ventricular infarction
- Fluid overload

JVP waveform In sinus rhythm, two waves are visible: the 'a' wave before the carotid pulse and the 'v' wave after it (**Figure 2.7**). Pathologies include an absent 'a' wave due to atrial fibrillation (AF; **Table 2.18**).

Guiding principle

The internal jugular vein drains directly into the right atrium, and so is a barometer of right atrial and CVP.

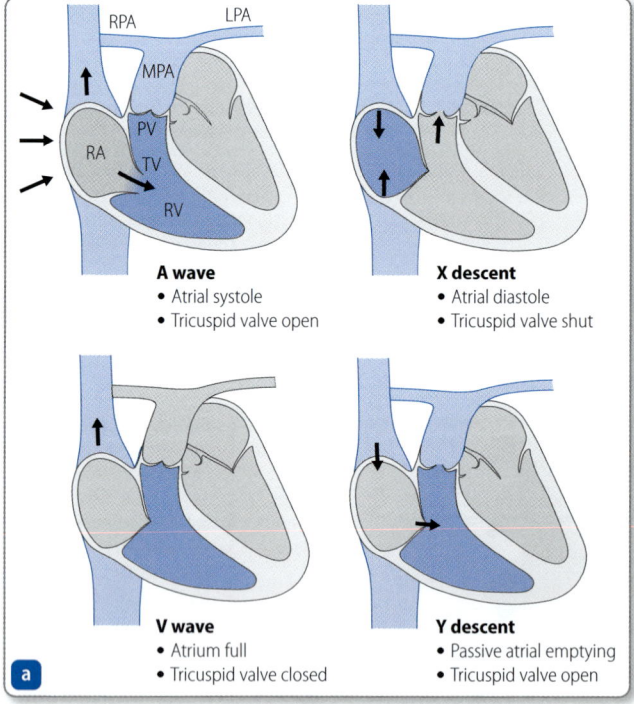

Figure 2.7 The jugular venous pulse (JVP) waveform (a) The waveform and its relation to the cardiac cycle. (b) The JVP and its relation to ECG, heart sounds and carotid pulse. LPA, left pulmonary artery; MPA, main pulmonary artery; RA, right atrium; RPA, right pulmonary artery; RV, right ventricle; TV, tricuspid valve. *Continues opposite.*

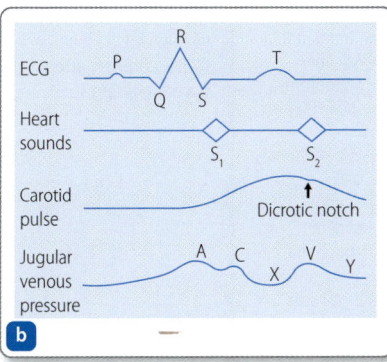

Figure 2.7 Continued.

Wave	Descent	Meaning	Physiology	Pathology
A		RA systole	Retrograde venous flow	Big in TS and absent in AF
C		RV contraction	TV bulges into RA	–
	X	RA diastole	TV pulled down by RV	–
V		RA diastole	Venous filling of RA	Big in TR
	Y	TV open	Fall in RA pressure	Deep in CP
AF, atrial fibrillation; CP, constrictive pericarditis; RA, right atrium; RV, right ventricle; TS, tricuspid stenosis; TR, tricuspid regurgitation; TV, tricuspid valve.				

Table 2.18 Waves of the jugular venous pulse (JVP) and pathologies that affect them.

Chest

Inspection

Inspect the shape of the anterior chest, including pectus carinatum (pigeon chest) and excavatum (hollow chest), scars (**Figure 2.8**), masses, and observe its movement for regularity, symmetricity and speed.

> **Clinical insight**
>
> Inspection involves observing not just with the eyes, but also other senses. For example, noticing the metallic clicking sound of a metallic valve replacement.

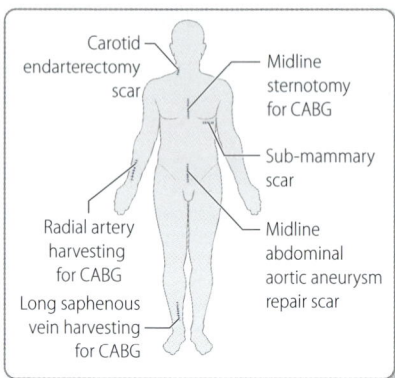

Figure 2.8 Surgical scars of cardiovascular surgery. CABG, coronary artery bypass grafting.

Palpation

Apex beat The apex of the heart is the most lateral and inferior part of the heart. It transmits a pulse – the apex beat – to the chest wall, usually in the 5th intercostal space (ICS) in the mid-clavicular line (**Figure 2.9**):
- Palpate the sternal angle; the 2nd ICS is lateral to this
- Count down to the 5th ICS and across to the mid-clavicular line on the left side
- With the index finger parallel to the ribs, feel the intercostal space for the forceful pulse
- Assess for abnormalities (**Table 2.19**)

Heaves Palpate the left parasternum with the right palm for a strong cardiac impulse, which can indicate right ventricular hypertrophy (RVH) due to pulmonary hypertension or pulmonary stenosis.

Thrills Assess the four valve areas (**Figure 2.9**) with fingertips for palpable murmurs; high-frequency vibrations.

Auscultation

Heart sounds Listen with a stethoscope to the four valve areas (**Figure 2.9**), with both the diaphragm (best for high pitch, e.g. aortic and mitral regurgitation) and the bell (better for low

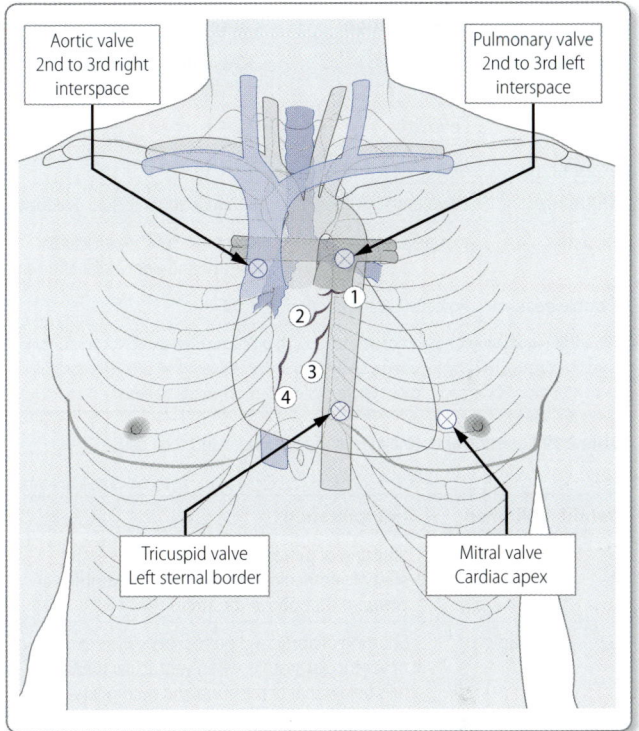

Figure 2.9 Location of the auscultation and palpation areas of the apex beat and heart valves. ①, pulmonary valve; ②, aortic valve; ③ bicuspid (mitral) valve; and ④ tricuspid valve.

pitch, e.g. aortic and mitral stenosis). While auscultating, palpate the carotid pulse to orientate where sounds are occurring in the cardiac cycle.

Heart sounds reflect the valves shutting: S1 and S2 are normally the most obvious (**Table 2.20**). S3 and S4 are 'added heart sounds' and can represent pathology.

Clinical insight

There is no direct correlation between murmur volume and the echocardiographic severity of the lesion.

Sign	Interpretation	Cause
Displaced	LV dilation	DCM, LV aneurysm, LVSD, chest wall deformities, and CLD
Tapping	Loud S1	MS
Heaving	LV pressure overload	AS, HTN, and LVH
Thrusting	LV volume overload	AR and iatrogenic fluid overload
Absent	Not palpable	Normal in 50%, dextrocardia, obesity, and pericardial effusion
Double beat	Forceful LA contraction	HCM

AR, aortic regurgitation; AS, aortic stenosis; CLD, chronic lung disease; HCM, hypertrophic cardiomyopathy; HTN, hypertension; LA, left atrium; LV, left ventricle; LVH, left ventricular hypertrophy; LVSD, left ventricular systolic dysfunction; MS, mitral stenosis.

Table 2.19 Common abnormalities of the apex beat and their cause.

Sound	Phonetic	Interpretation
S1	'lup'	Shutting of mitral and tricuspid valves at the start of ventricular systole, when the ventricular pressures rise above the atria
S2	'dup'	Shutting of aortic and pulmonary valves at the end of ventricular systole, when ventricular pressure falls below that of the aorta and pulmonary artery
S3	'lup-de-dup'	In diastole, between S2 and S1. Normal in children or young adults but can indicate rapid ventricular filling in heart failure
S4	'le-lup-dup'	Always abnormal, due to a stiff ventricle, normally secondary to left ventricular hypertrophy

Table 2.20 Heart sounds.

> **Clinical insight**
>
> A 'gallop rhythm' is the sound of all four heart sounds, S1 to S4 ('le-lup-de-dup') and is typically due to decompensated chronic or acute heart failure.

S2 split is when S2 consists of two separate sounds as the left ventricle typically contracts before the right ventricle: A2 when the aortic valve shuts, and P2 when the

S2 split	Pathologies	Mechanism	Split order
Normal inspiration split	None	Inspiration reduces intrathoracic pressure and increases venous return to RA, delaying P2	A2 occurs before P2
Abnormal expiration split	Electrophysiological pathology (e.g. LBBB), structural heart disease (e.g. aortic stenosis) or cardiomyopathy	Prolonged LV ejection	P2 occurs before A2
Abnormal inspiration and expiration 'fixed' split	ASD and VSD	Independent of ventilation, septal defects shunt blood from left to right circulation, down the pressure gradient, so that the RV ejection is delayed	A2 occurs before P2

ASD, atrial septal defect; LBBB, left bundle branch block; RA, right atrium; VSD, ventricular septal defect.

Table 2.21 Splitting of S2.

pulmonary valve does. This 'splitting' of S2 varies according to how it is affected by ventilation (**Table 2.21**).

Heart murmurs Murmurs are the sound of turbulent blood flow through heart valves, forward or backward. Forward murmurs reflect a narrowing; backward murmurs indicate valve incompetence (**Table 2.22** and **Figure 2.10**).

Pericardial rub This is a sign of pericarditis, when two layers of inflamed pericardium rub against each other, said to sound like the crunching sound of walking on fresh snow.

Stage of cycle	Murmur	Timing	Sound	Location	Radiation
Systole	AS	Ejection	Crescendo–decrescendo	2nd R ICS	Carotid
	MR	Pan	Blowing	5th L ICS	Axilla
Diastole	AR	Early	Decrescendo	2nd L ICS	Carotid
	MS	Mid	Rumbling	5th L ICS	Axilla

AR, aortic regurgitation; AS, aortic stenosis; ICS, inter-costal space; L, left; MR, mitral regurgitation; MS, mitral stenosis; R, right.

Table 2.22 Detection of heart murmurs.

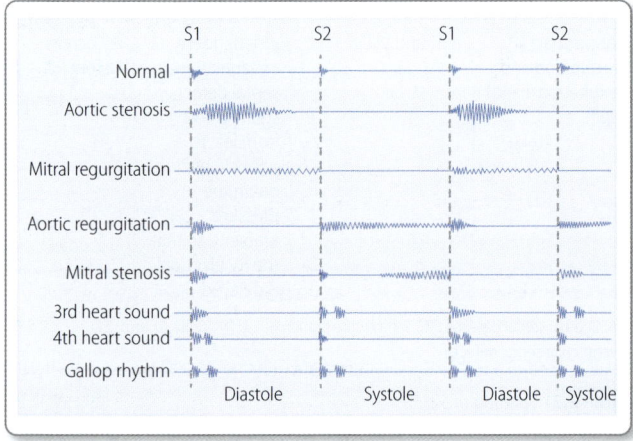

Figure 2.10 Normal and abnormal heart sounds.

Lungs

After auscultating the heart, ask the patient to sit forward and examine the lung bases, using inspection, palpation, auscultation and percussion.

Wheeze Cardiac asthma is a coarse, whistling sound heard during expiration due to obstruction of the small airways, this may be due to pulmonary oedema secondary to left ventricular failure.

Crepitations These are a crackling sound like Velcro, heard at the posterior bases of the lungs. It is a sign of pulmonary oedema, often secondary to left ventricular failure. The sound is most pronounced in inspiration as small airways and alveoli 'pop' open.

> **Clinical insight**
>
> Physiological (flow or innocent) murmurs are typically:
> - Soft
> - Heard all over the precordium
> - Pan-systolic
> - Absent on standing (i.e. with a decrease in venous return)

Stony dullness A lack of resonance on percussion – in the lung bases suggests pleural effusion, a sign of heart failure that also presents with reduced chest expansion and quiet breath sounds.

Lower limb

Inspection

Inspect the skin and large extensor tendons for yellow xanthomata (**Figure 2.11**), nodular cholesterol-rich deposits that are a sign of hypercholesterolaemia.

Ankle oedema Excess interstitial fluid, i.e. oedema, is caused by chronic disease that affects blood hydrostatic

> **Guiding principle**
>
> Heart failure is effectively a pump failure that leads to back-pressure and fluid leakage:
> - Left-sided failure – leakage in pulmonary circulation causes pulmonary oedema
> - Right-sided failure – leakage into interstitial space causing peripheral oedema (ankle and sacral oedema)
> - As right-sided failure worsens, leakage can occur into the abdomen causing ascites

or oncotic pressure or localised disease affecting fluid build-up

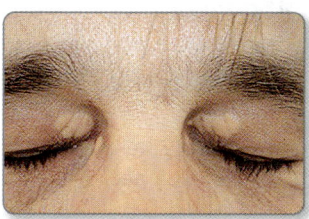

Figure 2.11 Xanthomata lipid deposits. Xanthelasma are small xanthoma around eyelids.

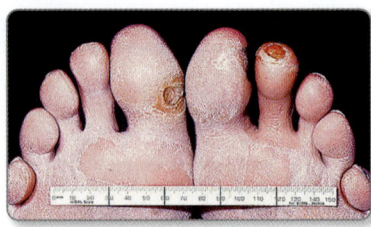

Figure 2.12 Arterial ulcers are usually deep, regular, painful, and have minimal exudate.

and return (see **Table 2.9**). Heart failure is a cause of bilateral pitting oedema, or sacral oedema in bed-bound patients, due to fluid retention from decreased hydrostatic pressure.

Ulcers Inspect the lower limb for ulcers (**Figure 2.12**); a sign of peripheral vascular disease (PVD). Arterial PVD is commonly due to diabetes, hypertension and smoking.

Palpation
Pulses Palpate the four pulses in each lower limb (**Figure 2.13**):
- Femoral artery
- Popliteal artery
- Posterior tibial
- Dorsalis pedis

Pulse absence suggests PVD due to atherosclerosis, typically with peripheral pulses lost first.

Calf tenderness Gently squeeze both calves to assess for pain due to DVT, which will also present with oedema, and possibly warmth, pain and erythema.

> **Clinical insight**
>
> The presence of atherosclerosis in the lower limb (peripheral vascular disease) reflects the likely presence of atherosclerosis in the carotid and coronary arteries, i.e. PVD indicates the risk of coexisting cerebrovascular and cardiovascular disease.

Abdomen
Examine the abdomen for fluid, and aortic or renal artery disease.

Inspection A distended abdomen may indicate ascites due to advanced right or biventricular failure, as back-pressure

Cardiovascular examination

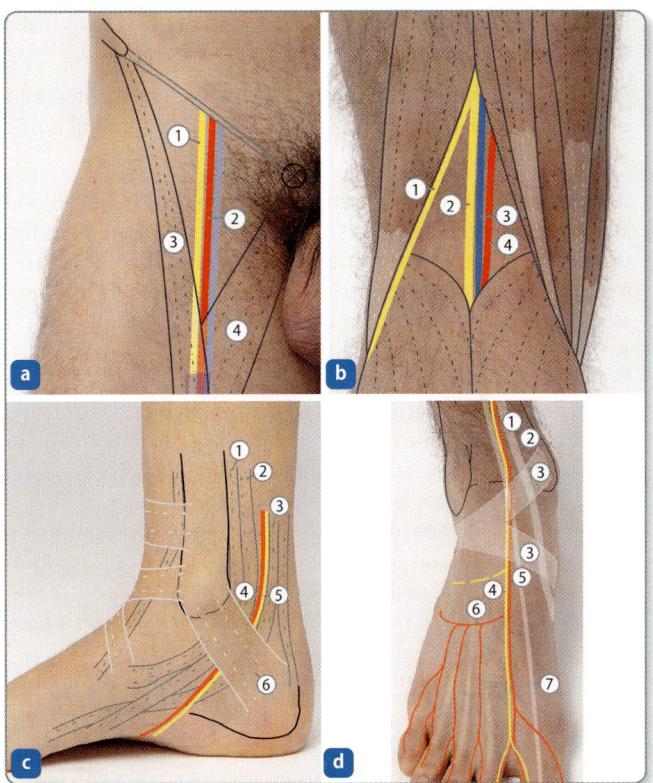

Figure 2.13 Pulses of the lower limb: the femoral, popliteal, posterior and anterior tibial arteries. (a) ① femoral nerve, ② femoral artery and vein, ③ sartorius, ④ adductor longus, ⊗ pubic tubercle. (b) ① Common fibular nerve, ② tibial nerve ③ popliteal vein, ④ popliteal artery. (c) ① Posterior tibial tendon, ② flexor digitorum longus, ③ flexor hallucis longus, ④ posterior tibial artery, ⑤ tibial nerve, ⑥ flexor retinaculum. (d) ① Anterior tibial artery, ② anterior tibial tendon, ③ inferior extensor retinaculum, ④ medial branch of deep fibular nerve, ⑤ dorsalis pedis artery, ⑥ arcuate artery, ⑦ extensor hallucis longus tendon.

in portal veins leads to fluid leak, though the vast majority is associated with liver cirrhosis or GI malignancy.

Palpation Palpate for the presence of a midline, central and possibly tender, pulsatile mass – a sign of abdominal aortic aneurysm (AAA).

Auscultation Listen for a renal artery bruit (turbulent blood flow) anteriorly at positions 9 and 3 o'clock, 5 cm from the umbilicus, otherwise posteriorly paraspinal at level of L2. This is a sign of renal artery stenosis, a cause of secondary hypertension and sudden pulmonary oedema.

Blood pressure

Blood pressure is an estimate of the force that blood is exerting against the walls of the large arteries. It is used to gauge disease severity in cases of blood loss and in aortic valve diseases, and to diagnose, monitor and manage hypertension.

Whether it is measured with an automated monitor or a sphygmomanometer and a stethoscope, the positioning of the patient and the cuff is the same:
- Ask the patient to remain still and rest their arm on a desk or similar
- Place the cuff around the patient's upper arm, approximately at heart-height
- Place the diaphragm over the brachial artery

If the measurement is being taken with a sphygmomanometer:

- Inflate the cuff until the radial pulse is obliterated
- Listen as the cuff is steadily deflated
- Record the pressure at which Korotkoff sounds of turbulent flow are heard – this is the highest, systolic blood pressure (SBP)
- Record the pressure at which they disappear – this is the lowest, diastolic blood pressure (DBP).

Pulse pressure

$$\text{Pulse pressure} = \text{SBP} - \text{DBP}$$

Pulse pressure (see **Figure 2.6**) is normally 40–80 mmHg.

Narrow pulse pressure Pressures < 40 mmHg occur if there is an increase in LV afterload (e.g. aortic stenosis, cardiac tamponade and cardiogenic shock) or a reduction in LV contractility (e.g. heart failure) causing a reduction in volume or speed of ejection of blood from the LV during systole.

Broad pulse pressure Pressures > 80 mmHg occur when there is a reduction in LV afterload (e.g. aortic regurgitation, pregnancy, fever, thyrotoxicosis, AV malformation and Paget's disease) causing a rapid dispersion of blood from the LV during systole.

Mean arterial pressure

$$MAP = DBP + (1/3 \text{ pulse pressure})$$

Mean arterial pressure is the average blood pressure throughout the cardiac cycle and represents the perfusion pressure supplying organs. It is normally 70–110 mmHg; <70 mmHg leads to tissue ischaemia, infarction and eventually necrosis.

Blood pressure symmetry

A difference of systolic blood pressure between arms of >20 mmHg is usually a sign of aortic dissection.

Fundi

Fundoscopy is performed in a darkened room with an ophthalmoscope to view the retinae.

Diabetic retinopathy

This can present with oedema (yellow exudate), retinal and vitreous haemorrhages and new vessels (**Table 2.23** and **Figure 2.14**).

Hypertensive retinopathy
Fundoscopy can reveal diffuse or focal vessel narrowing, microaneurysms, macroaneurysms, cotton wool spots, exudates and disc swelling (**Figure 2.15** and **Table 2.24**).

> **Clinical insight**
>
> The presence of retinal microvascular disease likely reflects microvascular disease in other organs.

Stage	Features
Early diabetic retinopathy	Microaneurysms, dot haemorrhages, blot haemorrhages, yellow exudate, and cotton wool spots
Preproliferative retinopathy	More severe
Proliferative diabetic retinopathy	New vessels
Diabetic maculopathy	Macular disease: exudate, haemorrhage, and oedema

Table 2.23 Stages of diabetic retinopathy.

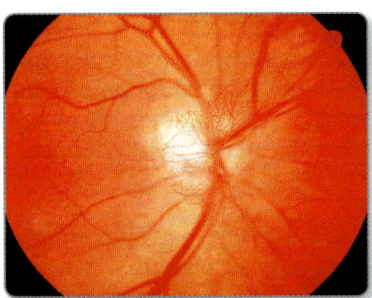

Figure 2.14 Proliferative diabetic retinopathy, with evidence of new vessel formation.

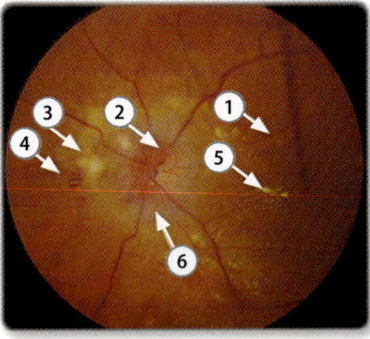

Figure 2.15 Severe, grade four hypertensive retinopathy: silver wiring (1); arteriovenous (AV) nipping (2); cotton wool spots (3); flame haemorrhages (4); hard exudate (5); optic disc oedema (6).

2.3 Investigations

Investigations support or refute the working diagnoses, determine disease severity and inform a management plan.

Grade	Sign	Pathophysiology
I	Silver/Copper wiring	Visible atherosclerosis; tortuous and shiny arterioles
II	Arteriovenous nipping	Venous constriction
III	Cotton-wool spots and flame haemorrhages	Retinal infarcts and bleeds
IV	Papilloedema	Compression of the central retinal vein swells the optic disc

Table 2.24 Grading of signs of hypertensive retinopathy.

Blood tests

Routine tests include:
- Complete blood count (CBC) to assess for anaemia, inflammation and infection
- Urea and electrolytes (U&E) to assess renal function
- Liver function tests (LFT)
- Clotting screen to assess for coagulopathies

> **Clinical insight**
>
> Natriuretic peptides are raised in hypertension and:
> - Renal failure
> - Pulmonary embolus
> - Myocardial infarction
> - Sepsis
> - Extreme exercise

Cardiac biomarkers Cardiac biomarkers are molecules released into the blood when myocardial cells are damaged (**Figure 2.16** and **Table 2.25**). They are measured as soon as possible after a suspected cardiac event, e.g. chest pain and suspected MI; dyspnoea and suspected heart failure, to obtain a baseline level.

Lipid profiles

Inherited or acquired raised serum lipids are a risk factor for vascular disease. Concentrations are measured in a venous blood sample after overnight fasting.

Low-density lipoprotein (LDL) Often called 'bad cholesterol' in conversations with patients, this carries cholesterol from the

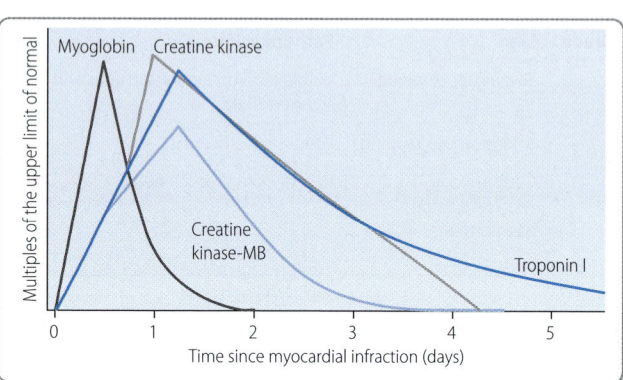

Figure 2.16 Cardiac biomarkers.

Biomarker	Definition	Cardiac subtypes	Released	Measure second level	Comment
Troponin	3-unit protein involved in muscle contraction	I and T	Myocardial damage	3–6 hours after height of pain	
Creatine kinase	Enzyme in high – energy cells; catalyses ATP to ADP	CK-MB	Myocardial damage	72 hours after height pain	Doubling suggests MI. CK-MB is sensitive but not specific for MI
Myoglobin	Muscular form of haemoglobin (Fe-based porphyrin ring that binds O_2)		Myocardial damage	2 hours	Sensitive but not specific for MI
Natriuretic peptides	Small proteins that cause sodium and water excretion	BNP and precursor NTpro-BNP	Myocardial stretch		Support a diagnosis of heart failure

ATP, adenosine triphosphate; ADP, adenosine diphosphate; MI, myocardial infarction; BNP, brain natriuretic peptide; NTpro-BNP, N-terminal pro-brain natriuretic peptide.

Table 2.25 Cardiac biomarkers.

liver to the peripheries. It is associated with cholesterol deposition in arteries to form atheroma.
- Normally <2.5 mmol/L (<100 mg/dL)
- Elevated in pregnancy, corticosteroid use, hypothyroidism and cholestatic liver disease.

High-density lipoprotein (HDL) Often called 'good cholesterol' in discussion with patients, this is the major carrier from the peripheries to the liver and reduces cholesterol deposits in arteries. High levels are associated with a reduced risk of vascular disease.
- Normally >1.5 mmol/L (<60 mg/dL)
- Increased by exercise and modest alcohol consumption

Triglycerides (TGs) These are esters of glycerol and three fatty acids that transfer fatty acids and glucose between fat tissue and the liver. High levels increase the risk of vascular disease.
- Normally <1.5 mmol/L (<60 mg/dL)
- Increased in diabetes, renal failure, obesity and corticosteroids

Total cholesterol (TC) This includes LDL, HDL, VDL (variable density lipoproteins, estimated) and is normally <5 mmol/L (<200 mg/dL).

Electrocardiography

Electrocardiography (ECG) uses electrodes placed on the chest and limbs to measure the amount and direction of the heart's electrical activity.

Leads

A 'lead' is the term for both the physical electrode, and the abstract positional 'view of the electrical heart' that one or more leads represents. An ECG in clinical non-acute situations is recorded using 12 leads. A 3-lead ECG is used for monitoring, whereas defibrillator paddles can also function as leads to record an ECG in acute situations.

> **Clinical insight**
>
> Indications for ECG include chest pain, shortness of breath, palpitations, syncope, heart murmur, hypo-/hypertension and an irregular pulse.

The 12-lead ECG

A 12-lead ECG (**Figure 2.17**) is used to diagnose arrhythmias, electrolyte disturbances, myocardial disease, focal ischaemia and drug toxicity. The 12-lead signals are from six chest leads and six virtual leads created from four limb leads. Results should be interpreted in a systematic way (**Table 2.26**).

Chest leads

V1–V6 view the heart in the horizontal plane from front to back. They are unipolar; they record the difference in voltage between their location on the chest, and zero.

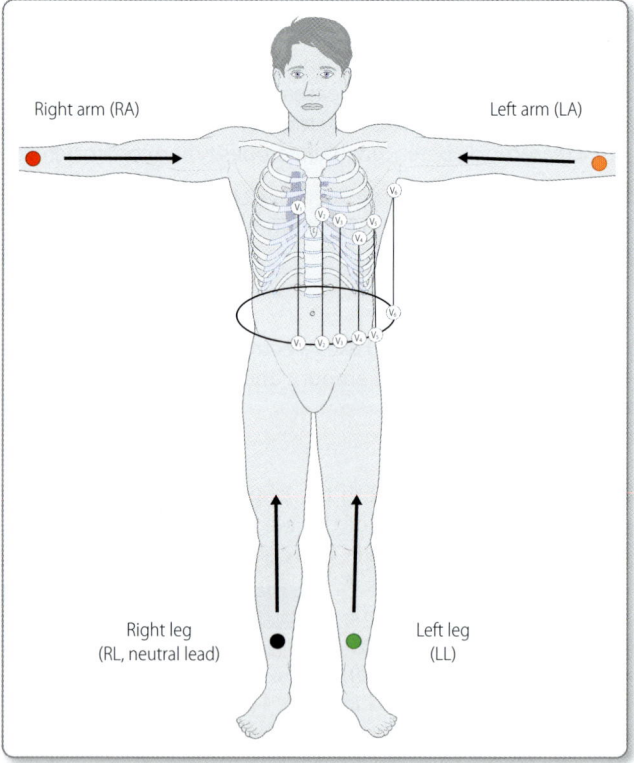

Figure 2.17 The 12-lead ECG.

Step	Observe
1	Patient's name, date of birth, and hospital number
2	Time and date of ECG
3	Speed and voltage of ECG
4	Cardiac axis – normal or deviated?
5	Heart rate (beats/min)
6	Heart rhythm – in normal sinoatrial rhythm, each QRS complex is preceded by a P wave
7	PQRST: Examine P wave, PR interval, QRS complex, ST segment, Q waves, QT interval and T wave in each lead

Table 2.26 Interpreting a 12-lead electrocardiogram (ECG).

Limb leads

The four limb leads view the electrical signal of the heart in the vertical plane (i.e. head to toe) and are colour coded:
- Left arm (LA) – orange
- Right arm (RA) – red
- Left leg (LL) – green
- Right leg (RL) – neutral/black

> **Clinical insight**
>
> ECG machines should be set to record at:
> - A speed of 25 mm/s: A large square (5 mm) represents 0.2 s and a small square (1 mm) is 0.04 s
> - A voltage of 0.1 mv/mm, so that 1 large square (5 mm) is 1 mv

Virtual leads

Limb leads are used to create the six virtual leads; virtual perspectives of the heart's electrical activity calculated from combinations of lead measurements (**Table 2.27**).

Unipolar leads Unipolar limb leads aVF, aVR and aVL record the electrical signal from one position, a limb, towards the centre of all three leads (**Figure 2.18**), looking at the heart in an axial plane.

Bipolar leads Leads I, II and III record the electrical potential difference between two leads and represent a view from the positive limb lead towards the negative.

Clinical essentials

Polarity	Lead	How is it calculated?	View
Unipolar	(aVF) augmented vector lead of the foot	LF – 0	From LF
	(aVR) augmented vector lead of the right arm	RA – 0	From RA
	(aVL) augmented vector lead of the left arm	LA – 0	From LA
Bipolar	I	aVR – aVL	From LA towards RA
	II	aVR – aVF	From LL towards RA
	III	aVL – aVF	From LL towards LA

LA, left arm; LF, left foot; LL, left leg; RA, right arm.

Table 2.27 Virtual ECG leads.

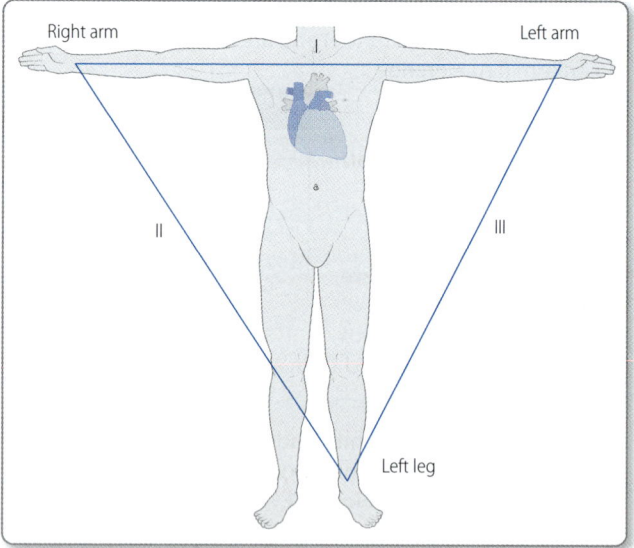

Figure 2.18 Einthoven's triangle – the right arm, left arm, neutral and left foot give three unipolar leads aVR, aVL and aVF, creating a triangle; the bipolar leads I, II and III are the potential difference measured between each. aVF, augmented vector foot; aVL, augmented vector left; aVR, augmented vector right.

The ECG shape

Electricity moving towards a lead causes an upward voltage deflection; and vice versa. The more directly it is moving towards the lead, the stronger the upward deflection. Most of the electrical impulse occurs during ventricular contraction – the QRS complex (**Figure 2.19**).

Cardiac axis

As the ECG deflection represents the amount and direction of the heart's electrical activity, the cardiac axis can be measured (**Figure 2.20**). It is normally –30 to +90° (11 o'clock to 5 o'clock) but can be deviated by disease (**Tables 2.28** and **2.29**).

Analysis of the ECG

An ECG trace is analysed for heart rate, rhythm and the shape, size and duration of characteristic deflections from the baseline, i.e. waves. Waves and the intervals between them give information about different aspects of heart function.

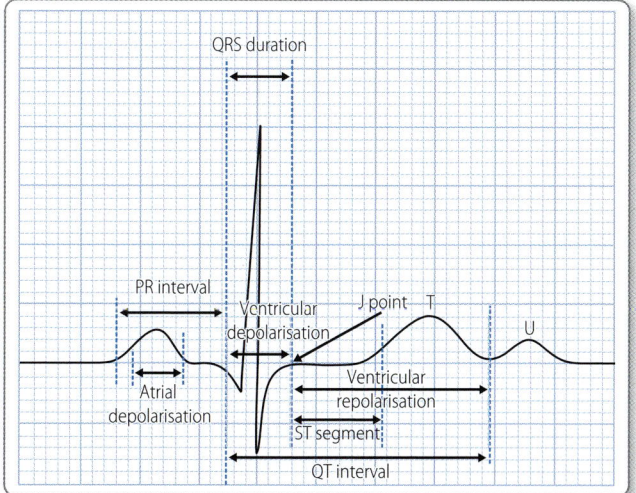

Figure 2.19 Waveforms and intervals of the ECG.

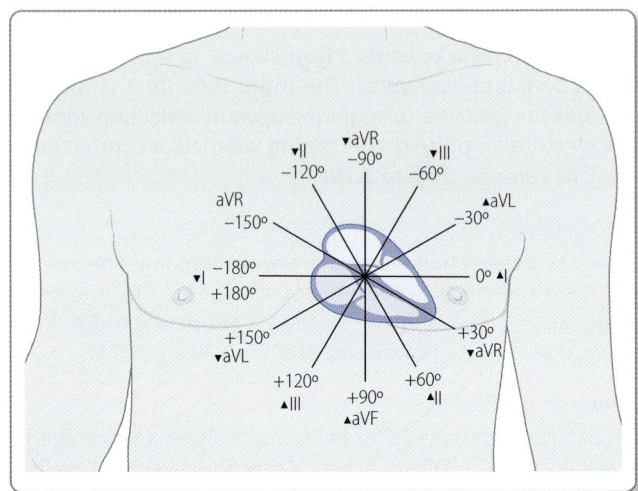

Figure 2.20 The cardiac axis. aVF, augmented vector foot; aVL, augmented vector left; aVR, augmented vector right.

Deviation	Examples
Right axis (+90 to +180°)	• Can be normal, especially in tall, thin individuals • Right bundle branch block (RBBB) • Right ventricular hypertrophy (RVH) • Pulmonary embolism (PE) • Cor pulmonale
Left axis (−30 to −90°)	• Left bundle branch block (LBBB) • Left ventricular hypertrophy (LVH) • Cardiac pacemaker • Left anterior hemiblock

Table 2.28 Cardiac axis deviation.

Heart rate The heart rate is best judged on the rhythm strip; the long lead II reading at the bottom. The rate in beats per minute (bpm) is the number of large squares between each QRS complex (the R–R interval) divided by 300.

Element	Definition	Morphology	Amplitude	Duration	Pathologies
P wave	Atrial depolarisation	Upward deflection before QRS	<0.2 mv (2 small squares)	<0.12 s (3 small squares)	P mitrale: Bifid wave due to LA enlargement P pulmonale: Tall, peaked wave due to RA enlargement
PR interval	Conduction through AVN and HPB	Region from start of the P wave and start of QRS	No deflection	0.12–0.20s (3–5 small squares)	<0.12 s = ventricular pre-excitation >0.20 s = AV block Depressed: Pericarditis
Q waves	Interventricular septum depolarisation (left to right)	Any negative deflection before R wave	<0.2 mV (2 small squares)	<0.04 s (1 small square)	>0.2 mV or >0.04 s = inert myocardium from MI
QRS complex	Ventricular depolarisation	Region from Q to the end of S	2.5–3 mv	<0.12 s (3 small squares	Axis deviation in LVH, RVH >0.12 s seen in BBB, paced ventricular rhythm, ventricular arrhythmia or ectopic beats
ST segment	Time between ventricular depolarisation and repolarisation	Region between S and T waves	No deflection	0.08–0.12 s (2–3 small squares)	ST depression = ischaemia ST elevation = infarction, pericarditis or LBBB

Table 2.29 ECG elements. *Continues overleaf.*

Element	Definition	Morphology	Amplitude	Duration	Pathologies
T wave	Ventricular repolarisation	• Positive deflections after each QRS complex • Inverted in AVR, V1 and V2 and any lead with negative QRS	<5 mm in limb leads, <15 mm in precordial leads	<0.2 s (5 small squares)	Inverted T waves in other leads suggest ischaemia or structural heart disease Tall and narrow T waves are seen in hyperkalaemia Tall asymmetrical T waves are seen in NSTEMI
QT interval	Ventricular depolarisation and repolarisation	Start of QRS to end of T wave. QT corrected (QTc) for heart rate = QT/square root of the RR interval (in seconds)	No deflection	QTc <0.40 s (10 small squares) in women and <0.45 s (11 small squares) in men	Prolonged QT is rarely genetic and commonly drug-induced. Risk of arrhythmias
U wave	Abnormal	Bifid small positive deflection immediately after T wave			Hypokalaemia
J wave	Abnormal	Positive wave just after QRS			Hypothermia

AVN, atrioventricular node; HPB, His-Purkinje bundle; LA, left atrium; RA, right atrium; LVH, left ventricular hypertrophy; RVH, right ventricular hypertrophy.

Table 2.29 *Continued*.

Rhythm In sinus rhythm, P waves (atrial depolarisation) are followed by QRS complexes (ventricular depolarisation) with a regular PR interval between them. Absence of this interval suggests an atrial arrhythmia, causing a tachycardia; or AV node disease, causing a bradycardia (**Table 2.30**).

> **Guiding principle**
>
> Atrial repolarisation is hidden by the much larger ventricular depolarisation (QRS complex).

BP and ECG monitoring

Hypertension and pathology affecting the ECG can be sporadic and change over time. It is therefore often necessary to monitor BP and ECG (**Table 2.29**) over periods of

> **Clinical insight**
>
> Enlarged Q waves represent a myocardial window of electrically inert myocardium (dead wall) due to MI, so that the electrical signal from the opposite active heart wall is detected.

Pathology	Disease	Pathophysiology	ECG signs
Atrial arrhythmias	Atrial fibrillation	No organised electrical activity	No discernible P wave
	Atrial flutter	Re-entrant circuit in the atria	Saw-tooth baseline, comprising flutter (F) waves before each QRS
Heart (AV) block	First degree	Delay in AV conduction	P wave before each QRS but the PR interval is prolonged
	Second degree	Some P waves not conducted by the AV node	• Mobitz type I: PR interval progressively prolonged until a P wave is 'dropped' • Mobitz type II: 2–3 P waves before each QRS
	Third degree (complete)	No conduction across the AV node; depolarisation originates in ventricles	Bradycardia with no relationship between atrial (P wave) and ventricular (QRS) electrical activity

AV, atrioventricular.

Table 2.30 Atrial arrhythmias and heart block on ECG.

time for diagnosis, to gauge disease severity or measure outcomes.

Ankle–brachial pressure index This is the ratio of the systolic BP in the arms (brachial artery) to the ankle (posterior tibial artery). A negative ABPI indicates PVD causing a relative decrease in leg blood pressure.

Ambulatory blood pressure monitor (ABPM) A portable sphygmomanometer measures BP at regular intervals, e.g. every 20 minutes, over a 24-hour period to diagnose hypertension and assess treatment.

24 hours, 48 hours, 7-day ECG, and implantable loop recorder A 3-lead ECG recorder (Holter monitor) is worn for 1–7 days; a matchbox-sized implantable loop recorder (ILR) can be used for up to 3 years.

Tilt table test This investigates autonomic dysfunction with postural changes, e.g. postural hypotension or postural orthostatic tachycardia. A patient is laid on a platform with ECG and BP monitoring as their posture is manipulated.

Exercise testing

Exercise tests are used to provoke symptoms and assess function.

6-minute walk test (6MWT) This is used to assess heart failure and preoperative fitness. It is the distance a patient can walk on a hard, flat surface; <500 m is abnormal.

Exercise tolerance test (ETT) In ETT, also known as the cardiac stress test, a patient exercises on a treadmill or exercise bike while BP and ECG data is recorded, before, during, and after exercise to a set target, such as maximal heart rate (maximum heart rate = 220 − age in years). It is used to:
- Diagnose CHD (when CT calcium scoring is not available) – a diagnosis is confirmed by observing horizontal ST depression in more than one lead
- Monitor rehabilitation after MI
- Detect arrhythmias

Cardiopulmonary exercise testing (CPET) This is the assessment of cardiorespiratory fitness and is used to assess the need for transplantation in heart failure and for preoperative risk assessment. The patient exercises while connected to an ECG, BP and breathing apparatus which records gas exchange and the exercise taken in terms of wattage. The maximal uptake of oxygen/kg of body mass/minute at peak exertion (VO_2) – is recorded (**Table 2.31**).

Imaging

Cardiac imaging is used to diagnose CHD, valve disease and to assess ventricular function. CHD is assessed with:
- An anatomical study, such as a coronary angiography, to locate the atherosclerotic lesion
- A functional study, such as stress echocardiography, to demonstrate the lesion's physiological consequences.

Chest radiography

Chest radiography is used to visualise changes in heart size and shape, thoracic vessels and lung fields, including signs of:
- Heart failure – cardiomegaly, pleural effusion, pulmonary oedema, pulmonary hypertension, ventricular hypertrophy
- Constrictive pericarditis – calcification of the pericardium
- Aortic dissection – widened mediastinum
- Pleural effusions – blunting of the costophrenic angles
- Remnants of interventions, e.g. sternal wires, artificial valves, LV-assisted devices and pacemakers.

VO_2 (mL/kg/min)	Patient groups
>70	Elite athletes
>50	Healthy active individuals
>30	Healthy sedentary individuals
<20	Pretransplant heart failure

Table 2.31 Cardiopulmonary exercise testing: typical VO_2 values for different patient groups.

Ultrasound

Ultrasound uses high frequency sound waves (>20 mHz) to visualise tissues and organs. The waves pass through less-dense structures such as blood and air but are reflected by denser structures such as muscle and bone. Reflections are detected by the transducer and transformed into a digital image. It is cheap, quick and involves no radiation.

> **Clinical insight**
>
> If there is cardiomegaly (i.e. a cardiothoracic ratio > 50% on a PA view) look for other signs of heart failure.

Carotid Doppler ultrasound This uses the Doppler effect of sound waves to visualise blood movement; the frequency is higher as it travels towards the transducer and lower as it moves away. It is used to locate and quantify the degree of artery narrowing due to atherosclerosis, particularly in the carotid arteries following a stroke or before a coronary artery bypass graft (CABG).

Abdominal ultrasound This is the first choice to assess for the presence, location and size of an AAA, but does not visualise the entire abdominal aorta.

Venous duplex ultrasound This is used to visualise venous anatomy and blood flow, e.g. in diagnosing DVT, typically in patients with a unilateral painful and swollen leg.

Echocardiography

Echocardiography uses ultrasound to assess the structure and function of the heart, particularly heart muscle and valves. Indications include breathlessness, heart murmur and syncope.

Transthoracic echocardiography Transthoracic echocardiography (TTE) uses an ultrasound probe on the thoracic wall.

Motion (M) mode Pulses are emitted in quick succession in a single plane, producing a one-dimensional image, a single, highly focussed 'cut' through the heart, with time on the X axis and the depth from the probe on the Y. It can show rapid and small movements well, and is best for fine measurements, such as left ventricular wall thickness.

Brightness (B) mode This is the most familiar echo mode, with width displayed on the X-axis and depth on the Y-axis. The fan-shaped beam projects across the heart, producing a cross-sectional tomograph from four viewpoints (**Figure 2.21**).
It is used to assess:
- Valve structure and function
- Ventricular function
- Chamber size
- Masses or structural heart disease
- Pericardial disease.

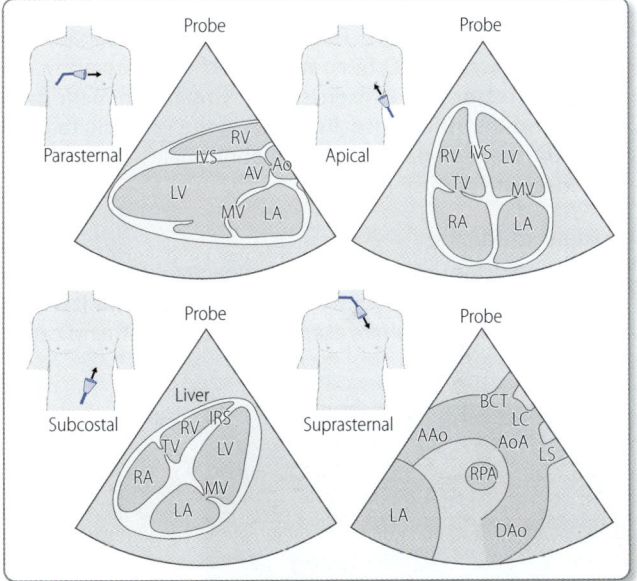

Figure 2.21 Echocardiography 'windows. (a) Parasternal next to the left parasternal border (b) apical at the LV apex (c) subcostal from under the diaphragm (d) suprasternal from the neck. Ao, aorta; AAo, ascending aorta; AoA, aortic annulus; AV, aortic valve; BCT, base of tricuspid valve; DAo, descending aorta; IRS, interatrial septum; IVS, interventricular septum; LA, left atrium; LC, left coronary artery; LS, left subclavian artery; LV, left ventricle; MV, mitral valve; RA, right atrium; RV, right ventricle; TV, tricuspid valve.

Doppler echocardiography Doppler echocardiography is used to estimate blood velocity and quantify the severity of stenotic and regurgitant valvular disease (**Figure 2.22**).

Three-dimensional (3D) echocardiography This is used to visualise structural heart and valve disease (**Figure 2.23**). Tissue resolution is limited compared to CT or MRI.

Trans-oesophageal echocardiography An ultrasound probe is inserted into the oesophagus to image posterior heart structures, including the aortic arch, mitral valve and left atrium. It is useful to visualise aortic dissection, mitral valve endocarditis and left atrial thrombus.

Stress echocardiography This is a functional investigation to induce and localise CHD, by combining echocardiography and a cardiac stressor such as exercise or a sympathomimetic drug (e.g. adenosine). It can visualise areas of the ventricle that fail to contract; a regional wall motion abnormality (RWMA) due to inadequate perfusion.

Nuclear medicine

Nuclear medicine uses intravenous radioactive contrast to visualise its uptake by tissues with a radiosensitive camera. It is used in patients with CHD, where exercise testing is contraindicated,

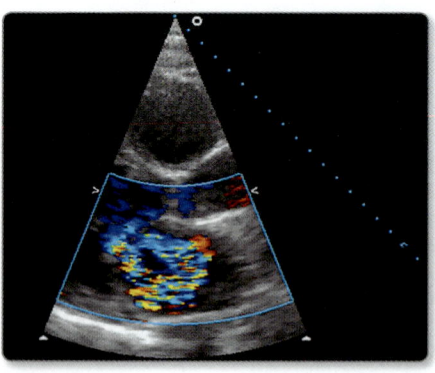

Figure 2.22 Echocardiogram demonstrating Doppler shift with colour flow mapping.

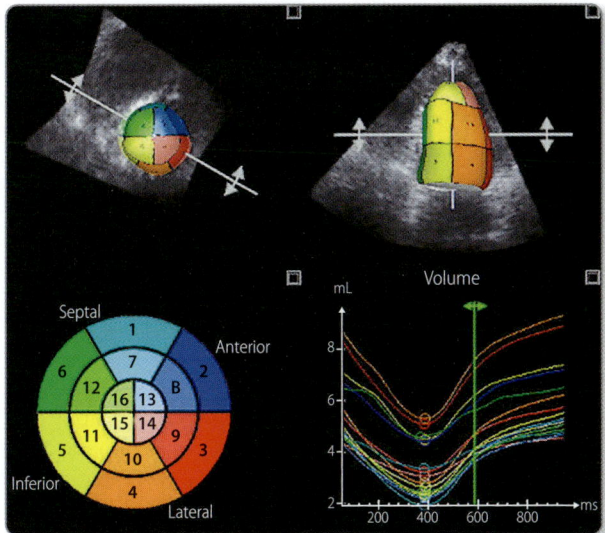

Figure 2.23 3D echocardiogram of the left ventricle. 3D, three-dimensional.

to compare blood flow before and after administration of a sympathomimetic drug (e.g. adenosine) (**Figure 2.24**).

Computed tomography

A computer tomography (CT) scan uses ionising X-ray radiation, reflected by tissues to varying degrees, to take tomographic (i.e. sectional) pictures of the heart and vessels. Axial sections are combined to create a 3D image. CT is used to diagnose CHD, and to visualise aberrant vessels and cardiac masses such as tumours.

Coronary artery calcium score As atherosclerotic lesions calcify as they age, a low-dose CT scan is used to quantify calcification in coronary arterial walls in patients with a low likelihood of CHD (<30%):
- Low (0 Agatston units) suggests that there is no CHD
- Moderate (1–400) indicates further imaging (CT angiography)
- High (>400) indicates invasive angiography

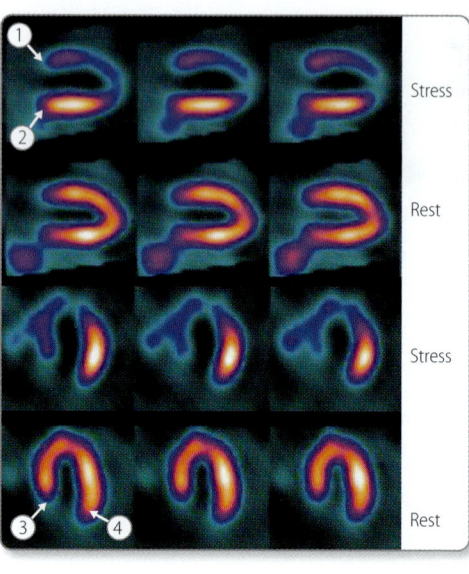

Figure 2.24 Cardiac nuclear medicine: A myocardial perfusion scan of a left ventricle (LV) showing a perfusion deficit in the anterior and septal LV walls not present at rest. This indicates reversible ischaemia from proximal left anterior descending (LAD) artery occlusion. ① Anterior wall; ② Posterior wall; ③ Septal wall; ④ Lateral wall.

Computed tomography coronary angiography (CTCA) This uses intravenous iodine contrast to visualise the coronary arteries. It is used to assess patients with a moderate likelihood of CHD (30–60%), and those post-CABG. It has a higher tissue resolution than CT calcium score or invasive angiography, and can visualise soft and unstable plaques.

> **Clinical insight**
>
> Calcium in arteries nearly always indicates atherosclerosis but gives no indication of plaque stability and therefore the risk of an acute coronary event.

Magnetic resonance imaging

Magnetic resonance imaging (MRI) uses a magnetic field at a specific resonance frequency to excite hydrogen atoms in the body. The resulting radio frequency signal emitted by the atoms is detected and converted into a two-dimensional (2D) image and combined 3D image (**Figure 2.25**). Cardiac MRI (CMR) is used to assess:

Investigations 143

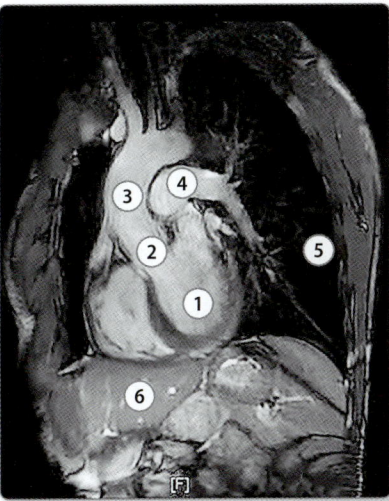

Figure 2.25 Cardiac magnetic resonance scan. (1) Left ventricle; (2) aortic value; (3) aorta; (4) pulmonary artery; (5) lung; and (6) liver.

- Cardiac volumes
- Right ventricular disease
- Congenital heart disease
- Post-MI scar tissue (with IV contrast)
- Coronary perfusion in CHD (with IV contrast)

Clinical insight

Cardiac MRI is invaluable in patients presenting with chest pain, ischaemic ECG changes, and significantly raised troponin but a normal angiogram, as it can visualise other causes such as acute cardiomyopathies.

Cardiac catheterisation

Catheterisation uses X-ray imaging and a catheter that injects contrast and senses blood pressures. It is used to investigate CHD, valve diseases, and pulmonary hypertension.

Catheter access The Seldinger technique of catheterisation involves:
- A guidewire is passed into the right radial or femoral artery
- A sheath is placed over the wire
- The short wire is replaced with a long one, which is pushed under X-ray guidance to the coronary area of stenosis and then exchanged for a catheter

- Radio-opaque iodine-based dye is injected through the catheter to visualise the vessels.

Left heart catheterisation (LHC) The LHC study includes coronary angiography, aortography and LV ventriculography, performed to investigate CHD and aortic valve disease.

Coronary angiography This uses contrast to visualise the patency and blood flow of the coronary arteries. It is normally performed in patients with a high likelihood of CHD (>60%), within <48 hours of a diagnosis of non-ST-elevation myocardial infarction (NSTEMI) or within 120 minutes of presentation of a STEMI.

Aortography A pigtail catheter is used to inject contrast in multiple directions and assess the aortic valve. Reflux of contrast from the aortic root into the LV, e.g. indicates aortic regurgitation.

Ventriculography A pigtail catheter is inserted into the LV and high-pressure contrast injection visualises the shape and regional contraction of the LV. It is used to localise LV myocardial death and assess mitral regurgitation.

If left ventricular end-diastolic pressure (LVEDP) is >30 mmHg, it indicates impaired relaxation of the LV, usually due to CHD or hypertension. After ventriculography, the catheter is pulled back across the aortic valve to detect any change in pressure due to aortic stenosis.

> **Clinical insight**
>
> Angiography takes <30 minutes and has a 0.1% risk of stroke, myocardial infarction or death and a 1% risk of bleeding, bruising, pseudoaneurysm and allergic reactions to contrast media.

> **Guiding principle**
>
> Pulmonary capillary wedge pressure (PCWP) access is via the right femoral or internal jugular vein to the RA, crossing the tricuspid and pulmonary valves and into the pulmonary artery.

Right heart catheterisation (RHC) The RHC study measures pressures in the RA, RV, pulmonary artery and pulmonary capillary bed.

It is performed to assess heart transplant recipients, suspected pulmonary hypertension and valve disease.

Pulmonary artery and capillary wedge pressure The pulmonary capillary wedge pressure (PCWP) is an estimate of the pressure in the LA, with pressures of the RA, RV and pulmonary artery measured enroute. The catheter is 'wedged' in a segmental or subsegmental branch of the right or left pulmonary arteries.

Pulmonary capillary wedge pressure, due to the high compliance of the pulmonary circulation, reflects the LA and, therefore, the LV filling pressure. A low PCWP (<5 mmHg) suggests the patient is fluid-depleted, and a high (>15 mmHg) that the patient is fluid overloaded.

2.4 Cardiovascular risk assessment

Cardiovascular risk assessment is the calculation of a patient's risk of CHD by the presence, absence or severity of key risk factors determined in the history, examination and investigations. Tools for risk assessment include online calculators and charts constructed from large-scale population studies.

Most calculators report a person's 10-year risk of an event; in most people a risk of 20% or over is considered high risk.

Uses

Formal risk assessment is a very useful tool in the primary prevention of CHD:
- In combination with the clinical context risk is used to guide treatment decisions
- It is proven to increase adherence to treatment and engage the patient in taking an often-asymptomatic disease seriously

Scores are used to judge when to use antihypertensive and lipid-lowering medication.

Risk factors

Risk calculators and charts usually consider the key risk factors for CHD, e.g.:
- Age

- Gender
- Smoking
- Diabetes mellitus or a measured blood glucose
- History of angina or MI in a first-degree relative
- Body mass index (BMI) in kg/m^2
- Systolic blood pressure
- Total and HDL cholesterol
- Ethnicity
- Presence of AF

These values are entered into the calculator, and it gives the 10-year risk of a CHD event.

Assessment tools

Risk calculators include the American College of Cardiology (ACC)/American Heart Association's (AHA) atherosclerotic cardiovascular disease (ASCVD), the Joint British Societies for the Prevention of Cardiovascular Disease's JBS3 and the National Heart, Lung and Blood Institute's CVRISK. Problems with calculators include:
- Risk overestimation in low-risk groups
- Underestimation in high-risk groups
- Inconsistencies between calculators

The inconsistencies can result in different treatment decisions, particularly if risk assessment is being used to determine therapy. This also has economic and public health implications and can lead to over-diagnosis and associated unnecessary anxiety and side effects from treatments.

When not to use risk assessment tools?

Risk calculators and charts are only of use in patients who do not have pre-existing cardiovascular disease, i.e. for primary and not secondary prevention, and who do not have a genetic predisposition, such as familial hyperlipidaemia.

2.5 Conservative management

Coronary heart disease is mostly a chronic result of lifestyle and diet factors. Conservative measures aim to reduce risk factors as a means of primary prevention, and decrease disease progression or recurrence in established disease.

Smoking cessation

Smokers are five times more likely to suffer from vascular disease than non-smokers; it is the leading preventable cause of CHD and PVD. Health professionals should regularly:
- Convey the risks
- Encourage smokers to quit
- Sign post-treatment options (e.g. nicotine replacement therapy in gum, patches or electronic cigarettes or hypnotherapy) and support services.

Exercise

Regular exercise helps to reduce many risk factors, including obesity, blood pressure and LDL cholesterol, and improves mood, cardio-respiratory fitness, HDL cholesterol and insulin sensitivity. It can reduce the risk of vascular disease by up to 50%.

All health professionals should regularly highlight the profound health benefits of exercise, with a target of 30–60 minutes of sufficient intensity to cause shortness of breath, 3–5 times a week.

Exercise can also help to reverse muscle wasting, and reduce angina, claudication and dyspnoea.

Alcohol

Alcohol guidelines in the UK advise daily maxima of 2–3 units for women and 3–4 units for men, as well as several alcohol-free days a week. More than this is considered 'harmful drinking'; can lead to alcohol dependence and its associated increased risks of, e.g. heart failure, alcoholic liver disease and some

> **Clinical insight**
>
> Obesity is an independent risk factor for CHD, hypertension, hyperlipidaemia, and diabetes. Those with central obesity have twice the risk of MI.

> **Clinical insight**
>
> 1 unit of alcohol = 250 mL beer/cider or 125 mL wine or 25 mL spirit.

cancers. A small amount of alcohol is known to reduce the risk of cardiovascular disease.

Health professionals should always assess alcohol intake and if patients drink to excess, advise them of:
- Associated risks
- A reduction in consumption
- Possible treatments, including medications, detoxification regimes, hospital admission, counseling and Alcoholics Anonymous.

Diet

A healthy, balanced and 'Mediterranean' diet rich in fruit, vegetables, grains, nuts, fish and unsaturated fats and low in red meat, sodium and saturated fat (**Figure 2.26**) helps to improve blood pressure and lipid profile and reduces cardiovascular risk by up to 30%.

Patients can be referred to dieticians who can advise on the practicalities of healthy eating.

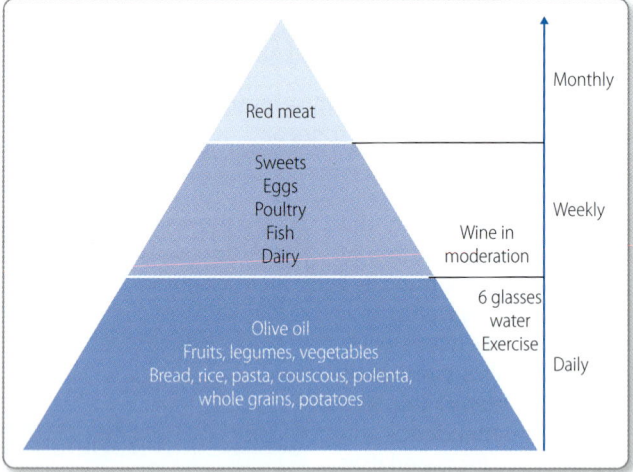

Figure 2.26 Healthy eating pyramid of a Mediterranean diet.

2.6 Medication

Patients must be made aware of:
- Why a drug is being initiated
- Possible side effects
- Monitoring requirements

Many cardiac medications require monitoring to maintain therapeutic levels and avoid harm. Warfarin is a notable example.

Lipid-lowering drugs

Hypercholesterolaemia is a total cholesterol >5 mmol/L (>200 mg/dL) or LDL cholesterol >3 mmol/L (>115 mg/dL). Medication is indicated if there is no response to conservative measures, or after a diagnosis of CHD or MI. Statins are the first-line agents used to lower LDL cholesterol (**Table 2.32**). Other lipid-lowering drugs, such as fibrates and bile acid

> **Clinical insight**
>
> Drug selection can be daunting; consult a pharmacist, national guidelines, hospital formulary or a senior colleague before prescribing an unfamiliar medication.

Drug group	Mode of action	Effect on cholesterol	Examples	Common side effects
Statins	Inhibit HMG-CoA reductase	Reduce LDL	• Simvastatin • Atorvastatin	• Muscle aches • Hepatic impairment
Fibrates	Activate PPAR receptors	Reduce LDL and TG	• Bezafibrate • Gemfibrozil	• Indigestion • Rash
Brush border lipase inhibitors	Inhibit gut absorption of lipid	Reduce LDL	Ezetimibe	• Diarrhoea • Headache
Bile acid sequestrants	Bind bile in the gut	Reduce LDL	Cholestyramine	• Diarrhoea • Constipation
Nicotinic acid	Activate adipocyte receptors	Reduce TG, LDL increase HDL	Nicotinic acid (niacin)	• Flushing • Itching

HDL, high-density lipoprotein; HMG-CoA, 3-hydroxy-3-methylglutaryl-coenzyme A; LDL, low-density lipoprotein; PPAR, peroxisome proliferator-activated receptor; TG, triglycerides.

Table 2.32 Cholesterol lowering medications.

sequestrants are not recommenced but may be used in statin-intolerant patients.

Statins
Statins (e.g. simvastatin and atorvastatin) reduce cardiovascular events and mortality in patients with CHD and reduce the likelihood of CHD in those with hypercholesterolaemia. They also improve endothelial function and maintain atherosclerotic plaque stability.

Other lipid-lowering drugs
Other drugs are generally not recommended in AHA/ACC or the National Institute for Health and Care Excellence (NICE) guidelines for CHD prevention but may be useful in some situations.

Fibrates There is no evidence that fibrates save lives in CHD, but they do reduce the risk of MI. They are used in patients intolerant to statins or in combination with statins when statin monotherapy is insufficient.

Brush border lipase inhibitors There is no evidence that brush border lipase inhibitors reduce cardiovascular mortality or morbidity. Ezetimibe is suggested by NICE as a second-line therapy for familial hypercholesterolaemia where patients are statin intolerant, or as combination therapy when statin monotherapy is insufficient.

Bempedoic acid: This is approved by NICE for managing hypercholesterolaemia in statin intolerant patients and also patients for primary or secondary prevention when targets are not met.

Bile acid sequestrants Bile acid sequestrants, also known as anion exchange resins, reduce the progression of, and mortality in, CHD. They may be used as an accessory drug with statins, if fibrates are contraindicated.

> **Clinical insight**
>
> Statins are metabolised in the liver by the cytochrome P450 (*CYP3A4*) enzyme system. Other chemicals that interfere with this (e.g. grapefruit, fibrates, and niacin) lead to elevated levels of circulating statins.

Nicotinic acid The broad-spectrum effects of nicotinic acid reduce CHD mortality, but its clinical use is limited by a high rate of side effects such as flushing, rashes and GI upset.

Anticoagulants

Anticoagulants inhibit blood coagulation (**Figure 2.27** and **Table 2.33**).

Coumarins

Coumarins are taken orally to reduce venous thrombosis in DVT or PE or prevent arterial thrombosis in patients with AF

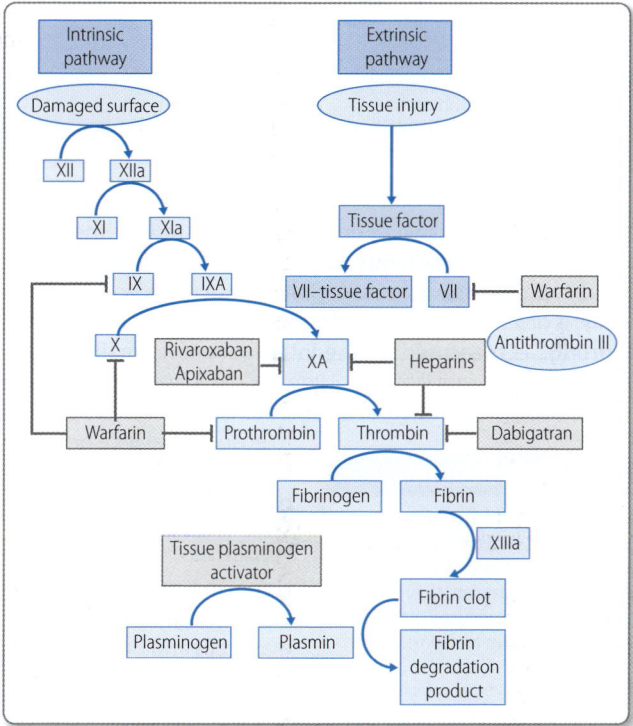

Figure 2.27 The clotting cascade and anti-coagulant drugs.

Types and mode of action	Side effect	Antidote	Indications
Coumarins: Inhibit clotting factors II, VII, IX, X, e.g. warfarin and phenindione	• Bleeding • Bruising • Osteoporosis • Hair loss	Vitamin K	AF, VTE, MHV
Heparins: Activate anti-thrombin III, e.g. enoxaparin and dalteparin	• Bleeding • Bruising • Hyperkalaemia • Thrombocytopaenia	Protamine sulphate	VTE, MI
Novel oral anticoagulants (NOACs): Inhibit thrombin directly, e.g. apixaban and rivaroxaban	• Bleeding • Bruising • Headache • Indigestion	N/A	VTE, AF

AF, atrial fibrillation; MHV, metal heart valves; MI, myocardial infarction; VTE, venous thromboembolism.

Table 2.33 Anticoagulants.

or metallic heart valves. For example, they reduce the risk of embolic stroke in patients with AF by 66%. The most widely used coumarin is warfarin. An initial dose (usually 5 or 10 mg daily) is given and daily blood tests monitor the patient's blood clotting, as measured by the international normalised ratio (INR). Once a target INR of 2–3 (ideally 2.5) is reached, a maintenance dose is continued, and INR is monitored every 2–4 weeks to ensure a balance between clotting risk (e.g. MI or stroke risk) and bleeding risk.

> **Clinical insight**
>
> Heparin-induced thrombocytopenia (HIT) arises in 3–5% of patients following administration of heparin. Antibodies to heparin bind to platelets causing activation, clumping, reduced platelet count and subsequent (paradoxical) thrombosis.

Heparins

Heparins are natural glycosaminoglycans found in mast cells and basophils that inhibit thrombosis. Synthetic heparins are used to prevent venous thrombosis in inpatients and the propagation of established thrombus in patients with DVT, PE or MI.

Low-molecular weight heparins (LMWH), e.g. dalteparin and enoxaparin, are administered subcutaneously, whereas unfractionated heparin (UFH) is given as a continuous intravenous infusion.

Novel oral anticoagulants

Unlike warfarin, the novel oral anticoagulants (NOAC) such as edoxaban, apixaban, dabigatran and rivaroxaban do not necessitate regular blood tests. They are approximately as effective as warfarin in a patient with DVT, PE or AF, and are used when warfarin is ineffective or when regular testing is difficult.

Anti-platelet drugs

Antiplatelet drugs (**Figure 2.28** and **Table 2.34**) inhibit platelet adhesion and aggregation and therefore thrombus formation.

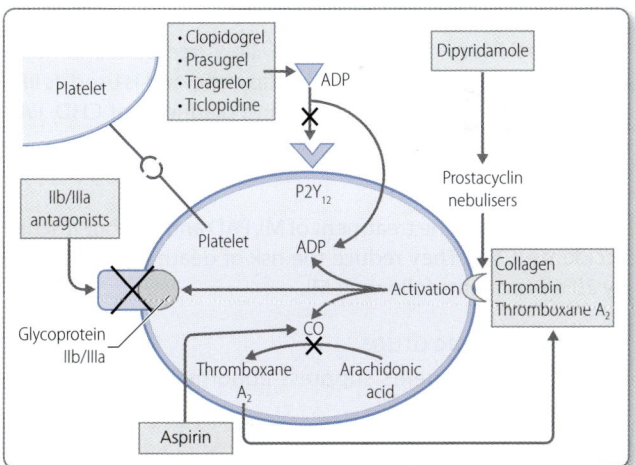

Figure 2.28 Mechanism of action of anti-platelet drugs. ADP, adenosine diphoshphate; COX, cyclo-oxygenase; GP IIb/IIIa, glycoprotein IIb/IIIa.

Drug or drug group	Mode of action	Examples	Common side effects	Indications
Salicylic acid	Inhibits platelet cyclo-oxygenase (COX) enzyme	Aspirin	• Bleeding • Bruising • Peptic ulceration • Gout	• CHD • Cerebrovascular disease • PVD
Thienopyridines	Inhibits platelet adenosine diphosphate (ADP)	• Clopidogrel Prasugrel Ticagrelor	• Bleeding • Bruising • Thrombocytopaenia • Dyspnoea	• MI • Cerebrovascular disease • PVD

CHD, coronary heart disease; PVD, peripheral vascular disease; MI, myocardial infarction.

Table 2.34 Anti-platelet medication.

They are used in the primary prevention and treatment of thrombotic CHD and PVD. They are more effective in the arterial circulation.

Salicylic acid
Salicylic acid (aspirin) is found in willow tree bark and many fruits. It is a minor analgesic and antipyretic, and is used as lifelong antiplatelet treatment following diagnosis of CHD, PAD and MI. It reduces the risk of death in CHD by 30%.

Thienopyridines
These are used in the treatment of MI, PAD and cerebrovascular accidents (CVA). They reduce the risk of death and further MI by 20% in patients following MI.

Anti-arrhythmic drugs
Anti-arrhythmic agents suppress abnormal rhythms of the heart (**Table 2.35**).

Class I
Class I agents block the fast sodium channel of non-nodal cardiac myocytes which are responsible for the rapid depolarisation (Phase 0) of the action potential.

Medication

Drug class	Mode of action	Effect on cardiac AP	Examples	Side effects	Indications in CHD
IA	Inhibit fast Na$^+$ channel	Lengthened	Procainamide Disopyramide	Diarrhoea, nausea, headache, and dizziness	N/A
IB		Shortened	Lidocaine Mexiletine	Dizziness, bradycardia, hypotension, arrhythmia, and cardiac arrest	Ventricular tachycardia
IC		No effect	Flecainide Propafenone	Dizziness, nausea, dyspnoea, and arrhythmia	AF
II	Block β-adrenergic receptors	No effect	Bisoprolol Atenolol Propranolol	Bradycardia, heart block, bronchospasm, hyper-/hypoglycaemia, headache, and constipation	Angina, AF, ventricular tachycardia, and heart failure
III	Inhibit K$^+$ channel	Lengthened	Sotalol Amiodarone	Skin discolouration, thyroid dysfunction, corneal deposits, and long QT	AF and ventricular tachycardia
IV	Blocks Ca^{2+} channels	Shortened	Diltiazem* Verapamil†	Bradycardia, hypotension, dizziness, and headache	AF, AFL, and angina
V	Inhibits Na$^+$/K$^+$ ATPase	No effect	Digoxin	Anorexia, nausea, vomiting and tachy-/bradyarrhythmias	Atrial fibrillation/flutter
	Transient AV block	No effect	Adenosine	Dyspnoea, facial flushing, asystole, headache, and apprehension	Supraventricular tachycardias

*A benzodiazepine; † A phenylalkylamine. AF, atrial fibrillation; AFL, atrial flutter; AP, action potential; CHD, coronary heart disease.

Table 2.35 Anti-arrhythmic medication: The Vaughn–Williams classification, based on effect on cardiac myocyte action potential.

Class II

Class II agents (β-blockers) suppress atrial and ventricular arrhythmias, improve LV function in heart failure and reduce myocardial oxygen demand in CHD.

Mode of action Atenolol, bisoprolol and metoprolol antagonise $β_1$-adrenoreceptors, blocking sympathetic stimulation of the atrioventricular node (AVN). Carvedilol, labetalol, propranolol are non-selective and also target $β_2$-receptors causing bronchial muscle relaxation.

Class III

Class III agents (amiodarone and sotalol) are indicated in AF, ventricular tachycardia and ventricular fibrillation.

Mode of action These agents block cardiomyocyte potassium channels, lengthening the action potential and refractory period duration, preventing re-entrant arrhythmias.

Class IV

Class IV agents – calcium-channel blockers (CCBs) – are used for atrial tachycardias and CHD.

> **Clinical insight**
>
> Amiodarone has many side effects, some are due to its structural similarity to thyroxine; a daily dose of amiodarone (200 mg) accounts for 20 times the daily requirement of thyroxine (6 mg).

Mode of action CCBs block all cardiac calcium channels to decrease the sinus rate and cardiac contractility, prolong the refractory period, and slow conduction through the AV node.

Class V

These are used for atrial tachycardias but have no common mechanism.

Adenosine Adenosine is a purine nucleoside that acts on the A1 receptor subtypes leading to cell hyperpolarisation of both the SA and AV nodes, lengthening the refractory period. This temporarily blocks the AVN and prevents re-entry through the node, such as in SVT.

Digoxin Digoxin is a glycoside derived from foxglove (*Digitalis*) that inhibits the sodium/potassium adenosine triphosphate (ATP) pump in cardiac tissue. This increases intracellular sodium and calcium, slows SA and AVN conduction, and therefore ventricular contraction. It also augments cardiac contractility and is used in patients with heart failure.

Diuretics

Diuretics increase salt and water excretion (i.e. urine production) to lower blood pressure in hypertension and heart failure (**Figure 2.29** and **Table 2.36**). Most diuretics work by blocking different mechanisms of salt (Na^+ and/or K^+) reabsorption in the kidney.

Loop diuretics

Loop diuretics (e.g. furosemide) are the most powerful diuretics, leading to the excretion of 20% of filtered sodium. They are used to treat pulmonary and peripheral oedema in heart failure, but do not reduce mortality.

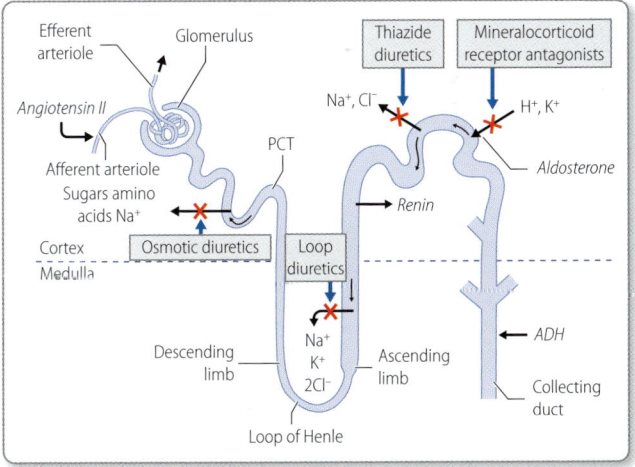

Figure 2.29 Diuretic drugs and their site of action at the loop of Henle. ADH, antidiuretic hormone; PCT, proximal convoluted tubule.

Type of diuretic	Mode of action	Location of action	Examples	Common side effects	Indications

Loop	Block Na+/K+/Cl-cotransporter	Thick ascending limb	• Furosemide
			  Bumetanide
				• Hyponatraemia
				  Hypokalaemia
				  Hyperuricaemia
				• Renal injury
					Heart failure

Thiazide	Block Na+/Cl-cotransporter	Distal convoluted tubule	• Bendroflumethiazide Metolazone	• Hypotension • Dizziness • Hyperglycaemia • Cholestasis	• Heart failure • Hypertension
Potassium sparing	Block epithelial Na+ channels	Collecting duct	• Amiloride Triamterene	• Hyperkalaemia • Dizziness • Rash	Hypertension
Mineralocorticoid receptor antagonists	Block aldosterone receptors	Distal convoluted tubule	• Spironolactone Eplerenone	• Breast tenderness • Hyperkalaemia	• Heart failure • Hypertension

Table 2.36 Diuretics.

Thiazide diuretics
Thiazide diuretics (e.g. bendroflumethiazide) are used in hypertension to reduce blood pressure by an average of 10/5 mmHg.

Potassium sparing diuretics
'Potassium sparing' diuretics (e.g. amiloride) do not increase potassium loss in urine and are used in hypertension and heart failure, normally as adjuncts to other diuretics.

Mineralocorticoid receptor antagonists Mineralocorticoid receptor/aldosterone antagonists (MRA's, e.g. spironolactone) are second-line potassium-sparing diuretics used in hypertension and heart failure. They reduce blood pressure by up to 17/10 mmHg and the risk of death by one-third in patients with chronic severe heart failure.

Mineralocorticoid receptor antagonists also decrease cardiac hypertrophy, fibrosis and arrhythmias and improve endothelial function by an unknown mechanism.

Antihypertensives
Antihypertensives lower systemic vascular resistance, and therefore blood pressure, in primary and secondary prevention of CHD and CVAs (**Table 2.37**).

Alpha-blockers
Alpha-blockers (e.g. doxazosin) are first-line agents that can decrease blood pressure by 11/7 mmHg. They block noradrenaline (norepinephrine) binding to α-1 adreno receptors in vascular smooth muscle, leading to dilation of arteries and veins.

> **Clinical insight**
>
> Alpha-blockers should be avoided in heart failure as they increase mortality.

Angiotensin-converting enzyme inhibitors
Angiotensin-converting enzyme (ACE) inhibitors (**Figure 2.30**) are first-line treatments of hypertension, heart failure, diabetic nephropathy and following MI. They reduce the risk of MI and CVAs by 11% in hypertension. Following MI, they reduce the

Drug	Mode of action	Examples	Common side effect	Indications in CHD
Alpha-blockers	Block α-1 adrenoreceptors	Doxazosin	• Dizziness • Urinary incontinence • Hypotension	Hypertension
Angiotensin converting enzyme inhibitors	Block conversion of angiotensin I to angiotensin II	• Ramipril • Enalapril • Lisinopril	• Dry cough • Hyperkalemia • Renal injury • Angio-oedema	• Hypertension • Heart failure • Diabetic nephropathy • Myocardial infarction
Angiotensin II receptor blockers	Block angiotensin II AT1 receptor	• Valsartan • Candesartan • Losartan	• Dizziness • Hyperkalemia • Renal injury • Angio-oedema	• Hypertension • Heart failure • Diabetic nephropathy • Myocardial infarction
Hydralazine	Direct peripheral vasodilation	Hydralazine	• Allergic reaction • Drug-induced lupus • Palpitations	• Hypertension • Heart failure
Calcium-channel blockers	Block L-type calcium channels	• Amlodipine • Felodipine • Nifedipine	• Dizziness • Flushing • Ankle/Gum swelling	• Hypertension • CHD

AT, angiotensin; CHD, coronary heart disease.

Table 2.37 Antihypertensives.

risk of death and heart failure by 25%, by reducing cardiac hypertrophy, progression of heart failure and proteinuria.

Angiotensin II receptor blockers

Angiotensin II receptor blockers (ARBs) are second-line agents used in hypertension and heart failure (**Figure 2.30**). They reduce the risk of MI by 10% in hypertension and death by

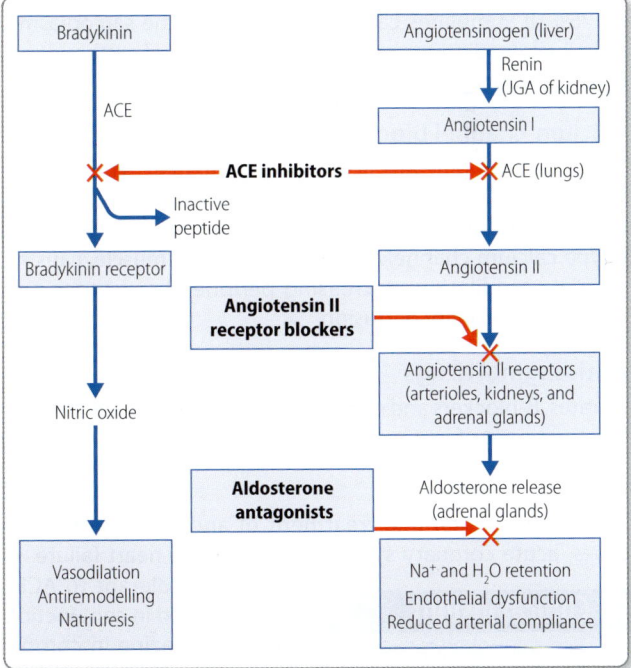

Figure 2.30 The mechanism of action of angiotensin-converting enzyme inhibitors (ACEIs) and angiotensin-II receptor blockers (ARBs). ACEIs block ACE converting angiotensin I (ATI) to angiotensin II (ATII) leading to inhibition of the renin–angiotensin–aldosterone system (RAAS). Less AT II leads to peripheral dilation, reducing cardiac pre- and afterload, improving endothelial function, reducing sympathetic tone and reducing blood pressure. ARBs inhibit the RAAS by blocking the ATI receptor of ATII leading to arteriolar and venous dilation. ARBs reduce cardiac pre- and afterload, improve endothelial function, reduce sympathetic tone and blood pressure. JGA, juxtaglomerular apparatus.

> **Clinical insight**
>
> Angiotensin-converting enzyme inhibitors cause a dry tickly cough in 20% due to build up of lung bradykinin, a peptide that causes pulmonary irritation and bronchoconstriction.

25% in severe heart failure, by reducing cardiac hypertrophy, progression of heart failure and proteinuria.

Hydralazine

Hydralazine is a second-line agent in hypertension and heart failure. It can reduce blood pressure by up to 25/17 mmHg and mortality in heart failure by 25%. It stimulates calcium release from the sarcoplasmic reticulum, leading to vasodilation, reduction of systemic vascular resistance and blood pressure.

Calcium-channel blockers (dihydropyridines)

The dihydropyridines are first-line agents to treat hypertension, and second-line in CHD, reducing blood pressure by 13/11 mmHg and the risk of MI by 11%, respectively. CCBs inhibit L-type calcium channels in vascular smooth muscle, causing arterial vasodilation, decreasing peripheral resistance and improving coronary perfusion.

Anti-anginal drugs

Nitrates, β-blockers and calcium-channel blockers are the first-line treatment of angina (**Table 2.38**).

Nitrates

Nitrates are a first-line treatment of angina, hypertensive crises, acute coronary syndromes and acute heart failure. In patients intolerant to ACEI, they are used in conjunction with hydralazine in chronic heart failure, leading to a 34% reduction in mortality.

> **Clinical insight**
>
> Calcium-channel blockers can exacerbate pulmonary and peripheral oedema.

Mode of action These are precursors to nitric oxide, a powerful localised venous and arterial vasodilator that reduces cardiac preload, afterload, myocardial oxygen demand and blood pressure. Side effects include headaches, dizziness, nausea, vomiting and hypotension.

Types and mode of action	Common side effects	Indications
FIRST LINE		
Nitric oxide donor; e.g. GTN, isosorbide	• Headaches • Dizziness • Hypotension	CHD
SECOND LINE		
Nitric oxide donor and potassium channel agonist, e.g. nicorandil	• Palpitations • Flushing • Gastric ulcers	• CHD • HF • MI
Funny channel agonist, e.g. ivabradine	• Flashing lights • Bradycardia • Dizziness	CHD
Sodium channel blocker, e.g. ranolazine	• Palpitations • Long QT • Indigestion	CHD
CHD, coronary heart disease; GTN, glyceryl trinitrate; HF, heart failure; MI, myocardial infarction.		

Table 2.38 Anti-anginal medication.

Nicorandil
Nicorandil is a second-line anti-anginal agent and is a nitric oxide precursor. Usage results in a 15% reduction in MI.

Ivabradine
This is a second-line anti-anginal agent used in patients with normal sinus rhythm and heart rate > 70 bpm. It reduces the risk of MI by 33% but does not reduce mortality. Ivabradine blocks the funny channel in the SA node, reducing heart rate.

Ranolazine
This is used to treat angina, likely by blocking the sodium dependent calcium channels. It has minimal effect on blood pressure and heart rate and no impact on MI or mortality but reduces anginal episodes by 1–2 per week.

2.7 Surgical management

Cardiovascular surgery is often high-risk, necessitating objective measures of risk before, during and after surgery: risk score, co-morbidity, functional status and cardiovascular fitness.

Percutaneous coronary intervention

In percutaneous coronary intervention (PCI), also known as angioplasty, a balloon is used to widen the lumen of a coronary artery narrowed by atheroma and stabilise the plaque (**Figure 2.31**).

Complications These include:
- MI – 3%
- Coronary dissection – 3%
- Death – 3%
- Stroke – 1%

Arterial bypass

Arterial bypass uses a synthetic or transplanted vessel to circumvent a section of blocked artery. It is indicated in patients with significant atherosclerotic lesions, particularly left main stem and triple coronary vessel.

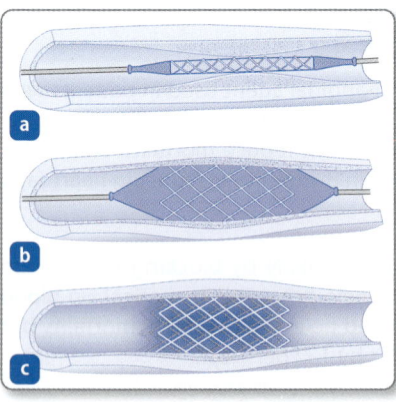

Figure 2.31 Percutaneous coronary intervention (PCI). (a) The stent is crimped over the balloon and guidewire. (b) Inflating the balloon expands the stent. (c) The stent in situ.

Procedure A coronary artery bypass graft (CABG; **Figure 2.32**) is performed under general anaesthetic and takes approximately 4 hours:

> **Clinical insight**
>
> Stents can be bare metal (cobalt–chromium alloy) or coated with drugs, such as sirolimus or paclitaxel, that prevent cell proliferation and thrombosis.

- The chest is opened via midline sternal incision (median sternotomy) a cardiopulmonary bypass is established with a heart lung machine (90 minutes) 'cardioplegia' – the heart is cooled with iced salt water, while a preservative solution is injected into the heart arteries
- The grafts are harvested (**Table 2.39**), washed and sewn proximal to the blockage, typically the aorta, and to the coronary artery distal to the blockage
- The patient is taken off bypass, the chest closed with wires and anaesthetic reversed

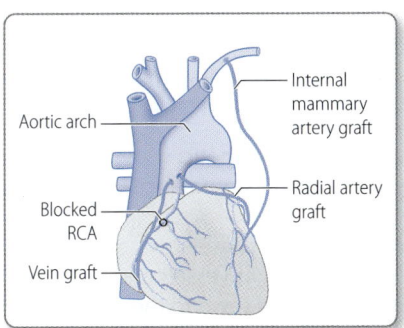

Figure 2.32 A triple coronary artery bypass graft. RCA, right coronary artery.

	Venous graft	**Arterial graft**
Example	Long saphenous vein of leg	Internal mammary of thorax
Length	Long	Limited
10-year patency	66%	90%

Table 2.39 Venous versus arterial coronary artery bypass grafts. Venous grafts are more prone to stenosis and deteriorate within 7 years in approximately half of patients.

Complications These include:
- Death: <1%
- Bleeding: 2%
- Thromboembolism: 1%
- Infection: 4%
- Myocardial infarction: 5%
- Temporary arrhythmias (e.g. AF): 25%

Arterial repair

Abnormal dilations, acute dissections and focal atherosclerosis of large arteries, such as an AAA (>5.5 cm) or carotid atherosclerosis (50–99%), are repaired under general anaesthetic.

Procedure For a carotid endarterectomy, e.g.:
- An incision is made over the carotid artery and a clamp placed above and below the blockage
- The artery is cut open and the atherosclerotic lesion removed
- The skin is closed and the anaesthetic reversed.

Heart transplantation

Heart transplantation is a life-saving treatment for end-stage heart disease.

Procedure Following a general anaesthetic:
- The chest is opened via midline sternal incision (median sternotomy)
- The patient is put on a bypass machine
- The heart is isolated from the major vessels and removed
- The donor heart is implanted and sewn to the vessels
- Finally, the patient is taken off the bypass machine, the chest is closed and the anaesthetic is reversed

Complications Complications include death, stroke, bleeding, thromboembolism, transplant failure, infection, MI and cardiac arrhythmia.

Valve repair/replacement

This is indicated in patients with symptomatic and severe valve disease not amenable to minimally invasive repair.

Procedure Following a general anaesthetic:

> **Clinical insight**
>
> Heart transplantation is limited by availability, e.g. around 200 were performed in the UK in 2013.

- The chest is opened via midline sternal incision (median sternotomy)
- The patient is put on a bypass machine and then the heart is then cooled
- The diseased valve is located and removed
- For repair of the mitral valve, stitches are used to repair the prolapsing leaflet and secure it to the valvular apparatus
- For replacement, a new tissue or metal valve is then sewn into place
- The patient is taken off bypass, the chest is closed and the anaesthetic reversed

Complications The complications include death, stroke, bleeding, thromboembolism, valve dehiscence, infection, MI and cardiac arrhythmia.

Myocardial repair and support

Certain myocardial defects are suitable for repair and/or the failing myocardium can be supported by the use of an artificial pump (**Table 2.40**).

Procedure	Indication	Purpose	Method
Left ventricular assist device	LV failure pre-transplant or post-MI	Assist myocardial recovery	Pump inlet is sewn to the LV apex and the pump outlet to the ascending aorta
Total artificial heart	End-stage heart failure	Complete replacement of heart function	Cardiac chambers are removed and the device attached to the great vessels
LV restoration therapy	LV aneurysm post-MI	Improves LV function	Diseased myocardium removed and the heart then closed
Septal repair	• ASD and VSD • If septum cannot be closed using a device	Separation of left and right circulation	Patch of bovine/native pericardium or Teflon is sewn into place

Table 2.40 Examples of myocardial repair and support.

Atherosclerosis

chapter 3

Atherosclerosis is a progressive process of atheroma formation – arterial wall lesions of white blood cells, lipid and cholesterol deposits and cell debris. These 'plaques' form in the intima of large and medium arteries, and can develop to include scar tissue, thrombosis and calcification.

All larger arteries develop atheroma as we age, but in excess it can cause hardening of the arterial wall (sclerosis) and narrowing of the lumen. The resulting obstruction restricts blood flow to cause ischaemia of downstream tissues. If the plaque becomes unstable and ruptures, thrombosis and thromboembolism can cause acute blockage and infarction of tissue.

Atherosclerosis is the underlying cause of most coronary and cerebral arterial disease; the two biggest killers in the western world. It is also accelerated by diabetes mellitus and underlies most peripheral vascular disease (PVD).

3.1 Clinical scenario

Painful and cold right foot

Presentation

Carol Newton is a 56-year-old store manager who presents to her local emergency department with a painful and cold right foot.

Diagnostic approach

Foot pain is common, and causes include PVD, gout, plantar fasciitis and ligament sprain. However, a cold foot suggests a problem with the blood supply. History should establish:
- Onset
- If it is worsening
- Associated symptoms, such as numbness and radiation of pain

Further history

The pain has been increasing for a couple of days, was not preceded by trauma, and has no focal tender point. It is worse when she lies in bed, causing her to hang her foot out of the bed. She is a lifelong smoker but has no other significant past medical history and takes no medications.

> **Clinical insight**
>
> The symptoms of acute limb ischaemia are the six P's.
> 1. Pain
> 2. Pulseless
> 3. Pallor
> 4. Perishingly cold
> 5. Paraesthesia
> 6. Paralysis

Examination

Other than having blood pressure of 155/95 mmHg, Carol's cardiovascular, respiratory and abdominal systems are all normal. She is afebrile, has normal oxygen saturation and blood glucose.

Her right foot is pale and pulseless, with a delayed capillary refill time of 6 seconds. The most distally palpable pulse is the femoral artery. Dorsiflexion and plantar flexion are difficult and painful when done passively.

Diagnostic approach

Lack of trauma or focal tenderness suggests the pain is unlikely to originate from the musculoskeletal system or a single structure. Night pain is common in lower limb ischaemia, because the raised limb decreases blood flow; lowering the foot increases flow and decreases the ischaemic pain.

Smoking and hypertension are major risk factors for atherosclerosis, increasing the likelihood of PVD. Accordingly, her delayed capillary refill time suggests impaired blood supply due to either the heart or the arteries.

The normal oxygen saturation, blood glucose and temperature rule out hypoxia, hyperglycaemia, hypothermia or overt sepsis as contributing factors, respectively. Cardiogenic or septic shock is unlikely as only one limb is affected, and she is not hypotensive.

A unilateral pulseless and cold foot confirms an arterial aetiology, likely distal to her palpable femoral artery.

Investigations
An electrocardiogram (ECG) and further blood tests (including full blood count and tests of renal and liver function) are done and are all normal.

The ankle-brachial pressure index (ABPI) is <0.5 (75 mmHg/ 155 mmHg).

Diagnosis
The diagnosis is acute lower limb ischaemia, as indicated by the unilateral painful, cold and pulseless foot and ABPI of <0.5, confirming a significantly lower blood pressure in her right foot than her arms. The foot pain at rest and delayed capillary refill indicate that tissue viability is threatened. Her difficulty in moving the foot means that urgent revascularisation is necessary.

> **Clinical insight**
>
> Patients with peripheral arterial disease are at higher risk of coronary heart disease (CHD) and cerebrovascular disease.

The blood tests are performed to obtain preoperative baseline values as blood loss and significant organ injury may follow any limb or life-saving operation.

Carol's condition is likely due to peripheral arterial atherosclerosis caused by cigarette smoking and worsened by uncontrolled hypertension.

3.2 Atherosclerosis

Atherosclerosis is the most common arterial pathology and underlies most diseases of ischaemia and infarction. Its features depend on the site affected, resulting from arterial constriction at the lesion and embolic disease. Treatment can be symptomatic relief of vasoconstriction, surgical removal of a thrombus, and stabilisation or bypass of the plaque. Primary and/or secondary prevention aims to treat symptoms and decrease risk factors.

Epidemiology

Atheroma begins to form as fatty streaks in late childhood and progresses with age. By the eighth or ninth decades, all medium and larger arteries have some degree of atheroma.

Atherosclerosis causes more deaths than any other pathophysiology.

Non-modifiable risk factors include age, sex and genetic predisposition (**Table 3.1**). Symptomatic disease is most common in males over 40 years of age.

Risk factor	Definition	Mechanism
Smoking	Tobacco smoke	Provokes endothelial damage and thrombosis
High blood cholesterol	• Age, sex, heredity, and diet affect cholesterol • High total cholesterol > 6.2 mmol/L (240 mg/dL) • High LDL cholesterol >3.4 mmol/L (130 mg/dL)	Increases cholesterol deposition in arterial wall
High triglycerides	>4.5 mmol/L (400 mg/dL)	Increases lipid deposition in arterial wall
Hypertension	>140/90 mmHg	Provokes endothelial damage
Physical inactivity	• >4 hours sitting a day • <30 minutes exercise four times a week	Increases thrombosis and exposure of vascular endothelium to glucose, lipids and toxins and decreases cardiovascular muscle fitness
Diabetes mellitus	Most diabetics die from myocardial infarction secondary to atherosclerosis	Hyperglycaemia promotes endothelial and vascular connective tissue damage
Stress	History	Increased heart rate, blood pressure and circulating leucocytes
Obesity	BMI > 30 kg/m^2	Increases vascular workload
BMI, body mass index; HDL, high-density lipoprotein; LDL, low-density lipoprotein.		

Table 3.1 Risk factors for atherosclerosis and their contributory mechanism.

Aetiology

The lipid-rich, inflammatory cell and debris deposits of atheroma are a part of normal ageing (**Figure 3.1**). However, the process is accelerated in individuals with a family history of coronary artery disease or stroke, hyperlipidaemia, diabetes mellitus, smoking and hypertension.

Location

Haemodynamics – the physical forces of blood flow – affects where plaques tend to occur. Branched or curved sections of arteries, or areas where blood flow changes velocity or direction, are prone to atheroma. These areas have non-laminar flow with associated low shear stress, which promotes endothelial dysfunction and monocyte infiltration. Atheroma occurs most in the aorta, followed by the carotid, coronary, and iliofemoral arteries.

> **Guiding principle**
>
> '*Athere-*' is from a Greek word for 'gruel', a reference to the gross appearance of atheroma. '*Sclerosis*' is from the word 'skleros' meaning 'hard', describing the hardened fibrous cap of plaques.

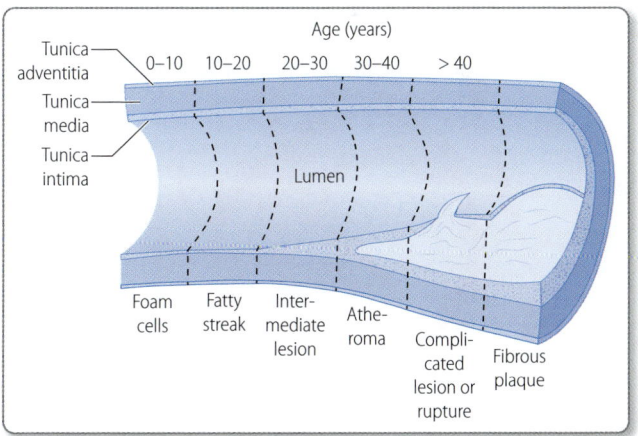

Figure 3.1 The progression of atherosclerosis.

Prevention

Prevention focusses on reducing modifiable risk factors with changes in lifestyle and medications (see Chapter 9). Lifestyle changes include cessation of smoking, regular exercise, weight loss if obese and control of diabetes and hypertension. A healthy diet is low in fat – especially saturated fat – salt, sugar, cholesterol, alcohol and high in fresh fruit and vegetables – and, therefore, antioxidants – and fibre.

Aggressive lowering of low-density lipoprotein (LDL) cholesterol can delay, stall and possibly even reverse atherogenesis.

Pathogenesis

Atherogenesis is generally considered a disordered response to endothelial injury, involving interactions between vascular endothelium, macrophages, smooth muscle cells, leucocytes and platelets (**Figures 3.1** and **3.2**).
- Endothelial injury occurs due to oxidised LDL, infections, toxins, free radical damage, hyperglycaemia or hyperhomocystinaemia, among others.

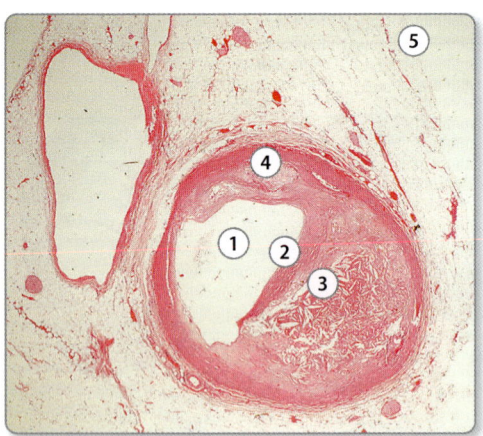

Figure 3.2 Haematoxylin and eosin staining of coronary artery (right) and vein (left). The artery shows a markedly diminished lumen ① due to atherosclerotic plaque on the right side. There is a fibrous cap ② overlying necrotic core matrix and cholesterol crystals ③. Some calcification is also present ④. Support fibrofatty tissue ⑤. Courtesy of Dr S.K. Suvarna.

- Vascular inflammation – monocytes in the blood adhere to and pass through the endothelium to infiltrate the arterial tunica intima and become macrophages, responsible for digesting debris and bacteria
- Foam cell formation and accumulation – macrophages consume oxidised LDL cholesterol to form foam cells, which promote inflammation (**Figure 3.3**)
- Foam cells proliferate to form the fatty streak – also known as intimal xanthoma – appearance of early atherosclerosis, along with T cells and smooth muscle cells
- Fibroproliferation occurs as activated smooth muscle cells and recruited fibroblasts produce extracellular matrix, i.e. scar tissue
- Scar tissue forms a fibrous plaque on the lumen side, covering the foam cells and deposits of lipid and necrotic cellular debris
- The plaque grows, stimulating neovascularisation of fragile vessels, and increasingly occluding the lumen.

Atherogenesis is generally progressive, but with periods of quiescence. Although it is a systemic disease, it manifests, usually at a late stage, with focal signs and symptoms. Symptoms develop as ischaemia progresses, or occurs acutely with plaque rupture or erosion, which can be catastrophic.

Plaque rupture Acute complications occur if the plaque ruptures or bleeds, promoting thrombosis and thromboembolism that can partially or completely block the artery (**Figure 3.4**). Rupture is predisposed by structurally unstable

> **Guiding principle**
>
> Vascular endothelial cells have important roles in atherogenesis, as key regulators of:
> - Haemostasis, by secreting antithrombotic (e.g. heparin sulphate) and, under stress, prothrombotic molecules
> - Blood flow, by secretion of vasodilators, e.g. prostacyclin and nitrous oxide, and when activated, vasoconstrictors (e.g. endothelin)
> - The immune response – when stimulated by injury, they attract leucocytes with chemokines and express surface adhesion molecules to allow entry to the vascular wall.

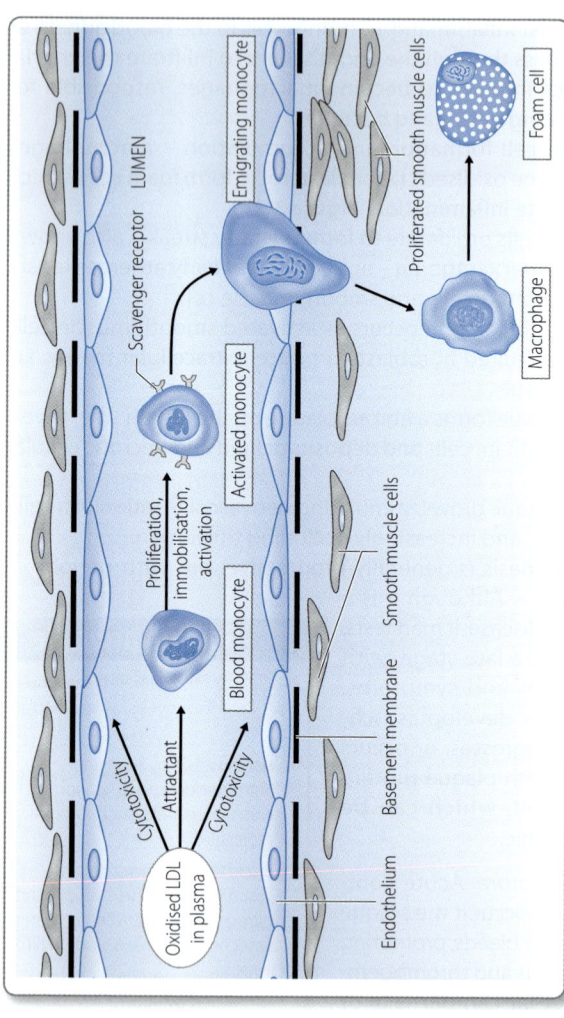

Figure 3.3 The formation of foam cells – the initiation of atherogenesis. LDL, low-density lipoprotein.

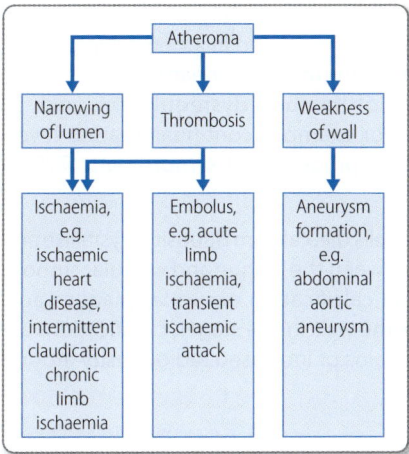

Figure 3.4 Complications of atherosclerosis.

fibrous caps and increasing size of the necrotic core. It is also associated with:
- Neovascularisation
- Intra-plaque haemorrhage/iron deposition in the lesion
- The presence of inflammatory enzymes
- Non-laminar blood flow
- Macrophage calcification

Atherosclerosis also weakens vascular connective tissue, increasing the risk of aneurysm formation and associated wall rupture.

Plaque erosion: Acute arterial occlusion can also occur when endothelium covering or near the plaque erodes to expose smooth muscle cells and extra cellular matrix. This initiates the clotting cascade and thrombosis, which can block the vessel at the lesion site or distally by thromboembolism.

Immune dysregulation: Vascular injury activates smooth muscle cells and endothelial cells to express inflammatory mediators, vasoactive compounds and surface adhesion molecules to recruit immune cells, i.e. monocytes/macrophages lymphocytes, dendritic antigen-presenting cells and fibroblasts. This immune response is dysregulated in atherosclerosis.

The involvement of immune cells means there is some overlap with diseases of immune dysregulation, such as autoimmune disease. For example, continually raised levels of C-reactive protein are predictive of symptomatic PVD in later life.

Calcification: As plaque cells die, calcium deposits crystallise and collect at the border between the plaque and vascular smooth muscle. This intramural calcification occurs as plaques age, decreasing elasticity of the wall. In late stages, calcifications are seen on CT images as halos of increased radiodensity around atheromatous plaques.

Clinical features

Atherosclerosis can occur in any medium or large artery and is mostly asymptomatic. It causes signs and symptoms by obstruction of blood flow at the site of atheroma or acute thromboembolic occlusion downstream (**Table 3.2**). Lesions

Site	Ischaemic pathology	Infarcted pathology
Coronary arteries	Angina	
Carotid arteries	Transient ischaemic attack	Haemorrhagic or ischaemic cerebrovascular accident
Cerebral arteries		
Iliofemoral arteries	Intermittent claudication	Impotence, persistent ulceration and infection of peripheries, necrosis, and gangrene
Mesenteric arteries	Mesenteric angina – epigastric postprandial pain	Haematemesis, haematochezia, diarrhoea, melena, nutritional deficiencies, and weight loss
Renal arteries	Renal artery stenosis; resistant hypertension	Kidney atrophy, necrosis, and renal failure

Table 3.2 The site of atherosclerosis and associated features of ischemic and infarcted pathology.

increase the risk of aneurysm or dissection of an artery. For example, an abdominal aortic aneurysm presents as an asymptomatic pulsatile abdominal mass but is at increasing risk of rupture and massive haemorrhage as it increases in size.

Ischaemic pain, such as leg claudication or angina, increases proportional to exertion, as the metabolic needs of tissues are not met by the limited blood supply. Conversely, it improves on rest.

Lesions may be evident on palpation as pulsatile, hardened masses, and bruits heard on auscultation due to turbulent blood flow.

All patients should be assessed for features of atherosclerotic risk factors, as most diseases are asymptomatic, and prevention is based on control of modifiable risk factors (**Table 3.3**).

Diagnostic approach

Diagnosis involves assessing for atherosclerotic risk factors, imaging of arteries to visualise lesions and loss of lumen patency, stress testing to indicate loss of blood flow as well as assessment of end-organ damage due to ischaemia or infarction.

> **Clinical insight**
>
> Atherosclerosis is a systemic disease; evidence of it in one artery usually indicates its presence in other arteries. For example, peripheral vascular disease (PVD) strongly suggests that there are similar lesions in the coronary arteries.

Risk factor	Clinical features
Smoking	History; tar-stained fingers or hair
High blood cholesterol/triglycerides	Xanthelasma and tendon xanthoma
Hypertension	BP > 140/90 mmHg
Sedentary lifestyle	History, overweight or obese
Diabetes mellitus	History, raised blood glucose, or HbA1c
Obesity	
HbA1c, glycated haemoglobin.	

Table 3.3 The main clinical features of risk factors for atherosclerosis.

Investigations

Atherosclerotic disease is investigated with blood tests to assess for risk factors or signs of end-organ damage, imaging to visualise the lesion and functional tests that gauge the ischaemic effect of the lesion.

Laboratory tests: A lipid profile assesses for hyperlipidaemia; high levels of LDL cholesterol are associated with increased atherosclerosis. Blood glucose and glycated haemoglobin (HbA1c) are measured to monitor for diabetes mellitus.

Some blood tests, such as cardiac enzymes, can indicate the timing and extent of tissue ischaemia or infarct. A raised white blood cell count is often found post-myocardial infarction.

Imaging: Doppler ultrasound is used to quantify the extent of atherosclerotic stenosis in the carotid arteries. Angiography can be performed in cerebral, coronary, peripheral, mesenteric or renal arteries to visualise the extent of narrowing. As contrast is injected into the circulation, the lumen is visible on X-ray, CT or MRI. CT is usually best as it is high resolution and quicker to perform than MRI.

CT calcium scoring quantifies the amount of calcification present within the coronary circulation, which correlates with plaque size. It does not show areas of soft plaque or thrombus.

Imaging can be essential for diagnosing and assessing end-organ damage from infarction. For example, a CT of the head is essential to investigate a suspected cerebrovascular accident.

Functional testing: Stress testing, such as the cardiac stress test, is used to assess the significance of a coronary stenosis and can indicate loss of function due to ischaemia.

Management

Primary and secondary prevention focusses on control of risk factors, including lifestyle changes and medication.

Symptomatic treatment, such as glyceryl trinitrate, relieves ischaemic pain. Revascularisation of the circulation is either by percutaneous intervention using stents or bypass surgery.

Lifestyle: Lifestyle changes reduce or control modifiable risk factors and are central to primary and secondary prevention:
- Smoking cessation
- Strict control of hypertension and diabetes
- Regular aerobic exercise, i.e. >30 min/day most days of the week
- A Mediterranean-style diet, rich in fresh fruit and vegetables. The widespread incidence means all patients should be encouraged to meet these targets, which also benefit general health and well-being.

As disease remains asymptomatic until a late stage, patients can be motivated by discussion of cardiovascular or cerebrovascular risk scores, and referral to fitness training, dietitians or other specialists.

Medication: Common medications include those to manage hyperlipidaemia, hypertension, diabetes mellitus and smoking cessation.

Surgery: Surgical treatments are indicated for patients with ongoing symptoms despite optimal medical management.

> **Clinical insight**
>
> Venous grafts used in heart bypass surgery also develop atherosclerosis.

Prognosis

Atherosclerosis is a multifactorial disease with a genetic predisposition, but lifestyle plays an equally important role. Patients present in many ways and symptoms do not clearly correlate with the level of atherosclerosis. Some patients remain asymptomatic throughout life, while for others the first sign may be sudden cardiac death.

Although primary prevention and medical and surgical symptomatic treatments are improving, there is no direct treatment of the underlying disease.

Hypertension

chapter 4

Hypertension is chronically and abnormally high arterial blood pressure.

Hypertension is the major risk factor for coronary heart disease (CHD), peripheral vascular disease (PVD) and cerebrovascular disease, by damaging arteries to cause arterial wall inflammation and atherogenesis. Globally, CHD causes a third of all deaths, and hypertension is believed to be responsible for at least 50% of these.

Most hypertension is primary (i.e. 'essential'), a result of multiple genetic and environmental factors that increase peripheral vascular resistance. Secondary causes include renal artery, vascular and endocrine disease.

As it is largely asymptomatic, diagnosis depends on regular opportunistic screenings.

4.1 Clinical scenario

Opportunistic blood pressure measurement

Presentation

Janet Johnson, aged 57 years, visits her primary care doctor for an annual review of her type 2 diabetes mellitus. Her doctor measures her blood pressure twice:
- 167/98 mmHg
- 170/95 mmHg

Diagnostic approach

Two blood pressure readings >140/90 mmHg indicate that Janet has hypertension. As she also has diabetes, she is at increased risk of CHD, PVD and cerebrovascular disease.

Further history

Janet is an office worker with a sedentary lifestyle. She eats processed foods, but little fresh fruit and vegetables. She smokes 20 cigarettes a day and drinks about 35 units of alcohol most weekends.

Her uncle and father both died from heart attacks in their late 50s.

Examination
Cardiovascular examination is normal except for her high body mass index (BMI) of 33 kg/m^2. Dipstick urinalysis shows glycosuria and proteinuria. Fundoscopic examination excludes signs of hypertensive retinopathy.

Diagnostic approach
It is clear from her family history, diabetes, smoking, poor diet, lack of exercise and age that Janet has a significant risk of cardiovascular disease, but investigations are indicated to establish a diagnosis, estimate her total cardiovascular risk and assess for end-organ damage:
- Ambulatory blood pressure monitoring (ABPM) for 24 hours for a more accurate assessment of her blood pressure
- Lipid profile to assess for hyperlipidaemia
- Kidney function tests including creatinine clearance or estimated glomerular filtration rate (eGFR) to assess for diabetic or hypertensive damage to glomerular blood vessels – either might be causing her proteinuria
- Heart function: A 12-lead electrocardiogram (ECG) is indicated to look for evidence of left ventricular hypertrophy (LVH) and signs of ischaemic heart disease (IHD). Echocardiogram to look for LVH along with systolic and diastolic function.

Fundoscopy is the easiest assessment of end-organ damage, and this was negative in her case.

Investigations
Janet returns a week later with her results (**Table 4.1**). These, along with her age, gender, diabetic status, smoking status and activity level are entered in the European Society of Cardiology HeartScore on-line cardiovascular risk calculator, which estimates her 10-year risk of death, stroke or heart attack to be 43%.

Test	Result
24 h ABPM	152/93 mmHg
ECG	Normal sinus rhythm
Urea and electrolytes	All in normal range
eGFR	82 mL/min/1.73 m^2
Total cholesterol	5.8 mmol/L (224 mg/dL)
HDL cholesterol	1.16 mmol/L (44.8 mg/dL)

ABPM, ambulatory blood pressure monitoring; ECG, electrocardiography; eGFR, estimated glomerular filtration rate; HDL, high-density lipoprotein.

Table 4.1 Janet's results.

Diagnosis

In view of her age and the lack of suspicious symptoms or signs, there is no need to investigate further for secondary causes; the diagnosis is essential hypertension. Although her 10-year risk is high, if her systolic blood pressure is normalised to 120 mmHg, her risk decreases to 32%. If she also stops smoking, becomes more active and reduces her total cholesterol to <5.2 mmol/L (200.7 mg/dL), this reduces to 17%.

A combination of lifestyle changes and drug therapy is required to reduce her blood pressure and the risk of IHD, cerebrovascular disease, end-organ damage and premature death.

> **Clinical insight**
>
> Online cardiovascular risk calculators use data from a large population but are only an estimate of an individual's cardiovascular risk. They can be a powerful clinical tool to help to convey the benefits of treatment to an asymptomatic patient.

4.2 Essential hypertension

Essential hypertension – also known as primary or idiopathic hypertension – is an increased systemic blood pressure in the absence of any identifiable pathological cause. It accounts for approximately 95% of all cases of hypertension, with the remaining 5% due to secondary hypertension.

It is important to be aware of local guidelines as definitions of hypertension as well as diagnostic criteria and treatment protocols vary.

Types

Hypertension is widely defined as a persistent systolic blood pressure of over 140 mmHg, a diastolic blood pressure over 90 mmHg, or both. Ideal blood pressure is under 120/80 mmHg. A systolic pressure between 120–140 mmHg and a diastolic 80–90 mmHg are considered 'high-normal'.

Hypertension severity is graded into stages (**Table 4.2**) to inform the treatment strategy, as the risk of cardiovascular events is proportional to severity. Overall cardiovascular risk also depends on the presence of other risk factors (**Table 4.3**).

Epidemiology

Hypertension is a global problem. Risk factors are associated with a western lifestyle (**Table 4.3**), but hypertension is most prevalent in low- and middle-income countries due to recent urbanisation (**Figure 4.1**).

Condition	Systolic blood pressure	Diastolic blood pressure (mmHg)
Ideal	<120	<80
High normal hypertension	120–139	80–89
Stage 1 hypertension	140–159	90–99
Stage 2 hypertension	160–179	100–109
Stage 3 hypertension	≥180	≥110
Accelerated hypertension	Same as stage 3 hypertension but with signs of grade 3 or 4 retinopathy	

Table 4.2 The stages of hypertension. Precise boundaries differ depending on the methods and guideline used. Repeated elevated measurements are needed to establish a diagnosis of hypertension as outlined in **Figure 4.2**.

	Risk factor	Mechanism
Modifiable	Obesity	Multifactorial, but obesity is associated with increased activity of the sympathetic nervous system, renin, angiotensinogen, angiotensin II and aldosterone
	Increased salt intake	Increased salt intake increases serum osmolality, which triggers increased water retention and peripheral vasoconstriction
	Excessive alcohol intake	Chronic excessive alcohol consumption is associated with hypertension, but the mechanism is not fully understood
	Sedentary lifestyle	Regular aerobic exercise is associated with healthier blood pressure
	Nicotine (smoking)	Nicotine causes increased cardiac output and peripheral vasoconstriction
Non-modifiable	Family history of hypertension	Multifactorial and heterogenous, but there is a polygenic influence
	Advanced age	Reduced arterial compliance
	African–Caribbean heritage	Reduced renin, increased sensitivity of blood pressure to salt and impairment of salt excretion all result in expansion of blood volume
	Male gender (<50 years)	Men and women are equal overall, but men are affected at a younger age, possibly due to excess of other risk factors

Table 4.3 Modifiable and non-modifiable risk factors for essential hypertension.

African-Caribbean populations have a higher prevalence of hypertension than white and Asian populations due to a genetic tendency towards low renin levels, increased sensitivity to salt and impairment of salt excretion. Furthermore, people of African descent have a greater tendency to develop cardiovascular disease, especially stroke.

Aetiology

Essential hypertension is due to multiple factors that cause widespread constriction of arterioles and small arteries which increase peripheral vascular resistance. Hypertension is

Hypertension

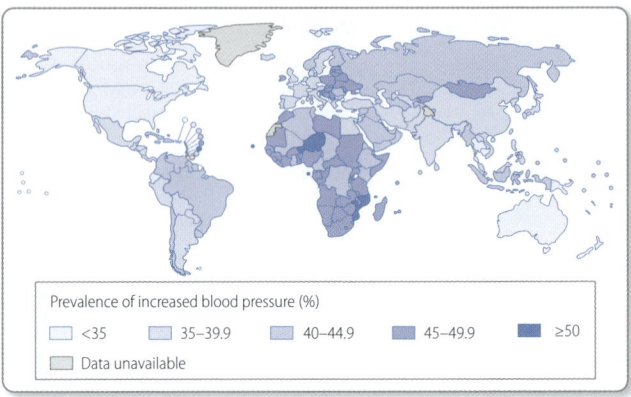

Figure 4.1 The global burden of hypertension. High-income countries have a lower prevalence of hypertension, and low- and middle-income countries have a higher prevalence. Raised blood pressure is defined as a systolic blood pressure ≥ 140 mmHg and diastolic blood pressure ≥ 90 mmHg or using medication to lower blood pressure. Redrawn with permission from World Health Organisation (WHO). Raised blood pressure, 2008. Geneva: WHO, 2008.

> **Clinical insight**
>
> The history and examination should be tailored to the individual patient. For example, signs of aortic coarctation should be sought in a young patient with severe upper body hypertension, but essential hypertension is far more likely in an 80-year-old with high overall cardiovascular risk.

more common in those with affected family members and multiple genes are implicated.

Factors may include genetic, environmental or even behavioural traits that affect blood pressure regulation. Factors that affect the renin–angiotensin–aldosterone system (RAAS) are particularly important. As hypertension progresses, excessive activation of sympathetic (adrenergic) nerves and the RAAS is usually seen.

Clinical features

Blood pressure should be measured whenever possible to detect hypertension as it is usually asymptomatic unless severe. Diagnosis requires multiple careful readings (**Figure 4.2**).

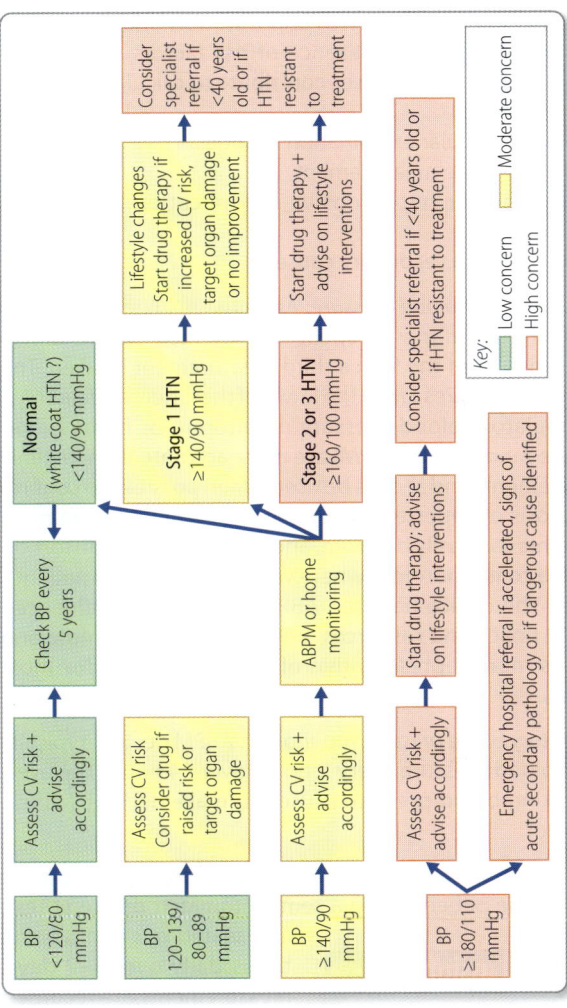

Figure 4.2 Diagnosis, investigation and management of hypertension. ABPM, ambulatory blood pressure monitoring; BP, blood pressure; HTN, hypertension.

The history should assess the duration and severity of hypertension and the presence of risk factors, including a family history. The responses contribute to calculating overall cardiovascular risk.

A full cardiovascular examination includes:
- Blood pressure measurement
- Assessing for hypertensive complications, including fundoscopy
- Detection of a secondary cause

Measurement of blood pressure: An initial reading of >140/90 mmHg should trigger a repeat measurement; if this differs significantly from the first, a third measurement is taken. The recorded blood pressure is the lower of the latter two readings.

Ambulatory blood pressure monitoring or home blood pressure monitoring (HBPM) are more accurate than in-clinic measurements and should be used, when possible, to confirm a diagnosis of hypertension or inform prognosis. More measurements can easily be taken, and they reduce the distortion of 'white coat syndrome', where values are raised by patient's anxiety. The choice between ABPM and HBPM is influenced by local policy and resources, but ABPM is more simple and perhaps more representative of what is 'normal' for most patients.

Ambulatory blood pressure monitoring: ABPM devices typically record blood pressure every 2 hours over 24 hours; the average waking blood pressure is used to make decisions about treatment.

Home blood pressure monitoring: HBPM recordings are usually taken by the patient using a semi-automated device at rest, in a seated position, several times daily over 5–7 days. Measurements are recorded in a blood pressure diary.

> **Clinical insight**
>
> Home blood pressure monitors are increasingly cheap and readily available. Self-measurement also helps to engage people in their own management, but patients must receive education and training on their use and interpretation.

Complications: Chronic hypertension may present with its complications, caused by atherosclerotic ischaemic

Organ system	Complication	Presentation
Cardiac	• Left ventricular hypertrophy • Diastolic heart failure • Arrhythmia (especially atrial fibrillation) ischaemic heart disease	• Forcible and displaced apex • Beat • Myocardial infarction and angina
Renal	• Hypertensive nephropathy • Renal insufficiency • End-stage renal disease	• Deranged kidney function tests
Cerebral	• Cerebrovascular accident • White matter ischaemia • Hypertensive encephalopathy (at very high blood pressure)	• Symptoms and signs of stroke • Impaired cognition or dementia • Altered mental state, seizures, tremor, myoclonus, and asterixis
Ophthalmic	Hypertensive retinopathy	Loss of visual acuity

Table 4.4 The complications of hypertension and their presentation.

damage to organ systems (**Table 4.4**). Damage can occur in major vessels, such as the aorta, or in arteries or arterioles. Fundoscopy, e.g. is the only direct way to assess arterial damage, and may show hypertensive retinopathy.

Detection of a secondary cause: Secondary hypertension is more likely in younger patients, resistant to therapy and accompanied by features of a primary disease. The most common causes are renal, vascular, endocrine, and neurological disease and drugs.

Investigations
Laboratory investigations are used to:
- Estimate cardiovascular risk, including assessment of diabetes and hyperlipidaemia
- Assess for evidence of end-organ damage in the heart, eyes and kidneys (**Table 4.5**)

Organ	Investigations	Looking for
Heart	12-lead electrocardiogram	Left ventricular hypertrophy and signs of ischaemic heart disease
Kidneys	Laboratory tests: • Urea and electrolytes • Creatinine clearance • eGFR	Impaired renal function
Eyes	Dipstick urinalysis	Proteinuria (including microalbuminuria) and haematuria (signs of glomerular damage)
	Fundoscopy	Hypertensive retinopathy

eGFR, estimated glomerular filtration rate.

Table 4.5 Investigations to assess for end-organ damage in hypertension.

- Identify secondary causes, especially in young patients with significantly raised or refractory hypertension. The presence of end-organ damage indicates a greater risk of cardiovascular events and death, and such cases need aggressive treatment and monitoring.

Blood tests: An elevated fasting blood glucose increases cardiovascular risk, whereas a normal result excludes diabetes. A lipid profile with raised total cholesterol, low-density lipoprotein (LDL) and triglycerides represents increased cardiovascular risk and may indicate treatment.

Urea and electrolytes are measured as raised urea and creatinine occur in renal impairment, which can both cause, and be a result of hypertension.

Urinalysis: Proteinuria is detected on dipstick testing or a 24-hour urine collection >150 mg/day. It occurs in renal disease and malignant hypertension.

Electrocardiography: LVH may be seen on ECG as tall R waves in chest leads V5 and V6 and correspondingly deep S-waves in leads V1–V4, reflecting thickened myocardium.

Imaging: Cerebrovascular and cardiovascular disease are common in older patients with hypertension. Cerebral computerised tomography (CT) or magnetic resonance imaging (MRI) is used to assess for small vessel ischaemic (white matter) changes or evidence of previous cerebrovascular accidents (CVA) in those with memory problems.

Echocardiography is a more sensitive technique to detect LVH than ECG and is particularly indicated in younger hypertensives.

Management

The European Society of Hypertension/European Society of Cardiology (ESH/ESC) 2013 guidelines, the UK's National Institute for Health and Care Excellence (NICE) 2011 and the American Heart Association/American College of Cardiology (AHA/ACC) 2007 guidelines all propose a stepped approach to treatment, with targets proportional to the patient's cardiovascular risk score, blood pressure and evidence of end organ damage (**Figure 4.2**). Those with established IHD, cerebrovascular disease or PVD are automatically classified as high risk and should be considered for secondary prevention of CHD. For others, a 10-year cardiovascular risk >20% is considered significant, and should be considered for primary prevention of CHD.

> **Clinical insight**
> Informing patients of their cardiovascular risk reinforces advice regarding lifestyle changes and may improve adherence to drug therapy.

Encourage all patients with high-normal or high blood pressure to aim for healthy lifestyle targets (**Table 4.6**). Antihypertensives may be considered in patients with high-normal blood pressure with a high cardiovascular risk or evidence of end-organ damage.

Stage of hypertension: Management depends on the stage of hypertension (**Table 4.2**):
- Isolated stage 1 hypertension – patients are first advised to make lifestyle modifications; antihypertensives may be necessary if the response to these changes is suboptimal
- Stage 1 hypertension with increased cardiovascular risk or end-organ damage, as well as those with stage 2 or

Risk factor	Target	Rationale
Salt intake	<6 g/day: Stop adding to food and avoid processed food	Excessive salt consumption increases blood pressure
Diet	Diet rich in fruits, vegetables, and reduced in saturated and total fat	Thought to have beneficial effects on the renin–angiotensin–aldosterone system, natriuresis, decreased adrenergic tone, and increased vascular relaxation
Weight	BMI < 25 kg/m^2	Obesity predisposes to hypertension
Exercise	30 minutes or more of aerobic exercise on most days of the week	A sedentary lifestyle predisposes people to hypertension and atherosclerosis
Alcohol intake	Men <3 or 4 units (24–32 g) and women <2 or 3 units (16–24 g)/day	• Alcohol consumption correlates with blood pressure • Excessive consumption may antagonise pharmacological treatment
Smoking	Stop	Smoking is a major risk factor for hypertension, IHD and stroke

BMI, body mass index; IHD, ischaemic heart disease.

Table 4.6 Targets for reducing blood pressure by lifestyle modifications.

3 hypertension, requires antihypertensives and lifestyle modification
- Stage 3 hypertension – drug therapy is started immediately, before further diagnostic testing, risk calculation or evidence of end-organ damage

Elderly patients: Although blood pressure increases with age as arteries naturally stiffen, treating hypertension is still effective, even in patients over 80 years of age.

Elderly patients taking antihypertensives require close monitoring for adverse effects, contraindications and polypharmacy-related interactions. Postural hypotension is common and can cause falls and reduced mobility.

Patients with diabetes mellitus: Hypertensive patients with diabetes mellitus are at additional risk of cardiovascular disease, retinopathy, renal damage and peripheral neuropathy, and the target blood pressure should be <130/80 mmHg. This is often difficult to achieve, but the benefits of control are greater than in non-diabetic patients.

Patients with coexisting diseases: Antihypertensive drug choice is influenced by the presence of coexisting diseases, due to contraindications or a combined benefit. Preferred drugs include:
- Ischaemic heart disease: Beta-blockers, angiotensin-converting enzyme (ACE) inhibitors and angiotensin II receptor blockers (ARBs)
- Heart failure: ACE inhibitors, ARBs and potassium-sparing diuretics such as spironolactone
- Renal impairment: Antagonists of the renin–angiotensin system (ACE inhibitors and ARBs) reduce blood pressure and proteinuria.

Pregnant patients: More than 10% of pregnant women experience hypertension during pregnancy, including new onset or exacerbation of existing chronic hypertension. It occurs due to hormonal and circulatory changes but may also indicate placental dysfunction.

Although usually benign, hypertension during pregnancy increases the risk of potentially fatal pre-eclampsia and eclampsia and requires specialist management.

Pre-eclampsia presents with worsening hypertension and proteinuria during pregnancy and can lead to seizures in late pregnancy: eclampsia.

> **Clinical insight**
>
> Metabolic syndrome is the association of at least three of:
>
> 1. Central obesity – the key feature
> 2. Insulin resistance (i.e. type 2 diabetes mellitus)
> 3. Hypertension
> 4. Dyslipidaemia – high serum triglycerides, and low high-density lipoproteins (HDLs)
>
> It is a powerful risk factor for cardiovascular disease and death and is increasing significantly, with 25–30% of US and western European adults affected. There is a genetic predisposition, but the main causes appear to be a poor and excessive diet and a sedentary lifestyle.

Antihypertensive drug therapy is limited by fetal side effects, but options include β-blockers (e.g. labetalol), methyldopa and hydralazine.

Lifestyle changes: All patients with hypertension require counselling about how and why to modify their cardiovascular risk (**Table 4.6**). This includes calculation and clear discussion of their overall cardiovascular risk. Referral may be useful for dietary advice, physical training or specialist smoking cessation services in patients that struggle to make positive changes without additional support.

Lifestyle changes may have other benefits, including increased general fitness and energy, improved self-esteem and can decrease the risk of other diseases such as lung cancer, colon cancer, and alcohol dependence.

Medication (Figure 4.3)

Antihypertensive drugs include:
- Angiotensin-converting enzyme inhibitors and ARBs
- Beta-blockers
- Calcium-channel blockers (CCB)
- Diuretics, chiefly thiazide and thiazide-like diuretics
- Alpha-blockers

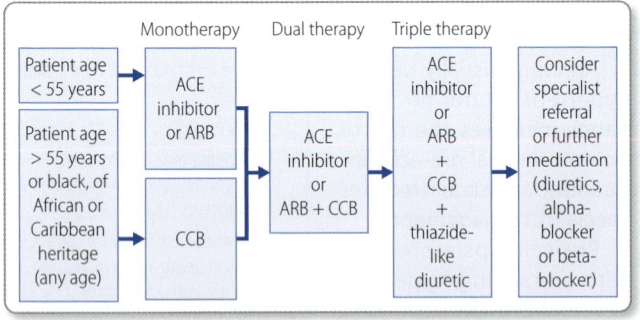

Figure 4.3 Pharmacological treatment of essential hypertension. ACE, angiotensin-converting enzyme; ARB, angiotensin II receptor blocker; CCB, calcium-channel blocker.

The ESH/ESC 2013, NICE 2019 and the AHA/ACC guidelines all advise a step-wise approach for escalating medication to reach BP targets (**Figure 4.3**):
1. *Step 1:* Monotherapy
2. *Step 2:* Dual therapy
3. *Step 3:* Triple therapy.

> **Clinical insight**
>
> Hypertension is more common in people of African descent, who tend to have low-renin, salt-sensitive hypertension that is less responsive to ACE inhibitor, ARB or β-blocker monotherapy.

Many patients require dual therapy. Drug choice when considering a third medication is very case-dependent, and diet and lifestyle factors should still be considered. If three drugs do not work, patient's adherence should be assessed. If non-adherence is identified, improved patient's education is required, with clear instructions on treatment regimen.

4. *Step 4:* If adherence is not a problem, the patient is considered to have resistant hypertension, indicating assessment for secondary causes, specialist referral and/or adding, for example:
- Spironolactone, another diuretic, α-blocker or β- blocker (NICE 2011)
- A long-acting thiazide diuretic (e.g. chlorthalidone), spironolactone or the diuretic amiloride (AHA 2008)
- An aldosterone-blocking diuretic (e.g. spironolactone), amiloride and/or the α-blocker doxazosin (ESH/ESC 2013).

The primary goal is tight control of blood pressure to prevent atherosclerosis. Drug regimen guidelines vary but drug choice is determined by:
- Effects on blood pressure
- Ethnicity
- Age
- Coexisting diseases
- Previous adverse effects
- Cost-effectiveness.

> **Clinical insight**
>
> Two potentially promising therapies for resistant hypertension are vagal nerve stimulation and renal denervation. Both lower blood pressure by influencing the balance between sympathetic and parasympathetic nervous activity.

Angiotensin-converting enzyme inhibitors and ARBs are ideal first-line drugs for patients with both hypertension and diabetes as they protect against the nephropathy that both diseases can cause. However, they are not first-line in elderly and African-Caribbean patients who often have low-renin hypertension but can be used in combination with a diuretic or the CCB in these patients as part of dual or triple therapy (see **Figure 4.3**).

Monitoring blood pressure targets: Blood pressure should be monitored regularly to achieve treatment targets of:
- <140/90 mmHg in individuals under 80 years
- <150/85 mmHg in those over 80 years
- <130/80 mmHg in patients with diabetes, high cardiovascular risk or renal dysfunction

Pressures should ideally be measured at least every 5 years in those with normal BP measurements.

Prognosis: The degree of end-organ damage and the level of cardiovascular risk determine prognosis. Every 20/10 mmHg increase in blood pressure doubles the risk of cardiovascular mortality.

4.3 Secondary hypertension

In approximately 5% of patients with hypertension, it occurs secondary to a specific underlying condition, such as renal artery stenosis (**Figure 4.4** and **Table 4.7**).

Clinical features

Secondary hypertension is usually differentiated from essential hypertension by the presence of features of the underlying disease (**Table 4.7**). Patients are usually under 40 years of age and present with:
- Unexpectedly severe hypertension
- Refractory hypertension
- Irregular features, such as weakness or profuse sweating
- Proteinuria or haematuria, suggesting renal disease
- Hypokalaemia not caused by diuretic use

Investigations

Investigations for a secondary cause are indicated based on clinical suspicion, on an individual, case-by-case basis. If a

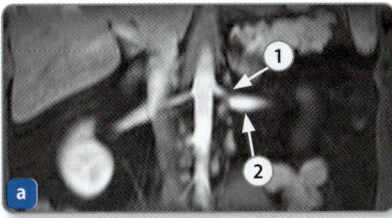
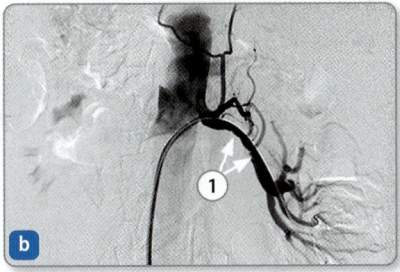

Figure 4.4 Renal artery stenosis. (a) Magnetic resonance angiogram showing left renal artery stenosis ① and post-stenosis dilatation ②. (b) Invasive angiogram showing multiple stenoses in the left renal artery ①. The dark tube in the descending aorta is the catheter, which is injecting contrast dye (black) into the artery.

Disease	Further information	Investigations
Chronic kidney disease	The most common cause of secondary HTN	Creatinine clearance or estimated GFR
Polycystic kidney disease	• Causes severe resistant HTN • Often autosomal dominant hereditability	• Renal ultrasound • Kidneys may be palpable
Renal artery stenosis	• Causes resistant HTN • Usually due to atherosclerosis	• Renal Doppler ultrasound, CT or MRI angiography
Pheochromocytoma	• Very rare cause of severe HTN • A catecholamine-secreting tumour	• (24-hour urinary collection) Catecholamines or their metabolites • CT or MRI to identify tumour

Table 4.7 Causes of secondary hypertension (HTN). *Continues overleaf*

Disease	Further information	Investigations
Primary hyperaldosteronism	• Causes HTN associated with hypokalaemia • Most commonly due to aldosterone-secreting adenoma (Conn's syndrome)	• Plasma K$^+$ aldosterone–renin ratio (increased) • CT or MRI to identify tumour
Cushing's syndrome	Caused by excessive exposure to corticosteroids or Cushing's disease – (due to ACTH-secreting pituitary tumour)	• Cortisol (24-hour urine collection) Dexamethasone suppression test • CT or MRI to identify tumour
Aortic coarctation	Causes of HTN due to congenital narrowing of aorta (usually close to the arch)	Echocardiogram or CT scan
Hormone replacement therapy, oral contraceptives, corticosteroids, NSAIDs, mineralocorticoids	Drug history is very important in hypertension	Drug history
Alcohol, nicotine or liquorice excess; drug misuse	Excessive use is associated with HTN	
Obstructive sleep apnoea	• Increasingly common cause of HTN associated with obesity • Morning headaches are common	• Overnight sleep studies (oximetry and polysomnography) • Collateral history from partner is useful
Pregnancy	HTN occurs in 10% of pregnancies	

ACTH, adrenocorticotropic hormone; GFR, glomerular filtration rate; NSAIDs, non-steroidal anti-inflammatory drugs.

Table 4.7 Continued

Type	Tests	Disease
Examination	Body mass index	Obesity
	Radiofemoral delay	Aortic coarctation
	Abdominal bruit	Renal artery stenosis
Blood tests	Estimated glomerular filtration rate	Renal impairment
	Parathyroid hormone	Hyperparathyroidism
	Thyroid-stimulating hormone	Hyperthyroidism
	Calcium	Hypercalcaemia (sometimes secondary to renal insufficiency)
	Potassium	Hypokalaemia in aldosteronism
	Aldosterone–renin ratio	Aldosteronism
24-hour urine	Cortisol Catecholamines Metanephrines	Cushing's syndrome Pheochromocytoma Pheochromocytoma
Imaging	Renal ultrasound (including Doppler)	Renal artery stenosis, polycystic kidney disease
Others	Sleep studies (if obese or history suggests obstructive sleep apnoea)	Obstructive sleep apnoea

Table 4.8 Investigations for secondary hypertension.

secondary cause is suspected but the cause remains unknown, a good general investigative work-up is outlined in **Table 4.8**.

Management

The underlying cause needs to be treated, and this may involve medication, surgery or even renal dialysis. Antihypertensive medication may also be required while the cause is being corrected; this may need to continue if blood pressure does not normalise.

Prognosis: Prognosis is determined by the underlying cause. Prompt diagnosis and treatment that successfully decreases the blood pressure indicates a good prognosis.

4.4 Hypertensive emergencies

Hypertensive emergencies are conditions that present with severe uncontrolled hypertension leading to end-organ damage. They include accelerated hypertension and hypertension associated with:
- Encephalopathy (usually >200/110 mmHg)
- Left ventricular failure
- Myocardial ischaemia or infarction
- Aortic dissection
- Cerebral haemorrhage
- Acute kidney injury (e.g. glomerulonephritis)
- Pheochromocytoma

> **Clinical insight**
>
> Rapid decreases in blood pressure should be avoided due to the risk of under perfusion of tissues, particularly the cerebrum.

Hypertensive emergencies can present with cerebral or pulmonary oedema, seizures, heart or renal failure. Urgent blood pressure reduction with close supervision is required in a secondary care setting. Intravenous glyceryl trinitrate or labetalol are used to reduce blood pressure above >220/120 mmHg or if there is dangerous secondary pathology.

The aim is to bring systolic blood pressure below 220 mmHg or diastolic blood pressure below 120 mmHg (or both) over 1–2 hours, and then <160/100 mmHg over the next 12–24 hours. The initial goal of therapy is to reduce mean arterial BP by no >25% (within minutes to 1 hour). If the patient remains stable, further reduce the BP to 160 mmHg systolic and 100–110 mmHg diastolic within the next 2–6 hours. Normal BP may be targeted over the next 24–48 hours.

Excessive falls in pressure may precipitate renal, cerebral, or coronary ischaemia and so should be avoided. Exceptions to this general rule are patients with aortic dissection, phaeochromocytoma crisis, and severe pre-eclampsia or eclampsia. Selected patients with spontaneous intracerebral haemorrhage may also require acute blood pressure lowering; careful titration in these patients is required to ensure continuous smooth and sustained control of BP.

Hyperlipidaemia

chapter 5

Hyperlipidaemia is chronic raised blood concentration of triglycerides (TG), cholesterol or lipoprotein. It is common but usually subclinical and discovered in screening blood tests of cardiovascular risk assessment.

It has inherited causes, including familial hypercholesterolaemia, and acquired causes such as diet and smoking.

Most types of hyperlipidaemia increase the risk and rate of atherogenesis, the deposition of lipid-laden macrophages in arterial walls. It is an important, but often readily treatable, risk factor for coronary heart disease (CHD). A recent study suggests 45% of myocardial infarctions are associated with hyperlipidaemia.

Lipid metabolism involves transport of lipoproteins that are pro- and anti-atherogenic. Hypertriglyceridaemia is not directly atherogenic but is associated with remnant lipoprotein particles.

5.1 Clinical scenario

Skin lesions and chest pain

Presentation

Bill Hansen, a 42-year-old man, presents to his primary care doctor concerned about chest pain and yellow 'blotches' that have appeared on his ankles and posterior hand in the last few months. He smokes 20 cigarettes a day. He appears concerned but otherwise well and has body mass index (BMI) of 25 kg/m^2.

Diagnostic approach

His chest pain must be characterised, and his cardiovascular risk factors should be assessed.

Nodular lesions on the dorsal hand could be warts,

> **Clinical insight**
>
> Xanthomata lipid deposits occur in skin, e.g. as xanthelasma, when blood concentrations are high as the skin is an active site of lipid metabolism.

abrasions secondary to trauma or xanthomas – cutaneous deposits of foam cells and indicators of hyperlipidaemia.

Further history
Bill's chest pain is central, occurs on significant exertion and radiates to his left shoulder and elbow.

Bill's father had a fatal heart attack at the age of 48 years, and his grandfather died of a stroke at the age of 53 years.

Diagnostic approach
Bill's chest pain appears anginal, indicating blood tests including a complete blood count (CBC), urea and electrolytes (U&Es), thyroid function tests (TFTs) and liver function tests (LFTs), and an electrocardiogram (ECG) and a coronary CT angiogram (CTCA) and exercise/other stress test. Troponin levels are only measured if he has had chest pain within the preceding 24 hours.

His family history indicates that he may be at risk from early cardiovascular disease.

Examination
Cardiovascular examination reveals xanthoma tendinosum of the metacarpal and Achilles tendons, xanthelasma around the eyes, and tar-stained fingers. Auscultation reveals a left-sided carotid bruit. His peripheries are cold and no dorsalis pedis pulse can be detected in his left foot.

Diagnostic approach
Xanthomas are cholesterol deposits. Their presence often signals consistently excessive blood cholesterol levels. The carotid bruit likely reflects atherosclerotic narrowing and needs urgent assessment with duplex ultrasound to assess its extent and the risk of cerebrovascular accident. His absent dorsalis pedis pulses and cold feet likely indicate peripheral vascular disease due to femoral or iliac atherosclerosis.

With evidence of hyperlipidaemia and atherosclerosis, he has a high risk of cardiovascular disease. He is, therefore, referred to a cardiologist for ECG, CTCA and exercise/other stress test and blood tests to assess all cardiovascular risk factors.

Blood test	Value
Total cholesterol	9.6 mmol/L (370 mg/dL) – *raised*
LDL cholesterol	7.1 mmol/l (275 mg/dL) – *raised*
Triglycerides	3.5 mmol/L (310 mg/dL)
HDL cholesterol	0.8 mmol/L (30 mg/dL)
Glucose (non-fasting)	8.3 mmol/L (150 mg/dL)
Alanine aminotransferase	55 IU/L
Aspartate aminotransferase	65 IU/L
TSH	3.56 mIU/L
BUN, blood urea nitrogen; HDL, high-density lipoprotein; LDL, low-density lipoprotein; TSH, thyroid-stimulating hormone.	

Table 5.1 Bill's blood test results.

Investigations
ECG is normal. Exercise stress testing is positive, indicating probable coronary artery disease. His blood test results are given in **Table 5.1**.

Diagnosis
His angina and investigations suggest Bill already has coronary artery disease, and he is at very high risk of the clinical sequelae of this condition. His blood tests show very high total cholesterol and low-density lipoprotein (LDL) levels that are unlikely to be due to a secondary cause (e.g. diabetes, liver, renal or thyroid disease).

Bill is diagnosed with definite heterozygous familial hypercholesterolaemia according to the Simon Broome criteria. This is an autosomal dominant inherited hyperlipidaemia due to mutations in LDL receptor genes.

He is counselled about lifestyle and diet changes to lower his total cholesterol

> **Clinical insight**
>
> The World Health Organisation (WHO) estimated in 2002 that 60% of CHD in developed countries is attributable to a cholesterol level > 3.8 mmol/L (146.7 mg/dL).

and is also started on statins. He is also referred for genetic counselling to inform him of the inherited nature of the disease and ramifications of the diagnosis.

At 8-week follow-up, his total cholesterol has decreased to 6.4 mmol/L (250 mg/dL). He requires monitoring every 6 months for fasting lipid tests and clinical assessment and may need intervention for his carotid and coronary artery disease. With his relatively early intervention, his prognosis will be much improved but only if he maintains good control of his risk factors and stops smoking.

5.2 Hyperlipidaemia

Hyperlipidaemia is a significantly raised blood concentration of total cholesterol (e.g. >6.5 mmol/L or 240 mg/dL), lipoprotein or TG. Most forms are associated with an increased risk of atherosclerosis. It can be primary, with no identifiable cause, or it can occur secondary to diabetes mellitus, obesity, pancreatitis or renal disease.

Raised LDL is associated with increased atherogenesis, whereas raised high-density lipoprotein (HDL) is protective, as the former increases arterial wall lipid deposition and macrophage accumulation, and the latter decreases it.

Types

Types of hyperlipidaemia include:
- Hypercholesterolaemia – raised cholesterol
- Hypertriglyceridaemia – raised TG
- Chylomicronaemia – raised chylomicrons
- Dysbetalipoproteinaemia – raised intermediate density lipoproteins (IDLs) and TG and lowered HDL
- Mixed hyperlipoproteinaemia, raised very low-density lipoprotein (VLDL) and chylomicrons
- Combined hyperlipoproteinaemia – raised chylomicrons and TG.

Primary hyperlipidaemias are distinguished by the Fredrickson classification, based on separation of blood lipids by centrifuge or electrophoresis. Primary forms usually present with extreme lipid levels, family history and xanthoma, and patients should be referred to a specialist lipid clinic.

An increase in chylomicrons or VLDL leads to an increase in TG. An increase in LDL or IDL causes an increase in cholesterol.

> **Clinical insight**
>
> Dyslipidaemia refers to abnormal levels of lipids in the blood, including low levels of HDLs. Hyperlipidaemia is the most common dyslipidaemia and is usually due to a high fat diet and sedentary lifestyle.

Epidemiology

Nearly 31 million US adults have hyperlipidaemia with a total cholesterol ≥240 mg/dL (≥6.2 mmol/L). Approximately 40% of adults in the UK have high or borderline high LDL. It is closely associated with a Westernised diet and lifestyle. It is more common in men. Total and LDL cholesterol rises 20% from the age of 20–50 years. In the Prevalence of Dyslipidaemia in Urban and Rural India: The ICMR–INDIAB study; 79% had abnormalities in one of the lipid parameters.

Primary inherited hyperlipidaemias include familial combined hyperlipidaemia (FCH) and familial hypertriglyceridaemia, two of the most prevalent genetic disorders (**Table 5.2**). FCH is implicated in 10% of CHD patients.

Aetiology

Lipids are transported as lipoproteins, of which there are five types based on size and density:
1. Chylomicrons carry lipids from the intestine to the liver, muscle and adipose tissue
2. VLDLs TGs from liver to adipose tissue
3. Intermediate density lipoproteins are not usually detectable
4. Intermediate density lipoproteins carry lipid around the body
5. HDLs collect peripheral lipid and take it to the liver

Size is important as this reflects a lipoprotein's role in metabolism and therefore disease. As metabolic pathways interconnect lipoproteins, the amount of one type is affected by the concentration of others. Each is associated with a different

Type	Raised elements	Example	Approximate prevalence
I	Cholesterol, TG and chylomicrons	Familial hyperchylomicronaemia (decreased lipoprotein lipase or apolipoprotein (apo) CII)	1/1,000,000
IIa	Cholesterol and LDL	Familial hypercholesterolaemia (loss of LDL receptors)	• Homozygous – 1/1,000,000 • Heterozygous – 1/500
IIb	Cholesterol, TG, LDL and VLDL	Familial combined hypercholesterolaemia	1/200
III	Cholesterol, TG and IDL	Familial dysbetalipoproteinaemia (apo E2 mutation) causing impaired VLDL clearance	1/10,000
IV	TG and VLDL	Familial hypertriglyceridaemia (increased VLDL synthesis or decreased breakdown)	1/100
V	Cholesterol, TG, VLDL and chylomicrons	Familial combined hyperlipidaemia (loss of lipoprotein lipase; increased VLDL synthesis)	1/50 – 1/200

apo E2, apolipoprotein E2; IDL, intermediate-density lipoprotein; LDL, low-density lipoprotein; TG, triglyceride; VLDL, very low-density lipoprotein.

Table 5.2 The Fredrickson classification of primary hyperlipoproteinaemias.

level of atherogenesis (i.e. cardiovascular risk). For example, raised LDL is associated with an increased risk, a high level of chylomicrons is not associated with increased risk, and HDL decreases cardiovascular risk.

Moderate or severely raised TG levels are substantial risk factors for cardiovascular disease and long-term mortality, although the high levels of type I hyperlipidaemia are, surprisingly, not associated with increased atherogenesis.

Primary

Primary causes are genetic (see **Table 5.2**) or idiopathic.

Secondary causes

Hyperlipidaemia can occur due to other causes including systemic disease or drugs (**Table 5.3**). The most common cause is poor diet and a sedentary lifestyle, which may be associated with metabolic syndrome including type II diabetes mellitus. There is a normal increase in blood lipid concentrations following a meal – postprandial

> **Guiding principle**
>
> All cells can make cholesterol, but liver cells are the most active. It is also consumed in the diet, particularly egg yolk, cheese, butter, liver, oily fish and many processed foods.

System	Disease	Pathophysiology	Lipid profile
Endocrine disorders	Diabetes mellitus	Increased production and reduced removal of TG	↑ TG ↓ HDL
	Hypothyroidism	Decreased LDL receptor activity	↑ LDL, TC ↓ normal TG
Renal disorders	Nephrotic syndrome	Increased LDL production, reduced VLDL clearance	↑ TC, LDL ↑ normal TG
	Renal failure	Impaired TG breakdown	↑ LDL, TG ↓ HDL
Drugs	Adrenal steroids	Increased hepatic fatty acid synthesis	↑ LDL and HDL
	Thiazides	Likely due to decreased insulin sensitivity and/or reflex RAAS and SNS activation	↑ TC, LDL and TG
	Anticonvulsants	Likely via hepatic enzyme induction and increased cholesterol absorption	Raised TC, TG and HDL
	Oral contraceptives	Increased hepatic VLDL production	↑ LDL, HDL and TG
	Alcohol	Inhibits chylomicron breakdown	↑ TG and HDL

Table 5.3 Causes of secondary hyperlipidaemia. *Continues overleaf.*

System	Disease	Pathophysiology	Lipid profile
Hepatic disease	Obstructive liver disease	Reduced hepatic lipoprotein metabolism	↑ Free cholesterol and LDL ↑ normal HDL
	Hepatitis		↑ TG, LDL ↑ TC, HDL
Storage diseases	Gaucher disease	• Liver malfunction due to glucocerebroside accumulation • Low insulin causes hypertriglyceridaemia	↓ HDL
	Von Gierke disease	Low HDL	↑ TG ↑ normal TC
	Systemic lupus erythematosus	• Liver malfunction due to glucocerebroside accumulation • Low insulin causes hypertriglyceridaemia	Normal TC, LDL, TG ↓ HDL
Other	Obesity	Increased free fatty acids to liver reduces apoB breakdown, increases TG release by lipoproteins	↑ TG ↑ normal TC and LDL

apoB, apolipoprotein B; LDL, low-density lipoprotein; TG, triglyceride; VLDL, very low-density lipoprotein.

Table 5.3 *Continued.*

hyperlipidaemia. A high fat, low-fibre diet leads to increased circulating lipoproteins and TGs and a sedentary lifestyle means that levels stay raised for longer.

Clinical features

Most patients are asymptomatic, and hyperlipidaemia is diagnosed by blood tests. Xanthomas may be present in patients with very high lipid levels, usually indicating an inherited cause. These are subcutaneous usually raised, yellow-orange

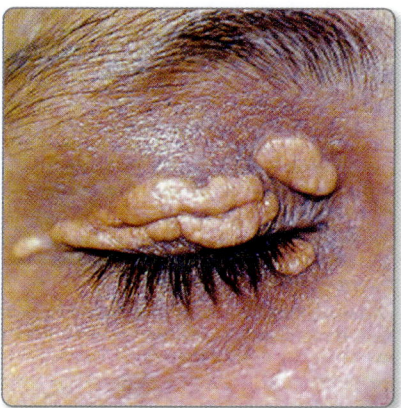

Figure 5.1 Xanthelasma. Yellowish papules and plaques of lipid-laden foam cells in xanthelasma palpebra.

or reddish-brown deposits of lipid-laden foam cells. They can be solitary or 'eruptive' collections:
- Xanthelasma around the eyes or on the eyelids, the most common form (**Figure 5.1**)
- Xanthoma planum is a flat deposit; this type of xanthoma occurs at various sites
- Xanthoma tuberosum on the elbows and knees
- Xanthoma tendinosum in tendons (e.g. Achilles' tendon); these xanthomas move with extension and occur later than other xanthomas

Deposits also occur in the stratum of the cornea, seen as a corneal arcus of grey-white rings.

Associated signs of atherosclerotic disease or hyperlipidaemic complications may be present (**Table 5.4**).

Diagnostic approach

Investigation and management of dyslipidaemias is always considered in the context of total cardiovascular risk. Primary prevention begins by identifying people likely to be at increased risk and performing a full formal risk assessment. Inherited and secondary causes must be ruled out. Management then focusses on reaching optimal levels or treatment targets, largely

System	Clinical feature	Pathogenesis
Cardiovascular	Decreased peripheral pulses or ankle/brachial index	PVD
Respiratory	Dyspnoea	CHD, congestive heart failure
Neurologic	Dementia and depression	Chylomicronaemia syndrome
Dermatologic	Xanthoma	Deposits of lipid-laden macrophages
Ophthalmologic	Corneal arcus	Oesterified cholesterol deposits
Gastrointestinal	• Upper right abdominal tenderness • Hepatomegaly	Liver disease

CHD, coronary heart disease; PVD, peripheral vascular disease.

Table 5.4 Clinical features associated with hyperlipidaemia and associated atherosclerosis.

of LDL or non-HDL cholesterol, proportional to the patient's individual total cardiovascular risk. There is a large overlap in international guidelines, for example:
- The American Heart Association and American College of Cardiology (AHA/ACC) (2013)
- The European Society of Cardiology/European Atherosclerosis Society (ESC/EAS) (2011)
- The National Institute for Health and Care Excellence guidelines (NICE) (2014; see **Figure 5.2**).

Once identified at risk, an initial lipid profile is taken. Secondary causes and familial hypercholesterolaemia must be considered and tested for before therapy commences for primary prevention of CHD. Suspect familial hypercholesterolaemia in a patient with a family history

> **Clinical insight**
>
> Non-fasting blood lipid measurements slightly overestimate CHD risk with a higher TG and lower HDL concentrations. However, the NICE 2014 guidelines consider them sufficient for screening and convenient for patients.

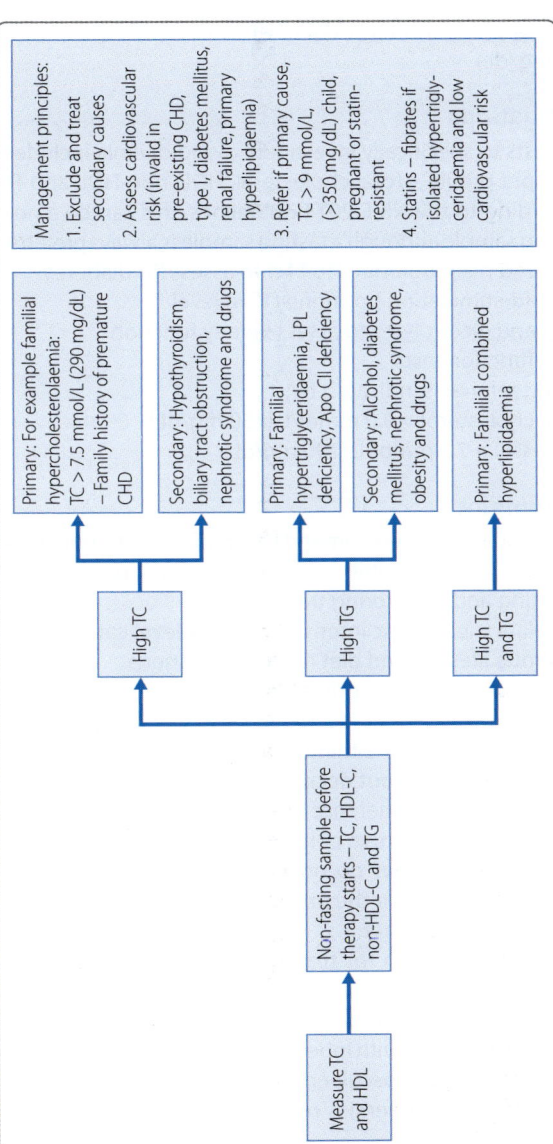

Figure 5.2 Investigation and management principles of hyperlipidaemia, based on the UK's National Institute for Health and Care Excellence (NICE) 2014 guidelines. apo, apolipoprotein; CHD, coronary heart disease; HDL, high-density lipoprotein; LPL, lipoprotein lipase; TC, total cholesterol; TG, triglyceride.

of early CHD, xanthoma and a total cholesterol >7.5 mmol/L (>290 mg/dL).

Investigations

Blood tests to specifically investigate dyslipidaemia include:
- Full lipid profile – total cholesterol, HDL, non-HDL and TG. According to the NICE 2014 guidelines, this can be a non-fasting sample although a fasting sample is always preferred
- Glycated haemoglobin (HbA1c) to assess for diabetes
- Thyroid-stimulating hormone (TSH) level
- Urea and electrolytes to assess kidney function
- Liver function tests

Specialist referral is indicated by:
- Total cholesterol > 9.0 mmol/L (350 mg/dL)
- Non-HDL > 7.5 mmol/L (290 mg/dL)

Management

All recent guidelines recommend key management principles:
- Consider absolute total cardiovascular risk of patient when initiating and monitoring treatment
- Correlate therapeutic intensity with risk level category
- Continue lifestyle and diet recommendations
- Focus on achieving optimal levels of LDL and non-HDL (**Table 5.5**)
- Use statins as first-line therapy if lifestyle modifications are insufficient, or without delay in secondary prevention
- Address issues of adherence including clear communication and managing effective behavioural change

More recent guidelines do not recommend specific target levels of lipoproteins for the primary or secondary prevention of atherosclerotic disease.

As the main reason for treatment is to decrease cardiovascular risk, hyperlipidaemia is managed in context of total cardiovascular risk (**Table 5.5**). Standard risk assessment tools are not valid for those with inherited hyperlipidaemias or other causes of high cardiovascular risk.

The inherited lipidaemias respond best to different treatments (**Table 5.6**).

Patient's risk	Criteria		Optimal LDL
	Risk factors	CHD: 10-year risk (%)	

High risk	1. Known CHD
	2. CHD risk equivalents:
	  a. PVD
	  b. Cerebrovascular disease
	  c. Abdominal aortic aneurysm
	  d. Diabetes mellitus
	  e. 2+ risk factors
		>20	<1.8 mmol/L (<70 mg/dL) or a ≥50% reduction from baseline

Moderately high risk	2+ risk factors with CHD	10–20	<2.5 mmol/L (<97 mg/dL)
Moderate risk	2+ risk factors with CHD	<10	<3.0 mmol/L (<116 mg/dL)
Low risk	0–1 risk factor with CHD	<10	<3.0 mmol/L (<116 mg/dL)

CHD, coronary heart disease; HDL, high-density lipoprotein; LDL, low-density lipoprotein; PVD, peripheral vascular disease.

Table 5.5 Optimal lipoprotein levels according to overall cardiovascular risk. Based on the European Society of Cardiology/European Atherosclerosis Society (ESC/EAS) 2011 guidelines. Local risk assessment tools and guidelines should be used. Risk factors: smoking, hypertension (≥140/90 mmHg), HDL < 1.0 mmol/L (<40 mg/dL), age ≥45 years (men), >55 years (women), ischaemic heart disease (IHD) in first-degree relative [<55 years (men) and <65 years (women)].

Secondary hyperlipidaemia management must focus on treating the underlying cause, where possible. Lipid-lowering medication may also be needed. For example, patients with hypothyroidism should have their thyroid biochemistry corrected before starting lipid-lowering medication. Normalisation of thyroid function may be enough to treat the lipid abnormality.

Hyperlipidaemia

Type of primary hyperlipidaemia	Principal treatment
I	Diet
IIa	Diet, bile acid sequestrants, statins and niacin
IIb	Diet, statins, niacin and fibrate
III	Fibrate and statins
IV	Fibrate, niacin and statins
V	Niacin and fibrate

Table 5.6 Principal treatments for the inherited hyperlipidaemias.

Component	Examples	Frequency
Lean protein	Chicken breast and tofu	Every meal
High fibre and low GI carbohydrate	Vegetables, pulses, whole grains and fruits	Every meal
Nuts	Handful	Daily
Leafy greens	Cabbage and spinach	Daily
Highly processed foods	Processed sugar, high fructose corn syrup, trans fats and white flour	Avoid

Table 5.7 A recommended diet to lower blood triglyceride levels.

Diet and exercise

Initial treatment is lifestyle modifications including:
- Weight loss and exercise
- A diet with restricted saturated fat, trans fats and cholesterol (**Table 5.7**) and modest portion sizes
- Smoking cessation
- Limited alcohol intake.

Lipids are measured again after 3–6 months. If LDL is still raised, medication is considered.

Medication

Medications include 3-hydroxy-3-methylglutaryl coenzyme A (HMG-CoA) reductase inhibitors (statins), the routine first-line medication for primary and secondary prevention of CHD.

Non-statins are not recommended unless the patient is confirmed as intolerant to statins, statin therapy is ineffective, or an inherited hyperlipidaemia is confirmed (**Table 5.6**):

> **Clinical insight**
>
> Statin side effects include:
> - Elevated liver function tests
> - Myopathy – evident as increased muscle creatine phosphokinase (CPK)
> - Rhabdomyolysis (rare) – secondary to myopathy
>
> If a patient's CPK level is ≥5 times normal, stop treatment, check renal function, and monitor every 2 weeks.

- Fibrates – particularly useful to lower TG
- Bile acid sequestrants
- Niacin
- Omega-3 fatty acids – as fish oil supplements or purified forms as an adjunct to lifestyle changes

Lipid levels should be checked 8 weeks after starting or changing medication, until they are satisfactory. Once optimum levels have been achieved, lipids are checked annually.

5.3 Familial hypercholesterolaemia

Familial hypercholesterolaemia (FH) is an autosomal dominant condition that leads to extreme levels of LDL but normal TG. This increases the incidence of premature atherosclerosis and CHD. However, the risk is dramatically reduced if the condition is identified and treated. It is one of the most common inherited conditions.

Epidemiology and aetiology

Many different mutations have been identified. Most affect the *LDLR* gene on chromosome 19, which encodes the LDL receptor. Mutations lead to absent or significantly dysfunctioning LDL receptors (**Figure 5.3**).

Hyperlipidaemia

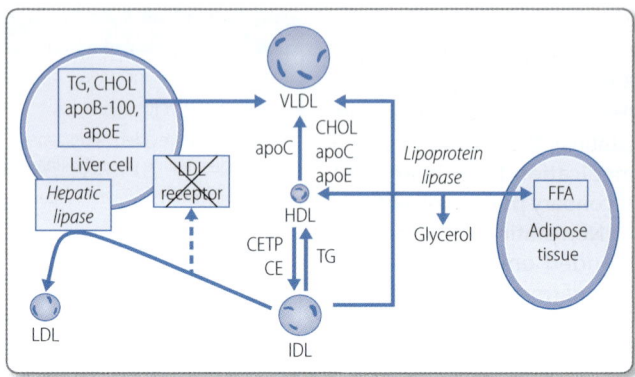

Figure 5.3 Familial hypercholesterolaemia most often involves dysfunctioning mutations of low-density lipoprotein (LDL) receptors. Intermediate-density lipoproteins (IDLs) are not taken up via LDL receptors on the liver, leading to increased LDL formation. apo, apolipoprotein; CE, cholesteryl ester; CETP, cholesteryl ester transfer protein; CHOL, cholesterol; FFA, free-fatty acid; HDL, high-density lipoprotein; TG, triglycerides; VLDL, very low-density lipoprotein.

Homozygous familial hypercholesterolaemia
Homozygotes have a mutation in both copies of *LDLR*, which leads to a more serious condition and a life expectancy under 30 years, if untreated. It affects one in a million people and presents in childhood with signs of atherosclerosis.

Heterozygous familial hypercholesterolaemia
One in 250/500 people have heterozygous familial hypercholesterolaemia, with a single mutant *LDLR* gene. Untreated, about 50% of men and 30% of women have clinical CHD by the age of 50 years. The majority remain undiagnosed until a cardiovascular event.

Clinical features
Features of cutaneous or vascular lipid deposits are earlier and more severe in homozygous disease.

Homozygous familial hypercholesterolaemia

Homozygotes present with signs of atherosclerosis in childhood: features of aortic stenosis, peripheral vascular or cerebrovascular disease, or, particularly, CHD. Nearly all homozygotes develop xanthoma, initially as dispersed flat lesions and evolving to xanthoma tendinosum and xanthelasma by the early childhood.

Heterozygous familial hypercholesterolaemia

Heterozygote children do not usually have signs but will likely have a parent with severe hypercholesterolaemia and a family history of cardiovascular disease.

Adults may present with:
- Long history of severe hypercholesterolaemia
- Angina or myocardial infarction, peripheral vascular or cerebrovascular disease
- 60% of those over 20 years who are untreated have xanthoma tendinosum on the Achilles or metacarpal extensor tendons
- Xanthelasma (**Figure 5.1**)

> **Clinical insight**
>
> Homozygous familial hypercholesterolaemia is associated with severe atherosclerosis in carotid, coronary, femoral and iliac arteries, highlighting the metabolic component of this inflammatory-metabolic disease. Patients have a four-fold risk of CHD.

Diagnostic approach

Familial hypercholesterolaemia is diagnosed according to the Simon Broome criteria (**Table 5.8**). The diagnosis is either definite or possible, depending on the presence of tendon xanthomas, family history of myocardial infarction, and serum cholesterol concentrations.

It is estimated that up to 90% of patients with FH are undiagnosed. Early recognition and treatment can vastly improve outcome.

Management

Patients are referred to a specialist lipid clinic. The target reduction in serum total cholesterol and LDL cholesterol is 50% of

Adult TC > 7.5 mmol/L (290 mg/dL) or LDL > 4.9 mmol/L (200 mg/dL) Or, Child (age < 16 years) TC > 6.7 mmol/L (260 mg/dL) or LDL > 4 mmol/L (155 mg/dL)	
And	
Xanthoma tendinosum in the patient, or a first- or second-degree relative Or, DNA evidence of a known mutation associated with family history	Family history of myocardial infarction (<60 years in a first-degree relative; <50 years in a second-degree relative) Or, Family history of increased total cholesterol > 7.5 mmol/L (290 mg/dL) in a first- or second-degree adult relative; >6.7 mmol/L (260 mg/dL) in a child or sibling younger than 16 years
↓ Definite FH	↓ Possible FH
LDL, low-density lipoprotein; TC, total cholesterol.	

Table 5.8 The Simon Broome criteria for the diagnosis of familial hypercholesterolaemia (FH). These are initial, fasting tests.

baseline values. All patients require lifestyle modifications, including:
- Smoking cessation
- Weight loss and exercise
- A diet with restricted saturated fat, trans fats and cholesterol. Homozygotes require intense lipid-lowering therapy with statins as first-line therapy. If lipid concentrations remain above the targets, a second agent (usually ezetimibe) is recommended.

Coronary heart disease

chapter 6

Coronary heart disease (CHD) – also known as ischaemic heart disease (IHD) or coronary artery disease (CAD) – is a reduction in blood supply to the myocardium, usually caused by atherosclerosis. Less common causes include non-embolic thrombosis, infective emboli, systemic vascular diseases and coronary artery dissection.

Coronary heart disease is the leading cause of death and serious illness in the developed world, and quickly becoming so in the developing world. In the UK, for example, CHD is responsible for 20% of male and 14% of female deaths. Worldwide it causes 12.8% of all deaths. Patients can be asymptomatic, or, if demand for oxygen exceeds supply, with central chest pain on exertion (i.e. angina). If an atherosclerotic plaque ruptures and occludes a coronary artery, patients are at risk of acute coronary syndromes (ACSs):
- Unstable angina
- Non-ST-elevation myocardial infarction (NSTEMI)
- ST-elevation myocardial infarction (STEMI)

Therapies focus on controlling risk factors, reducing myocardial oxygen demand, reopening blocked arteries and reducing blood coagulability.

6.1 Clinical scenario

Pain radiating across chest and down left arm

Presentation

Dan Taylor (58 years old) presents to the emergency department complaining of a central chest pain that radiates down his left arm. He has had the pain for 1 week, but it suddenly became worse this morning.

Diagnostic approach

Dan's chest pain should be characterised further, for example, using the Socrates mnemonic to differentiate the cause (**Table 6.1**).

	Ischaemic	Pleuritic	Musculoskeletal
Site	Central and retrosternal	Focal (single finger point)	Variable
Character	Heavy, tight and pressure	Sharp and 'stabbing'	Tender
Precipitating factors	Exercise, cold, heavy meals and stress (anything which increases physical demand on heart)	Deep inspiration and coughing	Movement, postural change and palpation
Relieving factors	Rest and nitrates (if stable angina)	Shallow breathing	Staying still or exertion
Radiation	Into jaw and arms and back	Rare	Rare
Other	Stable angina eases with rest and nitrates – ACS pain does not	Caused by friction between inflamed visceral and parietal pleural/pericardial layers	Tenderness to palpation common

Table 6.1 Characteristics of the main causes of chest pain.

Clinical insight

A 'silent MI' presents with little or no pain, but instead is often dismissed as indigestion, muscle sprain or trapped wind. This is more common in the elderly, diabetics and those with heart transplants.

Further history

Dan's past medical history includes CHD, hypertension, and hypercholesterolaemia. He suffers from infrequent angina on exertion, typically resolving with rest or use of glyceryl trinitrate (GTN) spray. However, rest or GTN have not worked for the last week. He dismissed the symptoms as indigestion and took an over-the-counter indigestion remedy to no effect. He is not nauseous or dizzy and has no palpitations.

Diagnostic approach

Episodic pain all week suggests that Dan may have unstable angina and a sudden deterioration may be due to a myocardial infarction, although differentials including pulmonary embolism or pericarditis must be excluded.

Patients with a history of angina are usually aware of what their 'normal' pain is. More persistent or severe pain suggests an ACS and immediate medical advice is needed.

Examination

On examination:
- Dan is dyspnoeic, pale and clammy
- His pulse is 90 bpm; regular
- His blood pressure is 110/60 mmHg
- The JVP is not raised
- The capillary refill time is 2 seconds
- His respiratory rate is 18 breaths/min
- His oxygen saturation is 95% on room air

On auscultation, his chest is clear, and heart sounds are normal. There is no peripheral oedema or fever. His chest pain is not reproducible on palpation and his abdominal examination is unremarkable.

Diagnostic approach

Dan's history suggests that his 'usual' angina has become unstable, and may have progressed to MI. Pallor and clamminess due to sympathetic activation are common in patients experiencing severe ischaemia and MI.

> **Clinical insight**
>
> Myocardial infarction often presents with normal examination findings, unless it has caused heart failure or an arrhythmia.

Investigations

A portable chest X-ray shows clear lung fields; an electrocardiograph (ECG) demonstrates convex ST elevation > 5 mm in leads II, III and aVF (**Figure 6.1**). Baseline blood tests including full blood count, renal function, liver function and troponin are all normal.

Diagnosis

Dan is diagnosed with STEMI, as evident on his ECG. ECG also suggests that it occurred in the right coronary artery as it is affecting the inferior myocardial territory (**Table 6.2**).

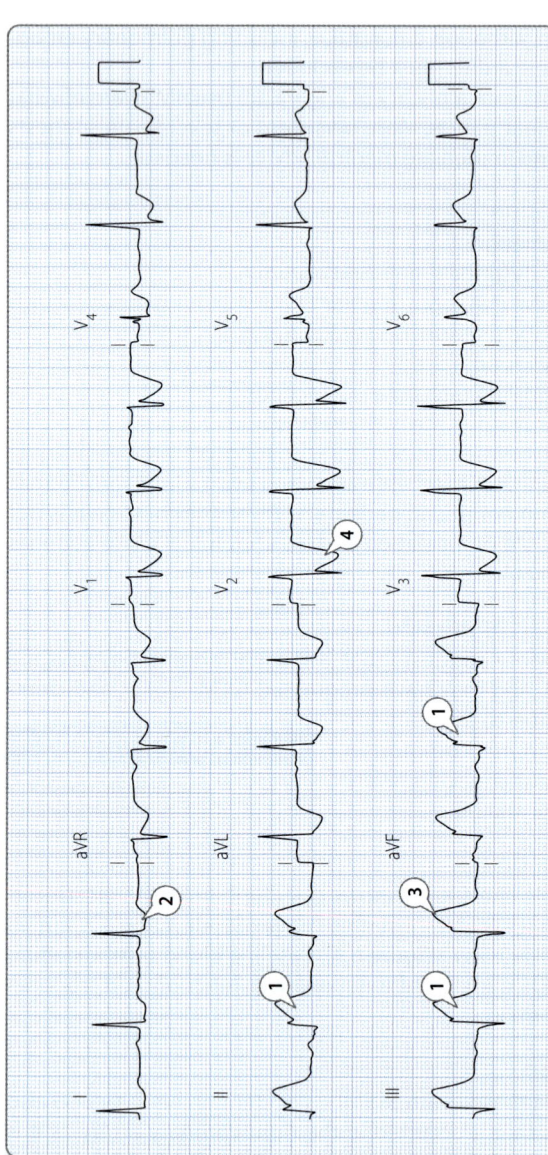

Figure 6.1 Mr. Bayliss' electrocardiograph demonstrating convex anterior ST elevation in inferior leads (II, III and aVF) ①, reciprocal changes ②, hyperacute T waves ③ and posterior extension of the infarction ④. aVF, augmented vector foot.

Site of infarct		ST elevation	Culprit vessel
Left ventricle	Anterior	V_1–V_4	Left anterior descending artery
	Septal	V_3–V_4	Left anterior descending artery
	Lateral	I, aVL and V_5–V_6	Left circumflex artery
	Inferior	II, III and aVF	Right coronary artery or left circumflex artery
	Posterior	V_7–V_9	Left circumflex artery
Right ventricle		V_1–V_2	Right coronary artery

Table 6.2 Localising infarcts by ECG changes. Note there is significant crossover.

He is transferred to the primary percutaneous coronary intervention (PPCI) centre for angioplasty to open the blocked coronary artery.

6.2 Angina

Angina (Greek *Ankhonē* 'strangling') is chest pain due to myocardial ischaemia, the most common presenting symptom of CHD. It is typically described as a 'heavy' or 'crushing' central chest pain on exertion and relieved by rest.

Stable angina only occurs on exertion; unstable angina also occurs at rest. It is graded by its severity and to what degree it limits activity (**Table 6.3**).

Epidemiology

There are over 20,000 new cases of angina a year in the UK. It affects 12% of men and 5% of women over 55 years in the UK, and approximately 2% of all adults globally.

Risk factors

Risk factors include those that are modifiable or non-modifiable – important to consider in prevention – and probable factors with unknown mechanisms (**Table 6.4**). The major factors are

Class	Definition
1	Angina only during strenuous or prolonged physical activity
2	Slight limitation, with angina only during vigorous physical activity
3	Symptoms with everyday living activities (i.e. moderate limitation)
4	Inability to perform any activity without angina or angina at rest (i.e. severe limitation)

Table 6.3 The Canadian Cardiovascular Society Angina Grading Scale.

Non-modifiable	Modifiable	Probable
Advanced age	High blood pressure	Obesity
Male gender	Diabetes	Poor diet
Personal history of coronary heart disease	Smoking	Chronic kidney disease
Family history of coronary heart disease	Hypercholesterolaemia	

Table 6.4 Modifiable, non-modifiable and probable risk factors for the development of coronary heart disease.

smoking, hypercholesterolaemia, hypertension, diabetes and a positive family history: a first-degree relative with premature CHD, i.e. diagnosed before the age of 65 years (**Table 6.5**).

Primary prevention focusses on controlling or reversing modifiable risk factors:
- Smoking cessation
- Strict control of hypertension and diabetes
- Regular exercise
- A Mediterranean-style diet, rich in fresh fruit and vegetables. Calculating the overall cardiovascular risk is an essential part of managing angina and preventing CHD.

Pathogenesis
Myocardial ischaemia can result from:
- Coronary vessel blockage

Type of chest pain	Non-anginal[‡]				Atypical angina[§]				Typical angina[ǁ]			
Gender	Male		Female		Male		Female		Male		Female	
Degree of risk[†]	Low	High	Low	High	Low	High	Low	High	Low	High	Low	High
Age (years) 35	3	35	1	19	8	59	2	39	30	88	10	78
45	9	47	2	22	21	70	5	43	51	92	20	79
55	23	59	4	25	45	79	10	47	80	95	38	82
65	49	69	9	29	71	86	20	51	93	97	56	84

[*]Low risk: No diabetes, smoking or hypercholesterolaemia.
[†]High risk: Diabetes, smoking or hypercholesterolaemia.
[‡]Non-anginal: One risk factor out of three (diabetes, smoking or hypercholesterolaemia) plus constricting discomfort on exertion or improved by rest.
[§]Atypical anginal: Two risk factors out of diabetes, smoking and hypercholesterolaemia.
[ǁ]Typical anginal: All three risk factors (diabetes, smoking and hypercholesterolaemia).

Source: Adapted from the National Institute for Health and Care Excellence (NICE). Chest pain of recent onset: assessment and diagnosis of recent onset chest pain or discomfort of suspected cardiac origin. London: NICE, 2013.

Table 6.5 Percentage likelihood of coronary heart disease, based on symptoms and risk factors.

- Coronary vessel vasospasm or constriction
- Decreased oxygen in blood.

Coronary heart disease results from atherosclerotic plaques impinging into the coronary arterial lumen inhibiting blood flow, leading to myocardial anaerobic respiration and compromised function. Angina arises when sensory nerve endings are stimulated mechanically and chemically (e.g. adenosine) in the coronary arteries and myocardium. The nerves travel to the first four thoracic spinal nerves (T1 to T4), the spinal cord, thalamus and then cortex. Pain increases as myocardial metabolic demand does.

Clinical features

Chest pain is typically central or retrosternal, and described as crushing or tight; 'like a band across the chest' and may radiate – or be solely localised to – the left arm, arms, the neck or jaw. Exacerbating factors include cold, exertion, large meals and stress. Relieving factors include use of GTN and rest.

> **Clinical insight**
>
> Stable angina is usually precipitated by exertion but quickly resolves (<10 minutes) with either rest or use of a glyceryl trinitrate spray. ACS is usually more severe, lasts longer and provokes more fear in the patient, or occurs at a lower threshold of exercise or stress.

Angina is often associated with dyspnoea, especially in cases of left ventricular systolic impairment resulting in pulmonary oedema.

Clinical signs

Signs of CHD risk factors may be seen:
- Glycosuria or complications of diabetes mellitus
- High blood pressure (i.e. hypertension)
- Tar-stained fingers (i.e. smoking)
- Xanthelasma (i.e. hypercholesterolaemia)

Investigations

Investigations aim to quickly distinguish angina from non-cardiac chest pain and ACSs. The American Heart Association (AHA)/American College of Cardiology (ACC) 2014 guidelines on the management of patients with non-ST-elevation myocardial

infarction recommend that patients with suspected angina or other ACS symptoms presenting to the emergency department have:
- A 12-lead ECG performed and are evaluated within 10 minutes of arrival
- High sensitivity troponin I or T blood levels measured at presentation and 3–6 hours post symptom onset
- If no ischaemic ECG or biomarker changes are present, non-invasive imaging within 72 hours
- Use of risk scores to guide management and assess prognosis

Less acutely, patients with suspected angina typically undergo ECG at rest, and graded exercise testing if angina is strongly suspected. If present, invasive coronary angiography is performed to investigate CHD severity.

The UK National Institute for Health and Care Excellence (NICE) guidelines help to assess the pre-test likelihood of CHD based on the patient's symptoms and risk factors (**Table 6.5**). Similarly, the AHA/ACC 2014 guidelines and European Society of Cardiology (ESC) 2011 guidelines on non-STEMI management both recommend use of the Global Registry of Acute Coronary Events (GRACE) data for calculating the risk of death or death/MI following an ACS (see www.outcomesumassmed.org/grace/).

Electrocardiography: ECG is typically normal in patients with CHD, unless they have had a prior myocardial infarction or there are signs of risk factors such as hypertension. Signs of current ischaemia include:
- ST-segment depression (**Figure 6.1**)
- T-wave flattening or inversion
- Left bundle branch block

Functional testing: Functional tests use exercise or drugs to precipitate signs of ischaemia:
- Exercise ECG
- Single-photon emission computed tomography (SPECT) scanning (also known as 'perfusion scanning')
- Stress echocardiography
- Magnetic resonance imaging (MRI)

They can help to differentiate scarred and ischaemic myocardium and can also indicate the site of the ischaemia.

Imaging: Coronary anatomy is assessed by coronary computed tomographic angiography (CCTA) and invasive angiography. CCTA is good at detecting atherosclerotic plaques and calcium in the coronary tree, but invasive angiography is better for assessing disease severity as its higher resolution results in less false positive results. Invasive angiography also allows treatment of the lesion during a single test.

Management

Treatment aims to reduce symptoms, slow CHD progression and reduce the likelihood of future ACS stroke events. Risk factor management for patients diagnosed with stable CHD is summarised in **Table 6.6**.

Risk factor	Recommendation
Smoking	Cessation via counselling and/or pharmacology
Blood pressure	Lifestyle modifications
	Target: <160/100 mmHg (<130/80 in diabetes or CKD)
	Regularly assess blood pressure
	ACE inhibitor* if CV risk is moderate or higher, or in presence of LVEF ≤ 40%, hypertension, diabetes or CKD
	ARBs for hypertensive patients who are ACEI-intolerant and have HF or a post-MI LVEF ≤ 40%
	ACE inhibitor/ARB combination therapy for HF due to left ventricular systolic dysfunction
	Aldosterone blockade (e.g. spironolactone) in patients post-MI, with no CKD or hyperkalaemia, who have LVEF ≤ 40%, and diabetes or HF, if hypertension not controlled by ACE inhibitor and β-blocker therapy
	Beta blockers* in patients post-ACS, or with left ventricular dysfunction or HF

Table 6.6 Summary of risk factor management in patients with chronic stable CHD. Based on the 2012 guidelines from the AHA and others on management of stable CHD. *Continues opposite*

Risk factor	Recommendation
Blood lipids	Diet: Reduce saturated fat intake (<7% of calorific intake) and trans-fatty acid intake (<1%) and total cholesterol < 5.2 mmol/L (<200 mg/dL)
	Plant sterols (2 g/day) or viscous fibre (10 g/day)
	Omega-3 fatty acids (1 g/day)
	Weight management/physical activity
	Regularly assess fasting lipid profile: • LDL target <1.8 mmol/L (<70 mg/dL) or use high dose statins • If LDL ≥ 2.6 mmol/L (≥100 mg/dL): Start lipid lowering medication and lifestyle modifications or intensify current treatment • High or moderately high-risk patients: Aim for LDL reduction of 30–40% • If TG 2.3–5.6 mmol/L (200–499 mg/dL), aim for non-HDL < 3.4 mmol/L (<130 mg/dL) • If TG ≥ 2.3 mmol/L (≥200 mg/dL), aim for non-HDL < 2.6 mmol/L (<100 mg/dL) After LDL-lowering therapy initiated, niacin or fibrates can lower non-HDL: • If TG ≥ 5.6 mmol/L (≥500 mg/dL): Fibrates or niacin to reduce risk of pancreatitis; aim for non-HDL <3.4 mmol/L (130 mg/dL) Drug combination helps to achieve LDL < 2.6 mmol/L (<100 mg/dL)
Physical activity	• ≤30 minutes five times a week • Exercise testing to guide exercise prescription • Cardiac rehabilitation after recent ACS, revascularisation or HF
Weight	• Assess regularly: Advise BMI maintained at 18.5–24.9 • Consider metabolic syndrome treatment strategies if waist > 89 cm (35 in) in women, >102 cm (40 in) in men • Initial goal: 10% reduction from baseline
Diabetes	• Aim for near-normal HbA1c • Aggressive treatment of other CV risk factors
Clotting	• Aspirin (75–150 mg/day)* • Additional anticoagulation with warfarin (requires INR monitoring)

*Indefinitely and unless contraindicated.
ACE, angiotensin-converting enzyme; ACS, acute coronary syndrome; ARB, angiotensin II receptor blockers; BMI, body-mass index; CKD, chronic kidney disease; CV, cardiovascular; HDL; high-density lipoprotein; LDL, low-density lipoprotein; LVEF, left ventricular ejection fraction; HF, heart failure; MI, myocardial infarction; TG, triglyceride.

Table 6.6 Continued

Medication

Symptomatic therapies reduce cardiac preload and afterload, and increase coronary dilation, by systemic and coronary vasodilation, whereas prognostic therapies improve outcome (**Table 6.7**). The 2012 AHA guidelines on management of stable CHD recommend initial symptomatic therapy of GTN and a β-blocker and adding/substituting a calcium-channel blocker or long-acting GTN if required.

Drug group	Mechanism of action	Example
Symptomatic drugs		
Nitrates	NO-induced coronary vasodilation	Glyceryl trinitrate (short acting) or isosorbide mononitrate (long acting)
Calcium-channel antagonists	Reduce intracellular calcium influx, therefore cardiomyocyte contraction	Nifedipine, nicardipine and amlodipine
Potassium-channel blockers	Relax coronary arteries	Nicorandil
Prognostic therapies		
Cardioselective β-blockers	Reduce sympathetic stimulation of the myocardium and reduce myocardial work	Atenolol, bisoprolol, carvedilol
Aspirin	Reduces platelet clotting function and atherosclerotic progression	
Statins	Stabilise existing plaques by reducing blood cholesterol	Simvastatin, atorvastatin and rosuvastatin
NO, nitric oxide.		

Table 6.7 Drugs used to treat angina.

Surgery

Patients with anginal pain despite optimal antianginal medication are considered for percutaneous coronary intervention (PCI), also known as 'angioplasty'.

Coronary artery bypass graft (CABG) is indicated in patients with severe disease – e.g. affecting all three vessels or with very tight stenosis of the left main stem – or where PCI is unsuitable.

Prognosis

2% of patients with angina will develop ACS every year.

6.3 Acute coronary syndromes

Acute coronary syndromes are a spectrum of CHD involving severe blockage of the coronary circulation. Like stable angina, they are caused by atherosclerotic deposits in vessel walls preventing sufficient blood flow through the lumen. However, they represent an acute change in the lesion(s) due to plaque rupture, acute thrombosis and/or embolism causing an actual or potential infarction. They all require immediate hospital admission.

Types

There are three main syndromes:
1. **Unstable angina:** Irregular, significant worsening angina that can occur at rest but with no evidence of infarction; a 'pre-myocardial infarction' condition
2. **Non-ST-elevation myocardial infarction:** Complete occlusion of a minor, or partial occlusion of a major, vessel causing infarction of a partial segment of the myocardium
3. **ST-elevation myocardial infarction:** Acute and complete obstruction in a main coronary artery causing infarction of a segment of the full width of the heart wall, severe pain and risk of sudden death.

Epidemiology

Acute coronary syndromes are rare in people under 35 years of age. In England, for example, there are 2,33,600 new cases of ACS per year; about 0.6% of people aged 35–74 years and 2.3% of people aged ≥75 years.

Approximate annual UK incidences:
- **Unstable angina:** 1.15 per 1,000
- **Non-STEMI:** 3 per 1,000 (also Europe)
- **ST-elevation myocardial infarctions:** 5 per 1,000

> **Clinical insight**
>
> Unstable angina can quickly progress to NSTEMI or STEMI and should be treated as an emergency.

Aetiology

In-hospital mortality is higher with STEMI than NSTEMI (7% vs. 3–5%), although long-term (4 year) mortality is twice as high with NSTEMI, as patients are often older with significant co-morbidities.

Aetiology, and therefore primary prevention, is as for atherosclerosis and angina. Although there is some influence of genetic predisposition, lifestyle/environmental factors contribute to most of the disease.

Pathogenesis

Acute coronary syndrome tends to occur when cardiac workload increases and causes an atherosclerotic plaque to obstruct blood flow. An unstable plaque may fissure and expose the underlying lesion to blood, stimulating platelet aggregation and coagulation. The resulting thrombosis (i.e. clot) may acutely obstruct the artery, causing a sudden reduction in blood flow to the myocardium.

Myocardial infarction – and myocardial cell death – occurs if ischaemia persists beyond 10 minutes. Unstable angina is ACS without infarction.

Clinical features

Acute coronary syndrome is a clinical spectrum, though all forms usually present with angina, dyspnoea and sympathetic activation (**Table 6.8**).

Symptom severity is usually: unstable angina < NSTEMI < STEMI. STEMI are the most likely to present with acute complications, including:

Diagnosis	Exertional central chest pain relieved by GTN		Electrocardiogram		Troponin concentration	
	Yes	No	Normal	Abnormal	Normal	Increased
Angina	✓		✓		✓	
Unstable angina		✓	✓		✓	
NSTEMI		✓		✓		✓
STEMI		✓		✓		✓

GTN, glyceryl trinitrate; NSTEMI, non-ST-elevation myocardial infarction; STEMI, ST-elevation myocardial infarction.

Table 6.8 Diagnosis of acute coronary syndrome based on symptoms, electrocardiogram and troponin concentration.

- Arrhythmia
- Cardiogenic shock
- Acute heart failure

Angina
Pain (see Figure 2.1) in ACS is usually more severe, longer lasting, provokes more fear or occurs at a lower threshold than stable angina.

Dyspnoea
The patient may feel breathless, particularly if there is pulmonary oedema from left ventricular systolic impairment.

Signs
Evidence of risk factors may be present.

Signs of sympathetic activation due to reduced cardiac output, i.e. pale and sweaty, may be seen in patients experiencing acute ischaemia/infarction.

Investigations
Investigations aim to quickly distinguish angina from non-cardiac chest pain and establish and distinguish ACSs. Patients with

> **Clinical insight**
>
> Myocardial infarction leads to sympathetic activation in response to the patient's pain, anxiety and reduced cardiac output.

suspected ACS should be risk assessed to guide treatment.

Acute coronary syndrome diagnosis requires the presence of typical ECG abnormalities (**Figure 6.2**); all patients presenting to hospital with chest pain require an ECG.

Acute MI is defined as evidence of myocardial necrosis in a clinical setting consistent with myocardial ischaemia. According to the ESC, diagnosis of acute MI requires a rise and/or fall of cardiac biomarker values (ideally troponin) with one or more value above the 99th percentile of the upper reference limit and with at least one of:

- Ischaemic symptoms
- New significant ST-T changes or left bundle branch block (LBBB)
- Pathological Q waves in the ECG
- A new regional wall motion abnormality seen on imaging
- Intracoronary thrombus seen on angiography

Chest X-ray

A chest X-ray is taken to exclude pulmonary oedema and aortic dissection.

Electrocardiography

Electrical evidence of arrhythmia may be present.

In unstable angina or NSTEMI, the ECG may show signs of ischaemia without ST segment elevation (**Figure 6.3**). STEMI, by definition, presents with ST elevation in a pattern that reflects the myocardial territory affected (**Figure 6.1**).

Blood tests

A full blood count, urea and electrolytes test and lipid profile are needed. Cardiac markers (e.g. troponin I or T, and creatine kinase) are increased in cases of MI but normal in unstable angina.

Acute coronary syndromes 239

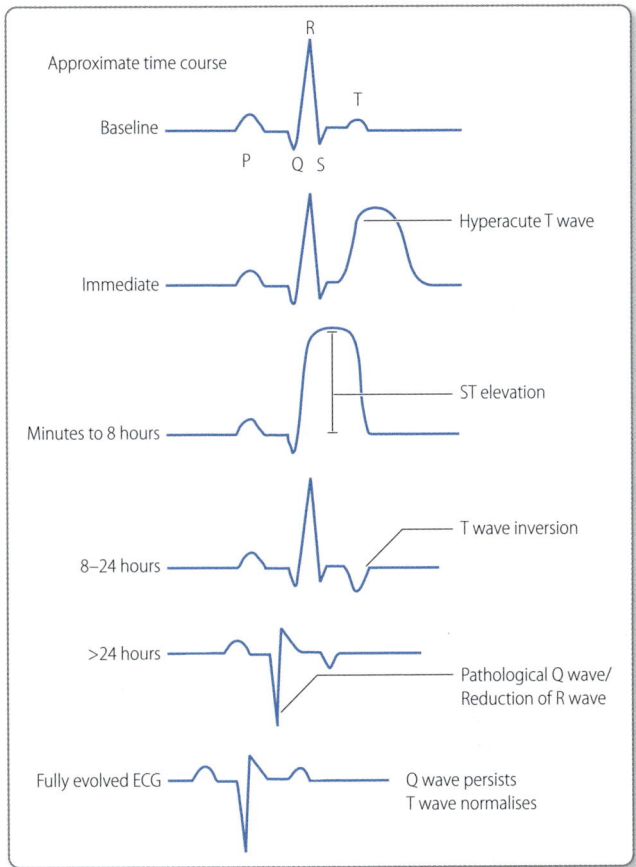

Figure 6.2 Time-dependent electrocardiograph signs of acute myocardial infarction.

Markers are measured at onset (if possible) and 3–6 hours after the onset of pain. The sole essential criterion for MI diagnosis is measurement of a value above the 99th percentile of the upper reference limit.

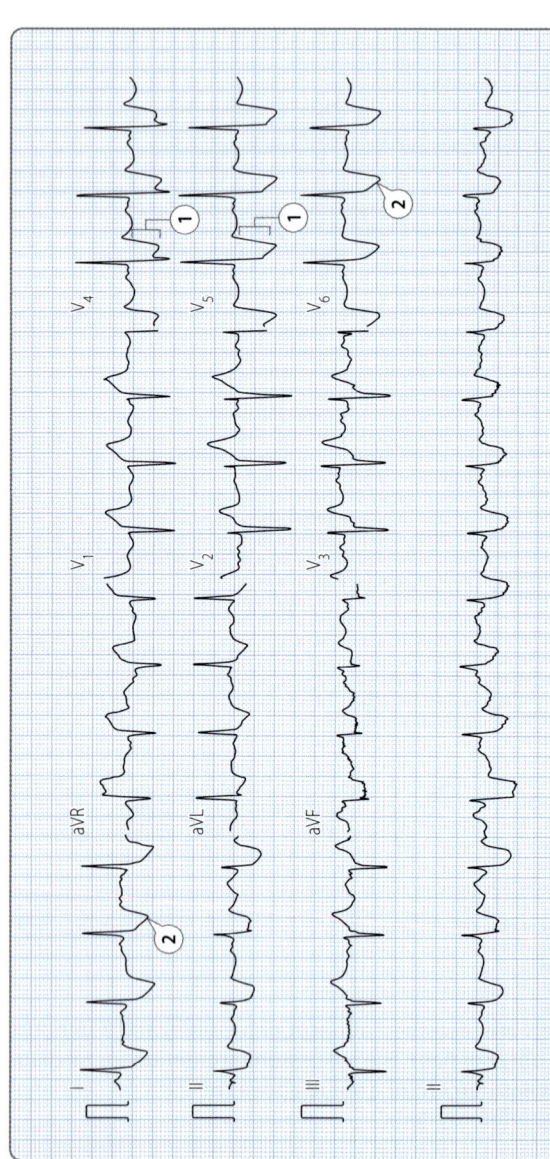

Figure 6.3 Electrocardiograph showing signs of significant myocardial ischaemia. Note the depression of the ST segments in leads I, II, aVF and V_3–V_6.

Coronary angiography

Angiography shows the nature and extent of the arterial narrowing (or narrowings). Revascularisation can also be performed during angiography, if indicated.

Management

An overview of MI management is given in **Figure 6.4**.

A central aim of managing angina or MI is to keep coronary plaques as stable as possible, using:
- Stents or grafts to reopen or bypass blocked arteries

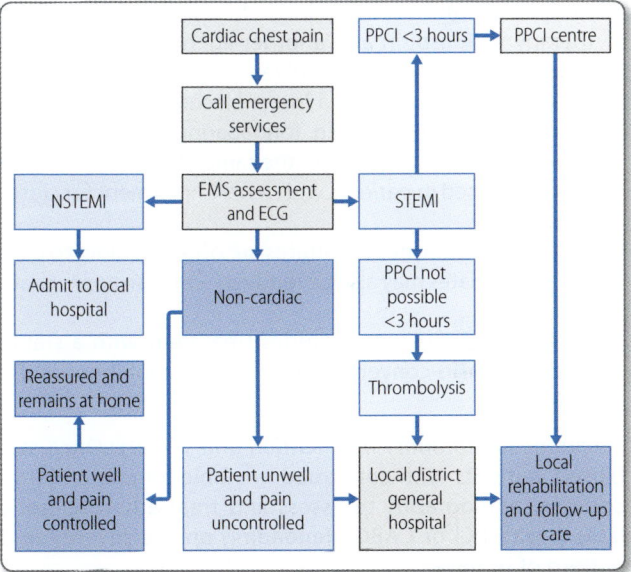

Figure 6.4 The management of myocardial infarction. ECG, electrocardiogram; EMS, emergency medical services; NSTEMI, non-ST-elevation myocardial infarction; PPCI, primary percutaneous coronary intervention; STEMI, ST-elevation myocardial infarction.
Source: Adapted from Boyle R. Mending hearts and brains – clinical case for change. London: Department of Health, 2006.

- Anti-platelet drugs to reduce thrombosis
- Anti-cholesterol drugs to reduce atherogenesis
- Drugs to reduce myocardial oxygen demand and dilate the coronary arteries

Lifestyle changes such as stopping smoking, reducing saturated fat intake and increasing exercise, are key in reducing the risk, and consequences, of future cardiac events. Losing weight and increasing unsaturated fat intake will also help to reduce symptom burden and improve functional capacity.

Unstable angina

Medication

- **Antiplatelet and antithrombotic therapy:** Dual antiplatelet therapy with aspirin and another agent (i.e. clopidogrel, ticagrelor or prasugrel) are given. Patients are started on an anticoagulant such as a low-molecular weight heparin or a factor Xa inhibitor (e.g. fondaparinux), unless cardiac catheterisation is planned for the same day. Unfractionated heparin is used in patients with renal impairment for closer monitoring
- **Analgesics:** Intravenous nitrates are often required to control pain; opiates may also be required – with an appropriate antiemetic
- Secondary prevention includes treatment with a statin, an angiotensin-converting enzyme (ACE) inhibitor and a β-blocker.

Percutaneous coronary intervention and surgery: Once stabilised, patients with confirmed unstable angina undergo coronary angiography to assess and treat atherosclerotic lesions with PCI or CABG, depending on the severity and pattern of disease.

Non-ST-elevation myocardial infarction

Medication

- **Antiplatelet and antithrombotic therapy:** As for unstable angina. Patients with ongoing pain and dynamic ECG changes are also given a glycoprotein IIb or IIIa inhibitor (e.g. tirofiban)

to maximise blood flow through a thrombosed blood vessel and minimise further clot formation
- **Analgesics:** As for unstable angina

Percutaneous coronary intervention and surgery: Patients with NSTEMI usually undergo coronary angiography within 72 hours of admission to assess lesions. Once the severity and pattern of disease have been determined, the decision is made to treat the lesions medically, with stent insertion (PCI) or with surgery (CABG).

ST-elevation myocardial infarction

It is essential that STEMI patients receive PCI as soon as possible.

Medication

- **Thrombolysis:** Can be used for patients who cannot quickly undergo PCI (door-to-balloon time < 120 minutes). Recombinant human tissue plasminogen activator is given intravenously as soon as possible (<12 hours from onset of pain). Patients need monitoring on a coronary care unit or equivalent ward. Contraindications to thrombolysis must be assessed before the drug is given.

> **Clinical insight**
>
> Criteria for PCI usually include chest pain <12 hours in duration (from the most severe pain) and ST-segment elevation of ≥1 mm in the limb leads and ≥2 mm in the chest leads, in two contiguous leads.

- **Antiplatelet therapy:** Patients are given aspirin 300 mg and another antiplatelet agent (e.g. clopidogrel 600 mg, ticagrelor 180 mg or prasugrel 60 mg according to local protocol) as soon as the diagnosis is made.

According to the 2013 ACCF/AHA and 2015 ESC guidelines, following a STEMI, all patients, assuming no contraindications, receive:
- **Aspirin:** Required lifelong
- **Additional antiplatelet agents:** Usually a P2Y12 inhibitor (e.g. clopidogrel, ticagrelor or prasugrel) for ≥1 year
- **Statins:** To achieve target cholesterol concentrations
- **Angiotensin-converting enzyme inhibitors and β-blockers:** To aid myocardial recovery

Percutaneous coronary intervention and surgery: PCI is the treatment of choice. Rarely, some patients may instead undergo CABG if PCI is not suitable or if they have had an MI despite previous PCI therapy.

Prognosis

30% of patients with unstable angina will have an MI within 6 months. The mortality of NSTEMI is 2% for those that reach hospital.

The mortality of STEMI is 4.4% for patients who reach hospital, although 30% of patients die before reaching hospital.

ST-elevation myocardial infarction patients may require subsequent coronary angiography to assess and treat further coronary lesions.

> **Clinical insight**
>
> Door-to-balloon time is crucial for treatment of STEMI. PCI should be done within 120 minutes of chest pain to achieve maximum benefit.

Once stable post-MI, patients require continued monitoring and treatment to assess and reduce risk of further ACS (see **Table 6.6**).

6.4 Complications of myocardial infarction

Myocardial infarction, necrosis and scarring can lead to loss or disorder of contractility, conduction and can increase the risk of thrombosis. Many patients also have cardiac arrest after the MI. Longer term; the key complication of MI is heart failure as scarred myocardium cannot contract and cardiac output is compromised.

Arrhythmia

Arrhythmias are common but usually resolve spontaneously as tissue heals:
- Paroxysms of non-sustained ventricular tachycardia (VT) (<30 seconds)
- Supraventricular tachycardia (SVT)
- Accelerated idioventricular rhythm
- Ventricular ectopic beats

Atrioventricular (AV) heart block is common in inferior territory infarcts as the posterior descending artery supplies the AV node. If it occurs due to an anterior infarct, this indicates extensive infarct territory, poor prognosis, and early pacing.

Clinical features
Patients may be asymptomatic or may experience syncope, palpitations or light-headedness. Signs include tachycardia, bradycardia and hypotension. Arrhythmia can be diagnosed from a cardiac monitoring system or ECG.

Management
Patients are best treated in a coronary care unit to diagnose and monitor arrhythmia promptly. Most resolve spontaneously within 48 hours. If not, and the patient is asymptomatic, monitoring is sufficient.

> **Clinical insight**
>
> Before starting cardiopulmonary resuscitation (CPR), confirm there is no 'Do not attempt resuscitation' order in the patient's medical notes.

The frequency of ventricular fibrillation or ventricular tachycardia can be reduced by administration of β-blockers. If either recurs after 48 hours, or if the patient is considered at high risk of future cardiac arrest (left ventricular ejection fraction < 40%), they may be considered for an implantable defibrillator. In inferior infarcts, asymptomatic, uncompromised AV block can simply be monitored, as it usually resolves spontaneously within 10 days. AV block due to an anterior infarct indicates more urgent temporary and then permanent pacing due to the poor prognosis.

Cardiac arrest
Cardiac arrest is the acute cessation of all or of effective heart contraction and is a dire emergency. Only 10% survive to be discharged.

It can occur due to an overwhelming MI, complications of an MI such as arrhythmia, or other acute or chronic heart or circulatory disease.

Clinical features

Four heart rhythms are seen:
1. **Ventricular tachycardia:** Regular rhythm, fast rate (>150 beats/min) and broad complexes
2. **Ventricular fibrillation:** Irregular rhythm, fast rate (>200 beats/min) and broad complexes
3. **Asystole:** No rhythm, no rate and no discernible complexes
4. **Pulseless electrical activity:** Any rhythm compatible with life but without a pulse

Only the first two are 'shockable via defibrillation'.

Management

Cardiopulmonary resuscitation must be started immediately, as the probability of survival decreases by 10% every minute:
- A ratio of 30 chest compressions (at a depth of 6 cm and a rate of 100 beats/min) to 2 rescue breaths (10 beats/min)
- During resuscitation, assess for and treat possible reversible causes. Drugs such as adrenaline (epinephrine) and amiodarone may be required
- Early defibrillation to restart the heart is crucial

Rupture of myocardial structures

Myocardial necrosis (particularly with severe infarcts) may result in rupture of an individual cardiac structure. This is less common when patients receive prompt and successful revascularisation.

Clinical features

Rupture of the left ventricular free wall causes collapse, shock and cardiac arrest (i.e. pulseless electrical activity) and is usually rapidly fatal. An echocardiogram may show a pericardial collection of blood. Immediate surgery is indicated, but few patients survive.

Post-MI ventricular septal defect (VSD) may result from rupture of the interventricular septum or rupture of a submitral valve papillary muscle causing mitral regurgitation. This presents with features of acute heart failure and a new pansystolic murmur.

Management

Suspicion of rupture requires immediate echocardiography and referral for urgent surgical repair.

Ongoing ischaemia or recurrent myocardial infarction

Post-MI patients may experience ongoing ischaemia (i.e. angina), a recurrent infarction in the same territory or in a new territory. Acute stent thrombosis can occur if a clot forms inside the new stent.

Clinical features

Patients often complain of chest discomfort and are monitored with daily ECG.

Acute stent thrombosis usually presents with severe pain and ST-segment elevation on ECG in the territory of the stented artery.

Management

Urgent coronary angiography and antianginal medication are indicated. Angiography may indicate CABG or PCI.

Left ventricular thrombus

Scarred or akinetic myocardium can lead to clot formation on the endocardial surface, with associated risk of stroke.

> **Clinical insight**
>
> After a myocardial infarction, be alert for signs and symptoms of heart failure and new murmurs.

> **Clinical scenario**
>
> Bruce Allan is a 67-year-old man who attends his 4-week post discharge check-up after a quadruple bypass.
>
> His scars have healed well, he has regained reasonable levels of fitness, but he complains of episodes of dyspnoea at rest, particularly when he bends forward.
>
> Two potential complications of CABG are pleural effusion – of which a small amount is normal and usually spontaneously resolving – and phrenic nerve damage. Bruce's chest X-ray shows the left side of the diaphragm almost 3 cm higher than the right – a sign of diaphragmatic hemiparesis.
>
> Unless the nerve damage is severe, recovery is usually good over a period of 6 months.

Clinical features

Left ventricular thrombus is more common after an anterior territory MI and is usually identified by echocardiography.

Management
Patients require long-term anticoagulation as the lesion of scarred myocardium is permanent.

Pericarditis
Patients suffering a full-thickness MI may experience pericarditis if the infarct-related inflammation involves the pericardial membrane.

Clinical features
Chest discomfort is the main symptom. Pericarditic pain is pleuritic in nature, and a pericardial rub may be heard on cardiac auscultation.

> **Clinical insight**
>
> A pericardial rub sounds like snow crunching underfoot.

Management
Anti-inflammatory medications such as high-dose aspirin or colchicine are indicated and echocardiography or cardiac MRI at diagnosis and at about 14 days later is required to identify and track a pericardial effusion.

Arrhythmias

chapter 7

An arrhythmia is an abnormal heart rate or rhythm due to an abnormal generation, conduction or propagation of electrical activity. They are a heterogeneous group of conditions, and may be inconsequential, or cause palpitations, syncope, cardiac arrest and death.

Coronary heart disease (CHD) is one of the principal causes of arrhythmias. Ischaemia causes electrochemical instability that can initiate or compound arrhythmias. Infarction causes cardiomyocyte necrosis and scar tissue formation that can block conduction and induce or encourage arrhythmias.

In patients with CHD, arrhythmia may precipitate ischaemia by increasing the metabolic demand of the myocardium. Some arrhythmias may cause thromboembolic disease. Occasionally, this can cause a blood clot to embolise to the coronary arteries causing occlusion and subsequent myocardial infarction.

Arrhythmias are categorised by heart rate, into bradycardias and tachycardias, and by the nature of the electrophysiological disturbance, for example, where the activity originates from or is localised to. Diagnosis can be difficult as many are paroxysmal in nature and there is often no correlation between symptom and pathological severity.

7.1 Clinical scenario

Lethargy and fainting

Presentation

Stan Goldman is a 72-year-old retired decorator with a long medical history of CHD, hypertension and type 2 diabetes mellitus, for which he takes diltiazem and metformin. He is seen in the outpatient clinic and gives a 4-week history of lethargy. He has 'fainted' several times and says that 'something just is not right'.

Diagnostic approach

Syncope (fainting) is a red flag symptom as it has serious potential cardiogenic and non-cardiogenic causes. More information is needed – most often from a collateral history – about its nature and frequency.

Further history

Mr. Goldman has fainted four times in the past month and has felt close to fainting many more times. He lacks energy and is tired all the time.

His daughter describes that he loses consciousness for a few seconds and quickly returns to normal. He has fainted while seated, and twice while standing, when he bruised and cut his limbs and head.

Examination

On examination:
- Blood pressure is 170/85 mmHg
- Radial pulse is 32 beats/min and regular
- Jugular venous pressure is not elevated, but every few seconds a large venous pulsation is seen rising up the neck
- He has a strong and non-displaced apex beat

The remainder of the cardiovascular and neurological examination is normal.

Diagnostic approach

His prompt recovery from loss of consciousness suggests syncope rather than seizure. Mr. Goldman's marked bradycardia could indicate reduced cardiac output leading to cerebral hypoperfusion syncope.

Orthostatic hypotension is unlikely as he has been syncopal while sitting. His occasional large venous neck pulsation indicate atrioventricular (AV) dissociation, suggesting complete heart block (CHB).

Investigations

Blood tests confirm normal thyroid function and serum electrolytes. An urgent electrocardiogram (ECG) shows an abnormal heart rhythm (**Figure 7.1**).

Clinical scenario

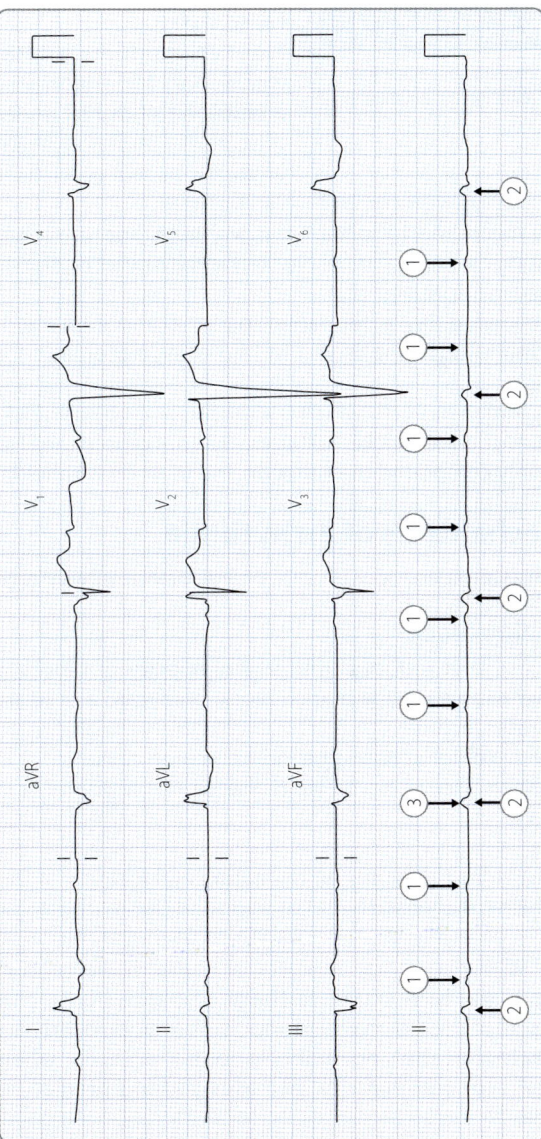

Figure 7.1 Mr. Goldman's electrocardiogram, showing features of complete heart block (CHB). QRS complexes ② and P waves ① are both regular but occur at different rates and are dissociated from each other. The QRS complexes are broad. ③ points to a 'hidden' P wave occurring at the same time as a QRS complex. aVF, augmented vector foot; aVL, augmented vector left; aVR, augmented vector right.

> **Clinical insight**
>
> Complete heart block occurs when the ventricles receive no electrical stimulus from the atria. Endogenous ventricular pacemakers begin to pace the heart at a slower rate and more unstable rhythm.

Diagnosis

The ECG confirms a CHB, warranting Mr. Goldman's admission to hospital under the care of a cardiology team until a permanent pacemaker can be fitted.

In the meantime, his diltiazem is withheld (because it is a rate-limiting calcium-channel blocker) and his heart rhythm is monitored in a specialist unit.

The following day, a permanent pacemaker is implanted. Mr. Goldman must not drive until he is asymptomatic for ≥4 weeks.

Mr. Goldman has CHD which is a risk factor for heart block. His calcium-channel blocker (diltiazem) has not caused the CHB but will only compound the situation and must be withheld.

7.2 Mechanisms of arrhythmia

Arrhythmias are aberrations of normal cardiac electrophysiology.

Conduction block

Any disease that reduces conduction velocity or blocks it altogether causes bundle branch block, bradycardia or heart block. Causes include:
- Ischaemia or infarction – the most common cause
- Infiltrative disease, e.g. amyloid disease
- Surgery
- Drugs

The clinical effect depends on the nature and location of the block, which is diagnosed by ECG rhythm and QRS morphology.

Ectopic beats

An ectopic beat is an 'extra' heartbeat (or 'extrasystole') initiated outside of the region where impulse formation is ordinarily generated, i.e. the sinoatrial (SA) node. They occur when cardiomyocyte automaticity increases causing premature discharge.

Occasional ectopics are normal but their frequency can increase due to:

> **Clinical insight**
>
> Drugs that reduce atrioventricular node (AVN) conduction velocity (e.g. Ca^{2+} channel blockers, β-blockers and digoxin) should be avoided in patients with significant conduction deficit as they may compound it.

- Ischaemia causing electrolyte derangement and sympathetic activation (**Figure 7.2**)
- Electrolyte derangement
- Sympathetic activation
- Myocardial stretch
- Drugs that disrupt the resting membrane potential and/or alter ion channel function

The more distal the site, the less co-ordinated its propagation through the conduction pathway. Atrial ectopics, therefore, cause abnormal P wave morphology on the ECG, whereas ventricular ectopics result in a broad QRS complex with abnormal morphology.

Re-entry

A conduction re-entry circuit is an alternative, abnormal route of cardiac conduction that loops back on itself. This can lead to

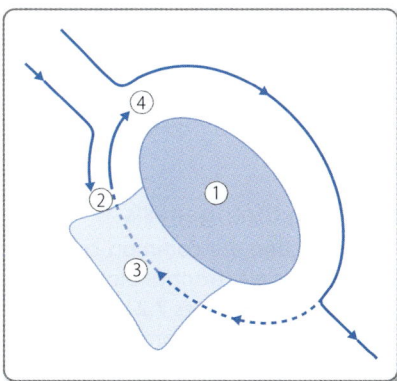

Figure 7.2 Re-entry. An impulse arrives at an area of scar tissue ①. It is blocked on one side ② but can pass on the other. Part of the signal then conducts retrogradely around the scar ③. If this conduction is slow enough (dashed line), by the time it reaches ④ the myocardium can be depolarised again, and the re-entry circuit continues.

a cyclic conduction of varying duration that disrupts the heart rate and rhythm. Re-entry circuits require:
- A circuit of conducting tissue
- An area of the circuit where conduction is unidirectional
- **Timing:** Conduction is slow enough to allow time for local cardiomyocyte repolarisation but is faster than the normal conduction pathway

A circuit is often instigated by scar tissue formation, most commonly the result of infarction (**Figure 7.2**). The property of electrophysiological timing means any factor that influences conduction velocity and/or repolarisation time will affect whether the re-entry occurs or not. Re-entry is a cause of supraventricular tachycardia (SVT) and ventricular tachycardia (VT).

Triggered activity and after depolarisations

Premature depolarisations can occur during phase 3 or 4 of repolarisation to cause an irregular heartbeat. An arrhythmia, e.g. torsade de pointes, can arise if these depolarisations recur regularly.

In the acute phases of ischaemia and myocardial infarction, triggered activity is increased (see **Figure 7.2**) which adds to the pro-arrhythmic milieu.

Early after-depolarisations (EADs) occur in phase 3 and delayed after-depolarisations (DADs) in phase 4. EADs are more common if phase 3 repolarisation is prolonged, for example, in long QT syndrome or with certain drugs. DADs are more common with increased cytoplasmic Ca^{2+} concentrations, as occurs in sympathetic activation.

Coronary heart disease arrhythmogenesis

Myocardial ischaemia and infarction are common causes of arrhythmias by disrupting cardiac electrophysiology and/or conduction pathways (**Table 7.1** and **Figures 7.2** and **7.3**).

Acute myocardial ischaemia is the most common cause of VT or fibrillation leading to sudden cardiac death.

Arrhythmias caused by myocardial infarction:

Arrhythmia	Prevalence	Timing/Mechanism	Significance
Ventricular tachycardia	• Non-sustained VT ~10% • Sustained VT ~1% • Polymorphic VT ~1%	• 2–10 minutes – altered cellular electrophysiology and re-entry • 10–30 minutes – catecholamine driven and increased automaticity • ≤72 hours (peak 12–24 hours) – increased automaticity, triggered activity, re-entry mechanisms • >72 hours – primarily re-entrant mechanisms	Immediately post-infarct, non-sustained VT is associated with a 2x risk of cardiac arrest. In the presence of LVSD, this increases to 5x. Sustained VT is uncommon in the peri-infarct period, it usually indicates previous MI/scarring. Polymorphic VT usually reflects ongoing or recurrent ischaemia. Prognosis like sustained VT. Both are associated with increased in-hospital mortality
Ventricular fibrillation	~3%	60% of episodes occur ≤4 hours and 80% ≤12 hours	Rapidly fatal without prompt defibrillation
Accelerated idioventricular rhythm	~40%	• Due to an ectopic ventricular focus firing at <120 beats/min but faster than the sinus node rate • Common in first 24 hours post successful reperfusion	Usually benign. Does not influence long-term prognosis

Table 7.1 Prevalence, mechanism and timing of arrhythmias occurring after myocardial infarction. *Continues overleaf.*

Arrhythmia	Prevalence	Timing/mechanism	Significance
Sinus bradycardia	~30%	Commonly within 1 hour	More common in inferior wall infarcts, secondary to hypervagotonia
Sinus tachycardia	~30%	Peri-infarct period, within 72 hours	Aggravates myocardial ischaemia. It can indicate underlying ventricular dysfunction
Supraventricular tachycardias	• AF ~ 10% • AFL ~ 5%	Mostly within 72 hours. AF occurring within 24 hours often associated with inferior infarction. AF occurring > 24 hours associated with anterior wall infarction and LVSD	AF is associated with increased in-hospital and long-term mortality, re-infarction, ventricular arrhythmias, cardiac arrest, shock, strokes and may reflect extensive CAD and insufficient reperfusion
AV conduction block	• 1st degree ~15% • 2nd degree ~10% • Complete ~ 5%	Most occur in peri-infarct period. AV block is more common in inferior wall infarcts reflecting hypervagotonia or damage to the AV node	AV block indicates a poorer prognosis in the context of anterior wall infarcts

AF, atrial fibrillation; AFL, atrial flutter; AV, atrioventricular; CAD, coronary artery disease; LVSD, left ventricular systolic dysfunction; MI, myocardial infarction; VT, ventricular tachycardia. Adapted from data from Ghuran AV, Camm J. Ischaemic heart disease presenting as arrhythmias. Br Med Bull 2001; 59:193–210.

Table 7.1 *Continued.*

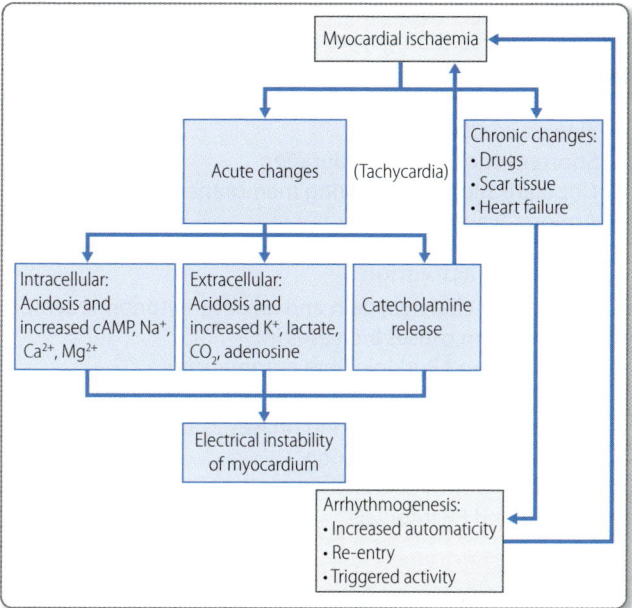

Figure 7.3 The pathophysiological mechanisms of arrhythmia in coronary heart disease. Catecholamines and arrhythmia itself can both exacerbate ischaemia by increasing the metabolic demands of the myocardium.

Ischaemia

Ischaemia causes evolving changes in electrochemistry inside and outside of cells. It is also associated with sympathetic activation, which is arrhythmogenic.

Electrochemistry

Extracellular changes include raised K^+ and adenosine concentrations, increased lactate and CO_2 production (and resulting acidosis), and catecholamine release. Intracellular changes include acidosis, elevated cyclic adenosine monophosphate (cAMP), Ca^{2+}, Mg^{2+}, and Na^+.

These changes alter ionic membrane transport, causing disruption of cardiomyocyte resting membrane and action potential including:
- Decreased excitability
- Slowed conduction
- Shorter action potential duration
- Depolarisation of the resting membrane potential
- Abnormal automaticity

Sympathetic activation
Triggered by ischaemia, pain and anxiety, autonomic sympathetic activation causes increases in:
- Junctional and Purkinje fibre automaticity
- Re-entry circuits during acute myocardial ischaemia
- After-depolarisations during phases 2, 3, or 4
- Risk of ventricular fibrillation.

It is associated with ECG changes in P wave morphology, and shorter QT and PR intervals.

Infarction
Myocardial infarction (MI) leads to cardiomyocyte necrosis, scar tissue formation (fibrosis) and sympathetic activation.

Fibrosis causes electrical conduction to slow or change route, increasing the risk of re-entry circuits and unsynchronised ventricular contraction.

7.3 Bradyarrhythmias

Bradycardia is a ventricular rate < 60 beats/min whereas a bradyarrhythmia is an inappropriately slow ventricular rhythm. They reflect a reduction in either electrical activity or conduction.

Myocardial ischaemia can produce a variety of conduction disturbances affecting any component or level of the conduction pathway. More chronically, CHD can cause fibrosis and dysfunction of the conduction tissues leading to a number of bradyarrhythmias.

Aetiology

Table 7.2 lists some common non-cardiac causes of bradycardia. Specific cardiac bradyarrhythmic syndromes include sinus node disease, heart block, atrial fibrillation (AF) and chronotropic incompetence. CHD is a major cause and should be considered in all patients presenting with bradyarrhythmia.

Sinus node disease

Sinus node dysfunction can cause:
- **Sinus pauses:** Temporary absence or delay of SA node impulse generation
- Sinus tachycardia
- Sinus bradycardia
- Atrial tachycardia
- Chronotropic incompetence
- Atrial fibrillation

Physiological	Sleep
	Athletic training (increased vagal tone)
Drug effects	Beta-blockers
	Calcium-channel blockers (dihydropyridine class)
	Amiodarone
Metabolic	Hypothyroidism
	Hypothermia
Electrolyte disturbance	Deranged potassium
	Deranged calcium
	Deranged magnesium
	Deranged sodium
Others	Increased intracranial pressure
	Obstructive sleep apnoea

Table 7.2 Common non-cardiac causes of bradycardia and bradyarrhythmia.

Tachy–brady syndromes are episodes of bradycardia and atrial tachycardia in the same patient and suggests sinus node disease.

Heart block

Heart block is impaired conduction between the atria and the ventricles. It is categorised by severity into 1st, 2nd and 3rd degree – or complete – heart block (**Table 7.3** and **Figure 7.4**). All cases of CHB require urgent specialist referral due to the increased risk of asystole. The slower the ventricular escape rate and the broader the QRS complexes, the more unstable the rhythm.

Atrial fibrillation

Atrial fibrillation can be associated with a bradycardic ventricular response, especially in the context of rate limiting drug therapy. The rhythm is irregular, but the rate depends on the ventricular response.

Degree	ECG features	Treatment
1st	Prolonged PR interval	Conservative
2nd	Prolonging PR interval culminating in a dropped ventricular beat (QRS complex)	Conservative
	Regularly more than one P wave to each QRS complex in a 2:1, 3:1 or 4:1 ratio; higher levels of block and variable block are also possible	Permanent pacemaker if symptomatic*
3rd (complete)	Complete atrioventricular dissociation: regular P waves, regular QRS complexes and no association between the two	Permanent pacemaker*

* If reversible causes are excluded.

Table 7.3 Types of heart block, their features on electrocardiography and treatment.

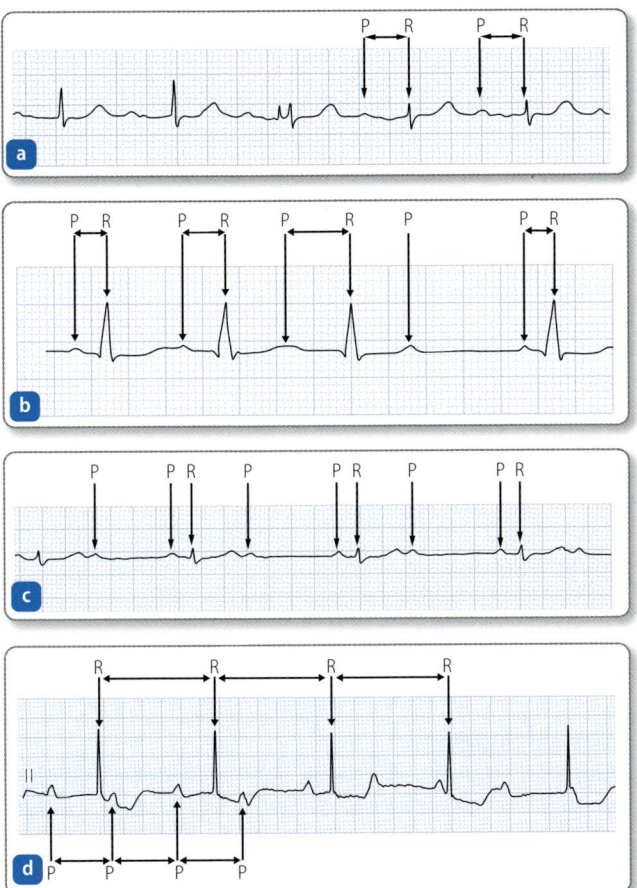

Figure 7.4 Electrocardiographic features of heart block. (a) 1st-degree heart block: A prolonged PR interval. (b) A 2nd-degree heart block (Mobitz type 1, Wenckebach block): Progressive prolongation of the PR interval culminates in a dropped QRS complex. (c) A 2nd-degree heart block (Mobitz type 2, with 2:1 block): There is an absence of the QRS complex after alternate P waves. (d) A 3rd-degree (complete) heart block: Dissociated atrial and ventricular activity.

Chronotropic incompetence

This occurs when a patient's heart rate fails to rise appropriately with exercise or physiological stress. It is often diagnosed with exercise ECG testing.

Chronotropic incompetence causes symptoms on exertion and may be the first sign of another bradyarrhythmia. If it is sufficiently symptomatic, a permanent pacemaker may be indicated.

Pathophysiology

Bradycardia is caused by conditions that reduce automaticity or block conduction tissues via infiltrative or fibrotic disease including:
- Coronary heart disease
- Age-related fibrosis
- Myocardial infiltration (sarcoidosis and amyloidosis)
- Rheumatoid conditions (systemic lupus erythematosus and rheumatoid arthritis)
- Congenital heart disease
- Electrolyte disturbance (e.g. hyperkalaemia)
- Hypothyroidism
- Excessive vagal tone
- Heart surgery

Clinical features

Bradycardia causes palpitations, light-headedness and dizziness (non-vertiginous). Systolic blood pressure (pulse pressure) is often increased in the early stages. Significant symptoms are unusual unless the heart rate is <45 beats/min. Severe bradycardia results in collapse and syncope.

Hypotension, cerebral hypoperfusion (resulting in confusion) and shock indicate cardiovascular decompensation, a late and dangerous sign.

Diagnostic approach

Diagnosis relies on ECG to 'catch' the arrhythmia when it occurs. Less frequent paroxysmal bradycardias can, therefore, be difficult to diagnose.

Investigations
Blood tests are done to exclude a biochemical cause (**Table 7.2**). A 12-lead ECG may detect more frequent bradyarrhythmias, otherwise, ambulatory ECG may be needed.

Management
Asymptomatic bradycardia is usually treated conservatively, unless there is a compelling reason to insert a permanent pacemaker such as CHB.

For symptomatic bradyarrhythmia, reversible secondary causes such as drugs should first be excluded. Otherwise, a pacemaker is usually indicated.

Pacemakers
Definitive treatment for symptomatic bradycardia is permanent pacemaker implantation (**Figure 7.5**). Implantation is not without risk (**Table 7.4**) and so requires that:
- Reversible causes have been excluded
- Symptoms are proven to be secondary to bradycardia
- Any infection is eradicated before insertion

Complication	Context
Pneumothorax	Occurs if a lung pleura is damaged during insertion
Bleeding	Post-procedural pocket haematoma – usually treated with a compression dressing in the first instance
Perforation	Can result in cardiac tamponade (i.e. compression of the heart by fluid build-up within the pericardial space), which requires emergency drainage
Infection	Treatment involves long courses of intravenous (IV) antibiotics and extraction of the pacemaker if this is unsuccessful (a risky procedure)
Lead displacement	Causes device to malfunction, requires lead repositioning

Table 7.4 Complications of permanent pacemaker insertion.

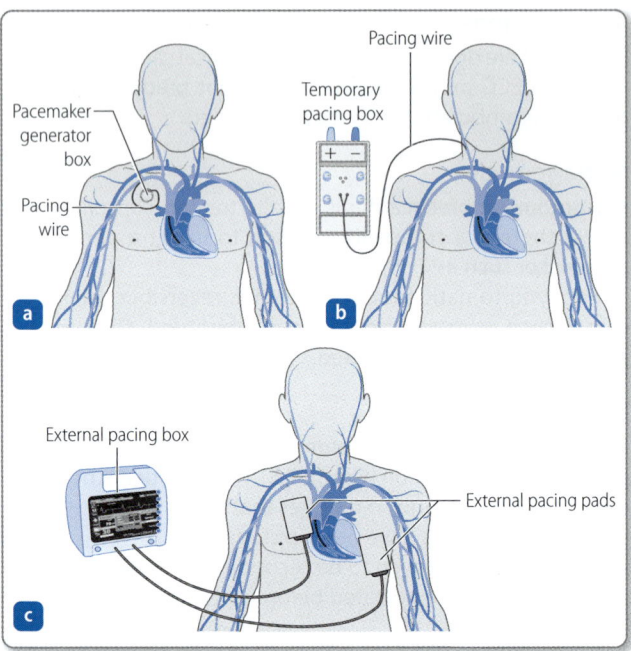

Figure 7.5 Pacemakers. (a) Permanent pacemaker. The lead is inserted into the right ventricle via a central vein and the generator box is inserted into a subcutaneous pocket. (b) Temporary transvenous pacing. A wire is inserted into the right ventricle under X-ray imaging through the jugular, subclavian or femoral vein. The wire is then connected to a generator box outside the body. (c) Transcutaneous pacing. Electrical activity is delivered through pads on the anterior chest wall.

> **Clinical insight**
>
> Rate-limiting drugs (e.g. calcium-channel blockers) should usually be withheld during symptomatic bradyarrhythmia.

Emergency and interim treatment

Severe bradycardia causing acute cardiac instability is an indication for temporary pacing or infusion with an intravenous (IV) chronotropic drug until a permanent pacemaker system can be implanted (**Figure 7.4**).

Transvenous pacing involves inserting a pacing wire into the right ventricular apex through a central vein and pacing the heart from an external power box. Transcutaneous temporary pacing is a non-invasive technique used in emergencies to manage severe symptomatic bradycardia and heart blocks.

An IV infusion of a positive chronotrope such as isoprenaline or atropine can be used (in specialist units with cardiac monitoring) to stabilise the patient once ischaemia is excluded.

Cardiac pauses

A cardiac pause is a transient cessation in cardiac electrical activity due to impulse conduction failure at the SA node, in the atrial myocardium or at the AV node (**Table 7.5** and **Figure 7.6**). The clinical features, diagnostic approach and management are like those for other paroxysmal bradyarrhythmias.

> **Clinical insight**
>
> Holter ECG monitoring usually lasts 24–72 hours and involves a 'patient symptom diary'. This allows clinicians to interpret the ECG in line with concurrent symptoms. Symptoms that occur during normal sinus rhythm do not respond to pacemaker insertion.

Type	Cause	Features
Sinus arrest	Temporary cessation of SA node impulse formation	• No evidence of atrial activity (i.e. absent P waves) • Duration is independent of the normal P–P interval
SA block	Transient failure of conduction across the atrial myocardium	Length of two or more times the normal P–P interval
AV block	Temporary block of AV node conduction	• Atrial depolarisation (P waves) may not be followed by ventricular depolarisation • A pause in cardiac output occurs before either AV conduction is restored or a ventricular escape rhythm occurs

AV, atrioventricular; SA, sinoatrial.

Table 7.5 Causes and features of cardiac pauses.

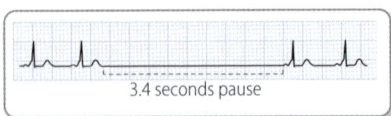

Figure 7.6 Electrocardiogram showing a cardiac pause of 3.4 seconds. The rest of the electrocardiogram shows normal sinus rhythm.

Clinical features
Pauses result in a pause in cardiac output that is usually asymptomatic but may cause palpitations, transient light-headedness and, occasionally, syncope.

Investigations
Pauses are best identified via Holter ECG monitoring.

Waking pauses lasting over 3 seconds are considered significant and require further investigation, especially when accompanied by symptoms.

7.4 Tachyarrhythmias

Tachycardia is a ventricular rate > 100 beats/min whereas a tachyarrhythmia is an abnormally fast ventricular rhythm.

Tachyarrhythmias are categorised by the duration of the QRS complex (**Table 7.6**).

Narrow complex tachycardias reflect organised, efficient electrical conduction originating from above the AV node. They are often stable and benign. Broad complex tachycardias may reflect an origin below the AV node (VTs) or a supraventricular origin with aberrant conduction, e.g. bundle branch block. VTs are less stable and can be associated with cardiac arrest.

Coronary heart disease is a major cause of supraventricular and ventricular arrhythmias both in the acute and chronic phases. Investigations for CHD should be considered in all patients presenting with tachyarrhythmias.

Supraventricular/narrow complex tachyarrhythmias
Supraventricular/narrow complex tachyarrhythmias are arrhythmias with tachycardia and a QRS duration < 120 ms.

Type	QRS duration	Origin	Electrical activity
Narrow complex (or supraventricular) tachyarrhythmias	≤120 ms	Above the AV node	Organised and efficient
Broad complex tachyarrhythmias	>120 ms	Below the AV node*	Unstable/ Disorganised and delayed depolarisation

*Unless supraventricular with aberrant conduction, e.g. bundle branch block.

Table 7.6 Narrow and broad complex tachyarrhythmias.

They can be asymptomatic or symptomatic. In an otherwise healthy heart, they are usually a relatively benign problem. AF is the most common type.

Modern catheter-based treatments that ablate the abnormal conduction tissue offer a high chance of a cure.

Epidemiology
Supraventricular tachycardias affect about 0.2% of the population.

Aetiology
Supraventricular tachycardias are categorised by the nature and location of the electrophysiological abnormality.

> **Guiding principle**
>
> Accessory pathways are embryological artefacts leaving conductible tissue through the fibrous cartilage that separates the atria and ventricles.

Atrioventricular nodal re-entry tachycardia
50% of SVTs are caused by a small re-entry circuit involving the AV node and surrounding atrial tissue. ECG characteristics of AV nodal re-entry tachycardia are shown in **Figure 7.7**.

Although the abnormality is present at birth (i.e. it is congenital), symptoms usually do not occur until young adulthood. Heart rates are usually 140–220 beats/min.

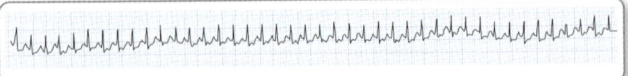

Figure 7.7 Electrocardiographic features of atrioventricular node (AVN) re-entry tachycardia. Note the tachycardia and narrow QRS complexes. The atria and ventricles depolarise almost synchronously so that P waves are hidden inside the QRS complexes.

Atrioventricular reciprocating tachycardia

Approximately 30% of SVTs are caused by an accessory pathway (AP), an abnormal electrical connection between atria and ventricle which may conduct in either direction (A-V or V-A). APs cause arrhythmia if the abnormal circuit usurps the normal conduction sequence. The resulting arrhythmia may be narrow or broad complex depending on the direction of conduction:

- Narrow complex tachycardia occurs when the circuit conducts down the AV node and septum in an antegrade (i.e. forward, normal or orthodromic) direction and the AP conducts from ventricle to atrium (**Figure 7.8**)
- Broad complex tachycardia results when the AP conducts from atrium to ventricle and there is retrograde (i.e. reverse or antidromic) conduction along the septum and through the AV node.

Accessory pathways are present from birth and usually manifest from childhood or adolescence.

> **Clinical insight**
>
> In atrioventricular reciprocating tachycardias, the breadth of QRS is determined by the direction of the circuit. Orthodromic conduction is antegrade down the septum and ventricles. Antidromic is more abnormal because conduction goes the 'wrong' way around the ventricles and the wrong way up the septum – this is inefficient and broadens the QRS.

Wolff–Parkinson–White (WPW) syndrome: This is when there is evidence of ventricular pre-excitation caused by an AP conducting in the AV direction. Premature ventricular excitation causes a shortened PR interval and a slurring of the R wave upstroke, i.e. a 'delta wave' (**Figure 7.9**).

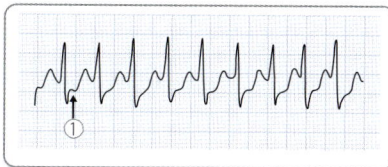

Figure 7.8 Electrocardiographic features of orthodromic atrioventricular reciprocating tachycardia. The atria are depolarised by the ventricles through an accessory pathway resulting in a retrograde P wave (arrow) after a narrow QRS complex.

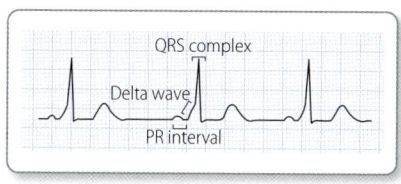

Figure 7.9 Electrocardiographic features of Wolff–Parkinson–White syndrome. The short PR interval and slurring of the QRS upstroke (delta wave) indicate early ventricular depolarisation through the accessory pathway during sinus rhythm.

WPW syndrome predisposes to atrioventricular re-entry tachycardia (AVRT) (and AF) but can be asymptomatic in up to 50%.

Atrial flutter

Atrial flutter (AFL) is a macro re-entry arrhythmia within the atria. Typical AFL circuits involve the cavotricuspid isthmus, atrial septum and the crista terminalis resulting in an atrial rate of around 300 beats/min. Atypical AFL circuits occur elsewhere in the atria, and usually associated with previous surgery or scarring. Flutter is usually episodic (but can be chronic) and presents with tachycardia of around 150 beats/min (when there is 2:1 block) and a classical saw-tooth appearance on ECG as seen in **Figure 7.10**.

> **Guiding principle**
>
> Despite atrial contractions of around 250–300 beats/minute in AFL, the AV node limits conduction to the ventricles, resulting in a ventricular rate of 75, 100 or 150 beats/minute, i.e. a value divisible into 300.

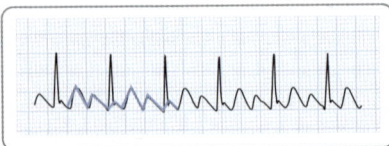

Figure 7.10 Electrocardiogram showing atrial flutter. Note the sawtooth baseline (blue) and narrow complex tachycardia (100 beats/min). There are three flutter waves to each QRS but the third is hidden within the QRS complex.

Atrial tachycardia

This SVT arises from increased automaticity, a macro or micro re-entry circuit, or both, in the atria. It causes a narrow complex tachycardia with an abnormal P wave shape.

Atrial fibrillation

Atrial fibrillation consists of fast, disorganised atrial impulses that – unlike other SVTs – causes an irregularly irregular rhythm. AF occurs with either a normal, slow or fast ventricular response rate.

Clinical features

Supraventricular tachycardias may be asymptomatic or cause:
- Fast, regular or 'fluttering' palpitations
- Shortness of breath
- Fatigue

Ischaemic chest pain and low blood pressure indicate myocardial compromise and require urgent (synchronised) direct current cardioversion (DCCV) to correct the arrhythmia.

Tachycardiomyopathy is heart failure due to persistent SVT. It develops over weeks or months. SVTs are much more often a complication of, and not the cause of, heart failure.

> **Clinical insight**
>
> 'Pre-excited atrial fibrillation' is a potentially dangerous complication of SVT. This is when AF is conducted via an accessory pathway to cause ventricular pre-excitation. It can quickly develop into ventricular fibrillation (i.e. cardiac arrest). Drugs that block the AV node are contraindicated in such patients, as these increase accessory pathway conduction.

Investigations
Diagnosis relies on defining the SVT on ECG and correlating it with patient symptoms. Ambulatory ECG monitoring may be required if episodes are infrequent.

Once diagnosed, investigations are used to identify the cause (**Table 7.7**).

Management
Supraventricular tachycardias causing cardiovascular instability should have urgent synchronised DCCV (**Figure 7.11**).

Ultimately, the optimal management is determined by the underlying cause. Drug therapy may reduce the chance of recurrence, whereas catheter ablation offers the possibility of a cure.

Vagal manoeuvres
Vagal stimulation may terminate the SVT quickly and simply. These include:
- The Valsalva manoeuvre – ask the patient to cough, bear down or blow hard into a 10 mL syringe
- Carotid sinus massage – after carotid bruit is excluded

Medication
Drugs that block AV node conduction (e.g. β-blockers and Ca^{2+} channel blockers) are effective in treating AV node re-entry

Investigation	Rationale
Echocardiography	Excludes structural heart disease and assess cardiac function
Thyroid function tests	Hyperthyroidism
Urea and electrolytes	Electrolyte derangement
Invasive electrophysiological studies	Characterise underlying pathophysiology
Investigations for CHD, e.g. coronary angiography	If ischaemia is suspected as a precipitant

Table 7.7 Investigations in supraventricular tachycardia.

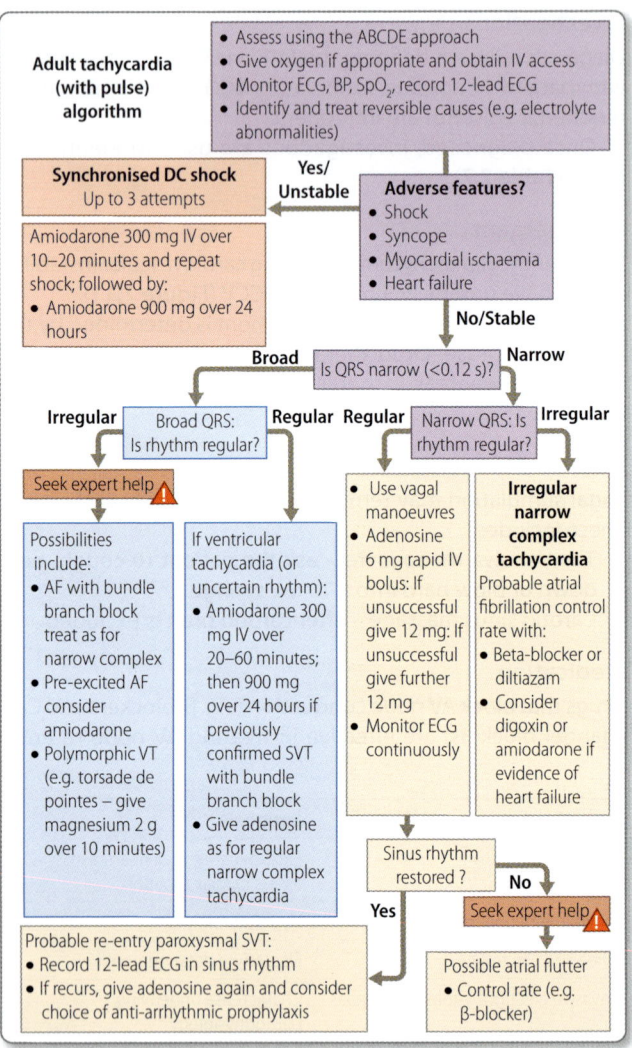

Figure 7.11 Advanced support guidelines for the management of tachycardia. AF, atrial fibrillation; BP, blood pressure; DC, direct current; ECG, electrocardiogram; IV, intravenous; SpO$_2$, oxygen saturation; SVT, supraventricular tachycardia; VT, ventricular tachycardia. Reproduced with the kind permission of the Resuscitation Council (UK).

and AV reciprocating tachycardias. They are contraindicated if ventricular pre-excitation is evident (e.g. in Wolff–Parkinson–White syndrome), because they increase the accessory pathway conduction causing pre-excitation. Instead, class 1 (flecainide, propafenone or disopyramide) or class 3 drugs (amiodarone) are favoured, as they reduce accessory pathway conduction.

Atrial flutter and atrial tachycardia respond poorly to drug therapy.

Catheter ablation
Either cryotherapy or radiofrequency ablation is the destruction of the abnormal circuit or electrical focus causing the tachycardia. It is delivered through intracardiac catheters and has a high success rate (>95%).

Prognosis
Although SVT may be worrying and difficult to treat, in an otherwise healthy heart, the prognosis is usually excellent.

Ventricular tachycardia
Ventricular tachycardia is a broad complex tachycardia originating in the ventricular myocardium. It is defined as ≥3 successive ventricular beats occurring at >100 beats/min.

Ventricular tachycardia is potentially life threatening

> **Clinical insight**
>
> Atrial flutter, like AF, often requires thromboprophylaxis due to increased stroke risk due to increased blood stasis.

> **Clinical insight**
>
> Always consider atrial flutter if the ventricular rate is 150 beats/minute. The atrial rate in flutter is always about 300 beats/minute, which is too fast for 1:1 AV node conduction.
>
> Ventricular rate usually occurs with 2:1 (150 beats/minute), 3:1 (100 beats/minute) or 4:1 (75 beats/minute) AV block.

> **Clinical insight**
>
> Not all supraventricular tachycardias (SVT) present with a narrow complex; some can present with broad QRS complexes:
>
> - Supraventricular tachycardias with abnormal conduction, e.g. atrial flutter with bundle branch block, can present with a regular broad complex tachycardia
> - Atrial fibrillation with a fast ventricular response and abnormal conduction (i.e. left or right bundle branch block) presents with an irregular broad complex tachycardia.

due to the risk of ventricular fibrillation, cardiac arrest, and sudden cardiac death.

Types
Ventricular tachycardia may be:
- Pulse-palpable or pulseless
- Non-sustained (<30 seconds) or sustained (>30 seconds)
- Monomorphic (with a consistent QRS appearance; **Figure 7.12**) or polymorphic (with a frequently changing QRS appearance; **Figure 7.13**)

Aetiology
Monomorphic VTs are usually caused by an abnormal re-entry circuit, often due to myocardial scarring secondary to CHD. Other causes include infiltration or cardiomyopathy.

Torsade de pointes is a polymorphic VT that occurs secondary to prolonged QT interval. It is therefore associated with the long QT syndromes, hypokalaemia and hypomagnesaemia, as well as the use of amiodarone, erythromycin and methadone.

Clinical features
Ventricular tachycardia is usually symptomatic. Symptoms include:
- Palpitations
- Presyncope – lightheadedness, blurred vision and weakness
- Syncope, i.e. loss of consciousness. This is a poor prognostic indicator
- Symptoms of heart failure in sustained VT

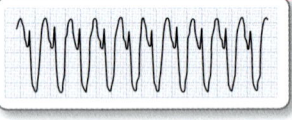

Figure 7.12 Electrocardiographic features of a regular broad complex ventricular tachycardia.

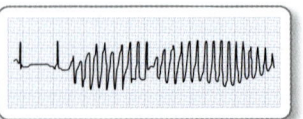

Figure 7.13 Electrocardiogram features of torsade de pointes, a polymorphic broad complex tachycardia. The complexes appear to twist around the baseline.

Patients are often agitated, anxious and fatigued.

History should also elicit symptoms of associated conditions, such as CHD and heart failure. Family history of arrhythmia or sudden cardiac death is also relevant.

If palpable, the pulse is usually rapid and weak. Pulseless VT presents with cardiac arrest. Signs of potential causes or complications should also be sought.

Investigations

Ventricular tachycardia is diagnosed by 12-lead ECG and must be distinguished from broad-complex SVTs (**Table 7.8**). About 85% of regular broad complex tachycardias are caused by VT. In patients with structural heart disease (including heart failure or

	Ventricular tachycardia (VT)	**SVT with aberrant conduction**
QRS complex	Very broad QRS: >160 ms	<160 ms
Axis	Extreme: −90° to −180°	Normal QRS axis (−30 – +90°)
Concordance	All chest lead complexes are positive, or all are negative	Not present
Fusion beats	Produced when a sinus beat fuses with a ventricular beat	Not present
Capture beats	Produced when a sinus beat 'captures' the ventricles to produce occasional 'normal'-looking beats	Not present
Bizarre QRS shapes	Present	Not present
AV dissociation	AV dissociation: regular P and QRS complexes but at different rates	Not present

AV, atrioventricular; SVT, supraventricular tachycardia.

Table 7.8 Typical ECG features of VT and SVT with aberrant conduction. The latter occurs when there is an SVT with abnormal and prolonged conduction between the atria and ventricles, e.g. bundle branch block.

> **Clinical insight**
>
> Accelerated idioventricular rhythms are ventricular in origin with a rate between 60 and 100 beats/minute. They are commonly associated with successful reperfusion following treatment for myocardial infarction. In this context, they usually resolve spontaneously.

CHD), around 95% of broad complex tachycardias are caused by VT. Therefore, in cases of doubt, the arrhythmia is treated as VT until proven otherwise.

Underlying cause
The underlying cause may be evident on ECG or cardiac magnetic resonance imaging (cMRI), which can show functional impairment or structural abnormalities, and coronary angiography may be used to diagnose CHD.

Electrophysiology
The mechanism of the arrhythmia can be identified through an invasive electrophysiological study. Multiple catheters are positioned within the heart and coronary sinus to detect the electrical activation sequence. This helps to determine the underlying electrical abnormality and guides ablation therapy.

Quantifying risk
Risk is determined by the presence or absence of structural heart disease, including heart failure and CHD.

Management
Emergency synchronised DCCV is required for any patient whose condition is acutely compromised, e.g. hypotension or ischaemia.

Once sinus rhythm is restored, the underlying cause is sought and treated where possible. This commonly requires alleviating ischaemia or optimising treatment of heart failure.

Torsade de pointes requires urgent DCCV to restore sinus rhythm. Correction of magnesium or potassium deficiency, or both, in addition to cessation of any QT-prolonging drugs reduces recurrence.

Medication

Drugs (e.g. amiodarone or β-blockers) may be used to reduce the frequency of VT in patients with a structurally abnormal heart. β-blockers and aldosterone antagonists may improve prognosis in the context of heart failure.

In patients with a structurally normal heart, drug therapy is often the only management necessary.

Surgery

If electrophysiological investigations identify an appropriate target, catheter ablation may be possible for monomorphic VT. Success rates are about 60–75%, and higher in the absence of structural abnormality.

Cardioverter defibrillators

Implantable cardioverter defibrillators (ICDs), after careful consideration, are used for primary prevention in patients with a high-risk condition (e.g. severe heart failure) and secondary prevention in patients with VT or VF causing syncope or cardiac arrest.

Implantable cardioverter defibrillators do not reduce the frequency of ventricular arrhythmia but attempt to restore sinus rhythm when it occurs.

Prognosis

The key prognostic factor is the presence of structural heart disease, including CHD and heart failure. VT in a structurally normal heart has a much better prognosis. In appropriate patients, ICD insertion has been shown to reduce mortality.

Ventricular fibrillation

In VF, the ventricular myocardium is devoid of any co-ordinated electrical or mechanical activity. Cardiac output ceases and cardiac arrest occurs (**Figure 7.14**). Immediate DCCV is indicated in all cases otherwise asystole and death quickly ensue. Survival is highly dependent on speed and quality of advanced

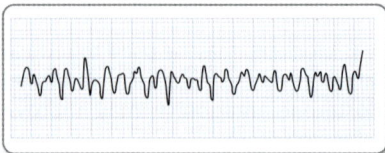

Figure 7.14 Electrocardiographic features of ventricular fibrillation. The rhythm, polarity and magnitude are completely irregular.

life-support treatment and defibrillation. Survival probability declines 2–10% per minute of delay of DCCV.

Ventricular fibrillation survivors and those deemed to be at high risk of VF are treated with ICD implantation.

7.5 Atrial fibrillation

Atrial fibrillation is an irregular, often rapid rhythm where the atria fail to contract efficiently, regularly or in co-ordination with the ventricles. It is the most common cardiac arrhythmia. Depending on the ventricular response rate, it can present with bradycardia, tachycardia, or a normal rate.

Atrial fibrillation is a major risk factor for thromboembolic disease, especially stroke, as it increases blood clotting due to stasis. AF often occurs in patients with CHD and may complicate the acute or chronic phases of myocardial infarction.

Types
Atrial fibrillation is classed according to duration:
- Paroxysmal (<7 days)
- Persistent (>7 days)
- Permanent (>7 days and resistant to therapy)

Epidemiology
Atrial fibrillation prevalence increases with age. It affects 1% of the general population and up to 10% of those over 80 years. Its true prevalence is likely higher than this as it is often asymptomatic and undiagnosed.

Aetiology
Atrial fibrillation can be:
- Lone, with no identifiable cause (10–15%)

- Valvular, often associated with prosthetic valves or rheumatic valve disease
- Secondary to other cardiac or non-cardiac disease that increases atrial stress (**Table 7.9**)

Excess alcohol consumption and drug misuse also predispose to AF. It is common in the acutely unwell or perioperative patients.

Pathophysiology

Fibrillation is a pattern of rapid, unsynchronised electrical activity, with no co-ordination of atrial electrical or mechanical activity. Conduction to the ventricles is irregular and haphazard, so the ventricular response rate is determined by the conductivity of the AV node and the His and Purkinje tissues.

The mechanisms of AF initiation and propagation are complex and not fully understood but involve structural and electrophysiological

> **Clinical insight**
>
> Atrial stress induces chronic myocardial, electrical and biochemical changes that initiate and propagate AF. In many patients with paroxysmal AF, the initiating electrical stimuli emanate from the pulmonary veins. This is the rationale behind pulmonary vein ablation (isolation) therapy in paroxysmal AF.

Common risk factors	Common investigative findings
- CHD (including previous MI) - Valvular heart disease - Heart failure - Advanced age - Obesity - Hypertension - Diabetes mellitus - Previous cardiac surgery - Smoking - Alcohol excess - Hyperthyroidism - Family history	- LVH (ECG or echo) - Dilated left atrium (echo) - Valve (particularly mitral) dysfunction (echo) - Systolic or diastolic dysfunction (echo) - Raised inflammatory markers (serum CRP/ESR) - Elevated white cell count

CHD, coronary heart disease; LVH, left ventricular hypertrophy; MI, myocardial infarction; VHD, valvular heart disease.

Table 7.9 Common risk factors for and investigation findings in atrial fibrillation.

alterations of the atrial tissue caused by a spectrum of pathological mechanisms including ischaemia, inflammation, increased metabolic demand and neurohormonal activation. AF is often the final common result of a variety of disease processes.

Clinical features

The clinical features of AF are often determined by the ventricular response rate. However, even AF with normal ventricular rate may be symptomatic with palpitations, lethargy, chest pain and dyspnoea. In otherwise asymptomatic cases, the first presentation can be with a cerebrovascular accident.

History should also include:
- Predisposing factors (e.g. family history, hypertension and lung disease)
- Stroke and bleeding risk
- Complications (e.g. heart failure and thromboembolic disease)

Signs include:
- An irregularly irregular pulse
- Those of predisposing factors (see **Table 7.9**)
- Complications, e.g. signs of heart failure or thromboembolic disease

> **Clinical insight**
>
> Atrial fibrillation is always 'fast': it is the ventricular response rate that can be slow, normal or fast.

> **Clinical insight**
>
> Atrial fibrillation predisposes blood clots, often in the left atrial appendage. These are best seen via trans-oesophageal echocardiography.

Investigations

Permanent AF is easily and quickly diagnosed by palpating an irregularly irregular pulse rhythm and performing an ECG (**Figure 7.15**). Paroxysmal AF usually requires Holter monitoring to record an episode.

Multiple investigations are necessary to exclude causes and guide treatment (**Table 7.10**). Trans-oesophageal echocardiography can also be done to identify or exclude left

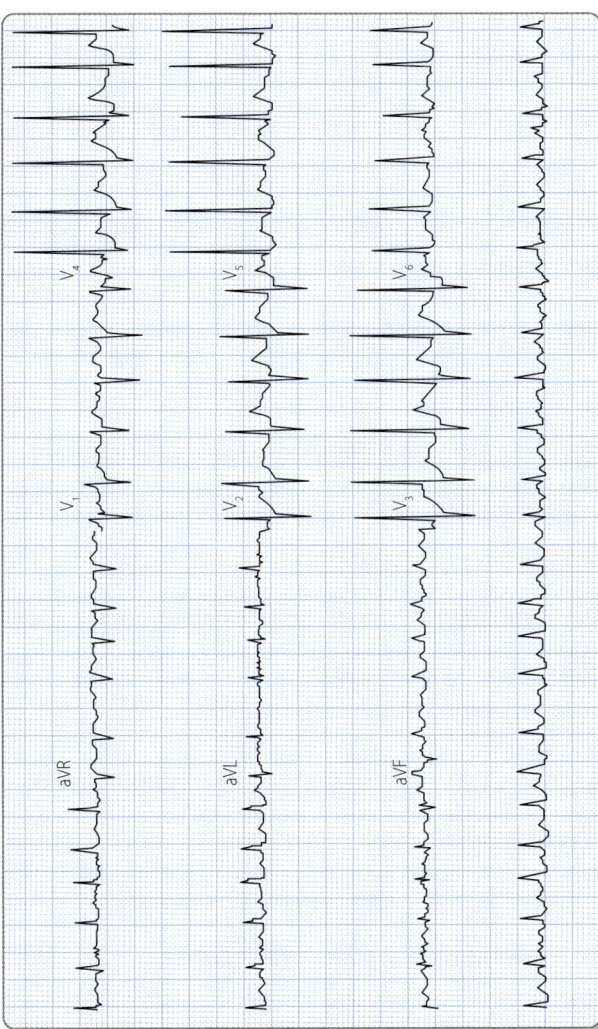

Figure 7.15 Electrocardiographic features of atrial fibrillation. The QRS complexes are narrow and occur irregularly. P waves are absent.

Test	Rationale
Thyroid function tests	To exclude hyperthyroidism
Coagulation screen	Required for patients considered for anticoagulation
Urea and electrolytes	To exclude electrolyte derangement
Liver function tests	To exclude structural heart disease

Table 7.10 Investigations indicated by atrial fibrillation.

atrial clot if DCCV is being considered in AF beyond 48 hours and before 6 weeks of anticoagulation is complete.

Management

The key aims are to reduce the risk of thromboembolic disease, control the ventricular rate and alleviate symptoms. The strategy depends on whether AF is acute, paroxysmal or permanent.

Anticoagulation: AF increases the risk of stroke five-fold. This risk is decreased by around two-thirds by oral anticoagulant therapy. Annual risk should be calculated using, e.g. the CHA_2DS_2-VASc score (**Table 7.11**). The patient's risk of bleeding, calculated with, e.g. the HAS-BLED score, must be balanced against the benefits of anticoagulation.

Rate control: The initial target is maintenance of a resting heart rate ≤ 110 beats/min, using a β-blocker, calcium-channel blocker or digoxin. A second agent can be added if control is suboptimal.

Digoxin is reserved for more sedentary patients because it can prevent increases in heart rate with exercise.

Management of acute atrial fibrillation

Emergency DCCV is required if there is significant cardiovascular compromise, regardless of AF duration. If AF occurs secondary to an acute systemic illness, the underlying cause is treated as a priority. If AF still persists, DCCV can be considered after ≥6 weeks of effective anticoagulation.

Factor	Category	Score if yes*
Congestive heart failure	Yes or no?	1
Hypertension	Yes or no?	1
Age (years)	<65	0
	65–74	1
	≥75	2
Diabetes mellitus	Yes or no?	1
History of stroke, transient ischaemic attack or thromboembolic disease	Yes or no?	2
Vascular disease	Yes or no?	1
Female sex	Yes or no?	1

*A total score of 0 indicates low annual stroke risk. Higher scores reflect increased risk. For example, total scores of 1, 2 and 3 equate to annual stroke risk of 1.3%, 2.2% and 3.2% respectively. A total score of 6 equates to a risk of 9.8%.

Table 7.11 The CHA_2DS_2-VASC score for estimating risk of stroke in patients with atrial fibrillation.

Management of paroxysmal atrial fibrillation

The frequency of paroxysms can be reduced by:
- Beta-blockers
- Class 1C drugs (flecainide or propafenone)
- Class 3 drugs (amiodarone or dronedarone)

> **Clinical insight**
>
> Novel oral anticoagulants (NOACs) include factor Xa and thrombin inhibitors.
>
> They are attractive because they appear to be as effective as warfarin in preventing venous thromboembolism in AF and do not require blood monitoring.

However, these drugs are limited by contraindications, complications and lack of efficacy in some cases.

Direct current cardioversion: DCCV can restore sinus rhythm, but reversion back to AF is common. Cardioversion carries a stroke risk and is avoided if AF lasts >48 hours. DCCV is done only if ≥6 or more weeks of effective anticoagulation has been achieved, or if a trans-oesophageal echocardiogram excludes atrial thrombus.

Atrial fibrillation ablation: In paroxysmal AF, electrical isolation of the pulmonary veins via catheter ablation can be used to prevent recurrence. This can provide long-term relief but is invasive and often requires multiple attempts.

Pill-in-the-pocket: This involves the patient taking a drug (usually a β-blocker, flecainide or propafenone) if symptoms suggest recent onset of AF. It is an effective strategy in some patients.

Permanent atrial fibrillation

When sinus rhythm cannot be restored, the primary aim is to reduce the risk of thromboembolism. Rate control is indicated if the ventricular response is fast.

Prognosis

The prognosis for AF is good if the risk of thromboembolism is minimised, and the rate is controlled.

Heart failure

chapter 8

Heart failure (HF) is a syndrome reflecting an inadequate circulation of blood due to impaired ventricular filling and/or ejection of blood. It has many causes and can be acute or chronic in nature. Coronary heart disease (CHD) is a common cause of both acute and chronic HF.

Heart failure has a complex pathophysiology, often involving multiple compensatory mechanisms. The cardinal features of HF are dyspnoea, fatigue and fluid retention. It also has many possible complications, including psychological, musculoskeletal, haematological, pulmonary, endocrine, endothelial, renal and hepatic dysfunction.

Echocardiography is used to assess both systolic and diastolic ventricular function and is the gold standard investigation for the diagnosis of HF. The underlying disease must be found and treated where possible.

8.1 Clinical scenario

Breathlessness at night, ankle swelling and cough

Presentation

Jeff Marks, aged 65 years old, presents to his local emergency department with a 6-month history of nocturnal breathlessness and cough. He previously felt that he merely had a series of colds but made an appointment after his wife noticed that his ankles had begun to swell.

Mr. Marks has three common presenting complaints: Shortness of breath, ankle swelling and cough (**Table 8.1**). Only heart, respiratory, renal or liver failure could cause all three simultaneously.

History

Mr. Marks' illness started 6 months ago with what seemed like a heavy cold. This increased in intensity, and he began experiencing a cough with white frothy sputum. He is not short of

Symptom	Questions to ask	Associated symptoms	Possible differentials
Shortness of breath	• Is it new? • Is it getting worse? Is it just at night or during the day too? Does it come on with exertion, the cold, heavy meals? How many pillows does he use? Does the cough wake him?	Wheeze, chest pain and dizziness	HF, CHD, COPD and pulmonary embolus
Ankle swelling	When did this come on? Is it on one or both sides? Did it start after injury or surgery? Has it happened before? How far does it extend up the leg, and is it worsening?	Pain, redness and distended veins	Heart, renal or liver failure, lymph oedema and deep venous thrombosis
Cough	When does the cough occur? Is it productive? If so, what is the colour and consistency of the sputum?	Green, frothy or blood stained	HF, infection, drug adverse effect, malignancy and anxiety

CHD, coronary heart disease; COPD, chronic obstructive pulmonary disease.

Table 8.1 Mr. Marks' presenting features.

> **Clinical insight**
>
> A patient's agenda must always be addressed, for example by considering:
>
> - Ideas: what do they think is going on, and why?
> - Concerns: what are their worries, and why?
> - Expectations: What do they want?

breath during the day but wakes up breathless during the night and has difficulty lying flat.

He started to worry when his ankles began to swell. Mr. Marks denies any palpitations, fever, weight loss or other symptoms.

His medical history includes:

- CHD – myocardial infarction treated with coronary artery bypass grafts (CABG) 5 years ago

- Hypertension
- Hypercholesterolaemia
- Type 2 diabetes mellitus

He has had no angina since his CABG. He takes aspirin, atenolol, simvastatin, metformin and gliclazide. He is a retired bank clerk and has never smoked and currently does not drink alcohol. His systems review is unremarkable.

Mr. Marks has multiple risk factors for HF: CHD, diabetes and hypertension.

Chronic obstructive pulmonary disease (COPD) is unlikely as he has never smoked nor worked in a dusty environment. The absence of chest pain suggests that the symptoms are not ischaemic in origin. The frothy white sputum strongly suggests pulmonary oedema. Symptoms specific to the pulmonary oedema of HF include:
- Paroxysmal nocturnal dyspnoea – waking up breathless during the night
- Orthopnoea - the inability to lie flat because of the resulting breathlessness

Examination
- Mr. Marks is apyrexial
- Heart rate - 110 beats/min
- Blood pressure - 100/80 mmHg
- Jugular venous pressure (JVP) is raised at 8 cm
- Capillary refill time is 2 seconds
- Respiratory rate is 20 breaths/min
- Oxygen saturation is 94% on room air

A laterally displaced apex beat is found on precordial palpation. On auscultation, there are crepitations and reduced air entry at the bases and normal heart sounds. His ankles are swollen with fluid (oedema) up to the mid shins.

Abdominal examination reveals moderate ascites and tender hepatomegaly.

Mr. Marks' tachycardia and hypotension indicate a reduced stroke volume due to impaired left ventricular function.

Tachycardia is a compensatory attempt to meet peripheral circulatory demand. His normal capillary refill time suggests demand is being met.

His raised JVP reflects right ventricular impairment and elevated central venous pressure (CVP), possibly secondary to left ventricular failure. Right ventricular impairment leads to a buildup of systemic fluid: ascites, ankle oedema and liver swelling. Left ventricular impairment leads to pulmonary oedema, evident as crepitations. Left ventricular failure leads to ventricular dilation, evident as a displaced apex beat.

The working diagnosis is congestive HF secondary to CHD.

Investigations

A chest X-ray shows cardiomegaly, pulmonary oedema and pleural effusions (**Figure 8.1**).

An electrocardiogram (ECG) shows sinus tachycardia.

Baseline blood tests include full blood count; lipid profile; blood glucose; and tests of renal, thyroid and liver function and are all normal except for elevated transaminases, hyperbilirubinaemia and hypoalbuminaemia.

Diagnosis

Mr. Marks is diagnosed with acute-on-chronic HF with reduced ejection fraction (HFrEF) syndrome caused by left ventricular

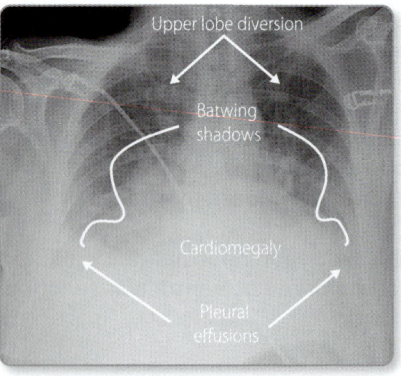

Figure 8.1 Chest X-ray showing the perihilar, batwing shadows of pulmonary oedema. The increased cardiothoracic ratio (i.e. cardiac silhouette is >50% of the total width of the lungs) indicates cardiomegaly. Pleural effusions are a common sign of heart failure but have many non-cardiac causes.

systolic dysfunction, most likely because of CHD. Ankle oedema, a displaced apex beat, and cardiomegaly are signs of chronic HF. His dilated, failing left ventricle has led to right-sided failure, as evident in the pulmonary oedema seen on X-ray and his associated breathlessness. This is an acute exacerbation of long-standing disease.

Tachycardia occurs as the autonomic system attempts to compensate for insufficient cardiac output by an increase in heart rate.

He is admitted to the coronary care unit for monitoring, intravenous diuretics and portable ECG to confirm the nature and severity of the left ventricular systolic dysfunction.

8.2 Chronic heart failure

Chronic HF is impaired ventricular filling and/or ejection with an onset over months to years. It is classified by:
- Time – acute versus chronic
- Anatomy – right versus left
- Physiology – systolic versus diastolic
- Aetiology – ischaemic versus non-ischaemic
- Genetics – inherited versus acquired
- Sequelae – low output versus high output

Anatomy – right versus left

Heart failure is categorised as to which side is affected. Congestive HF is when both sides are involved (i.e. biventricular HF). Rarely, isolated right ventricular failure occurs due to a massive pulmonary embolus or an inferior myocardial infarction.

Physiology – systolic versus diastolic

Heart failure is also categorised by ejection fraction as this reflects different pathophysiology and management:
- Heart failure with reduced ejection fraction represents a failure of systolic ejection function (50% patients)
- Heart failure with preserved ejection fraction (HFpEF) represents a failure of diastolic filling function (50% patients)

Functional classification: The New York Heart Association (NYHA) functional classification is useful to gauge the impact on the patient's life and monitor disease progress or improvement (**Table 8.2**).

Disease progression stages

The American College of Cardiology Foundation/American Heart Association (ACCF/AHA) 2013 guidelines provide criteria for staging HF disease progression (**Table 8.3**).

> **Clinical insight**
>
> Back pressure from left ventricular failure first affects the pulmonary system, causing pulmonary oedema. This leads eventually to right ventricular failure and backpressure in the systemic circulation.

Epidemiology

Heart failure affects about 1% of adults in Europe. Americans >40 years old have a 20% lifetime risk of developing HF. The average age of diagnosis is 76 years. HFrEF is more common in men and HFpEF in women.

Diagnosis is associated with a 5-year survival rate of 50%, which is worse than that for many cancers. HF is the most common cause of hospitalisation in over 65 years of age and is responsible for 5% of admissions.

Aetiology

Any significant mechanical, structural or electrical cardiac abnormality can cause HF (**Table 8.4**). Non-cardiac causes, such as haematological, endocrine, inflammatory, infective or malignant disease, increase physiological demand on the heart.

Class	Symptoms	Limitations	Example
I	None	None	Normal activity
II	Mild	Slight	Breathless on incline
III	Moderate	Moderate	Comfortable only at rest
IV	Severe	Severe	Breathless even at rest

Table 8.2 New York Heart Association (NYHA) functional classification of heart failure.

Chronic heart failure

Stage	Criteria	Example(s)
A	High risk without structural heart disease or symptoms	- Type 2 diabetes mellitus - Hypertension - Obesity - CHD - Family medical history
B	Structural heart disease without signs or symptoms	- Left ventricular hypertrophy - Previous myocardial infarction - Left ventricular systolic dysfunction
C	Structural heart disease with current or prior symptoms	Clinical HF
D	Refractory HF requiring specialist intervention	- Transplantation - Organ support - Palliation

Table 8.3 The American College of Cardiology Foundation/American Heart Association (ACCF/AHA) classification of the progression of the heart failure (HF).

Cause of heart failure	Example of underlying cause	Ventricle affected	Incidence
Vascular dysfunction	CHD	Left	Common
Rhythm disturbance	Atrial fibrillation	Both	Common
Valvular dysfunction	Mitral regurgitation	Left	Common
Lifestyle	Obesity	Left	Common
Pulmonary disease	Pulmonary embolus	Right	Intermediate
Idiopathic	Dilated cardiomyopathy	Both	Intermediate
Infective	Viral myocarditis	Both	Rare
Infiltrative diseases	Amyloidosis	Both	Rare

Table 8.4 Causes of heart failure. *Continues overleaf*

Cause of heart failure	Example of underlying cause	Ventricle affected	Incidence
Autoimmune disease	Hyperthyroidism	Both	Rare
Inherited	Atrial septal defect	Right	Rare
Drug adverse effect	Bleomycin chemotherapy	Both	Rare
Physiological state	Post-partum cardiomyopathy	Both	Rare

Table 8.4 *Continued*

> **Clinical insight**
>
> Encourage all cardiac patients to improve their lifestyle. Cardiovascular risk is reduced by stopping smoking, taking regular exercise and losing weight.

Heart failure with reduced ejection fraction: About 50% of HFrEF is a consequence of CHD, typically myocardial infarction. Non-ischaemic HFrEF are mostly due to idiopathic dilated cardiomyopathy secondary to toxic, metabolic, infectious, valvular or arrhythmic causes.

Heart failure with preserved ejection fraction

Heart failure with preserved ejection fraction typically arises from a combination of hypertension, CHD, type 2 diabetes mellitus and obesity.

Prevention

Primary prevention includes early recognition of and interventions to reduce cardiovascular risk factors, e.g. hypertension, type 2 diabetes mellitus, obesity and hypercholesterolaemia. The aim is to reduce the risk of myocardial infarction, which leads to HFrEF, and left ventricular hypertrophy (LVH), which leads to HFpEF.

Secondary prevention focusses on early recognition and intervention to reduce ischaemic injury and prevent adverse myocardial remodelling.

Chronic heart failure 293

Pathogenesis

Heart failure with reduced ejection fraction and HFpEF have different pathogenic mechanisms leading to distinct pathophysiology (**Figure 8.2**).

Heart failure with reduced ejection fraction: This is caused by an abnormality of systolic contraction, i.e. left ventricular systolic dysfunction. For example, myocardial infarction leads to cell death, tissue necrosis and scar formation. Scar tissue reduces stroke volume and disrupts the optimal length-tension relationship of the myocardium, according to the Frank–Starling law (**Figure 8.3**). In a healthy heart:
- Increasing venous return increases preload
- Increased myocardial stretch increases the number of actin-myosin interactions

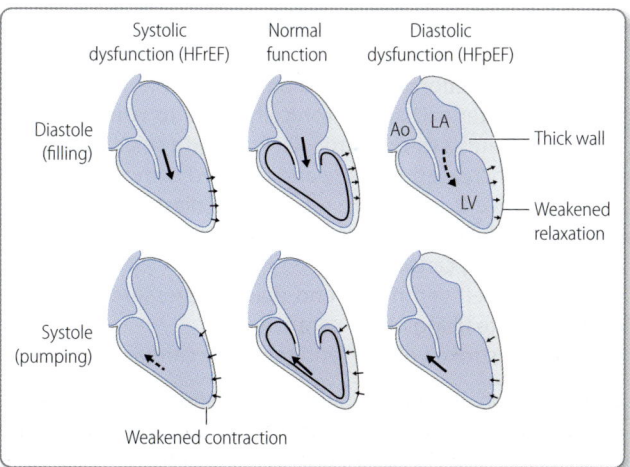

Figure 8.2 The pathophysiology of heart failure in the left atrium and ventricle. Heart failure with reduced ejection fraction (HFrEF) represents systolic dysfunction: reduced contraction of the heart during systole. Heart failure with preserved ejection fraction (HFpEF) represents diastolic dysfunction with reduced relaxation of the heart during diastole. Both lead to reduced stroke volume. Ao, aorta; LA, left atrium; LV, left ventricle.

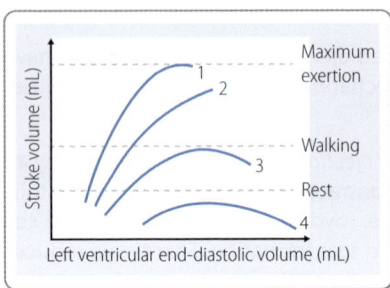

Figure 8.3 The Frank–Starling law. (1) healthy individual during exercise and (2) at rest; (3) heart failure; and (4) cardiogenic shock. Heart contractility (stroke volume) normally responds to increases in venous return (i.e. end-diastolic volume). This does not occur adequately in patients with heart failure.

- Increased end-diastolic volume
- Increased stroke volume

In the failing heart, after a certain point, the increased stretch only overstretches the myocardium beyond its optimum length-tension relationship, reducing its contractile force.

Heart failure with preserved ejection fraction: This is caused by an abnormality of myocardial relaxation, i.e. left ventricular diastolic dysfunction. Hypertension, for example, increases left ventricular afterload and chronically leads to compensatory LVH. This creates a thick ventricular wall and a small ventricular cavity. The increased stiffness and reduced compliance mean that the left ventricle fails to relax during diastole.

Myocardial fibrosis may also occur due to subclinical microvascular ischaemia, causing:
- Increased left ventricular end-diastolic pressure
- Inadequate filling of the ventricle
- Reduced stroke volume (and therefore cardiac output)

Compensation: Both HFrEF and HFpEF reduce cardiac output (**Figure 8.2**). This leads to up-regulation of the sympathetic nervous system and the renin–angiotensin–aldosterone system (RAAS), increasing cardiac output, total peripheral resistance, and blood pressure. This initially augments the failing heart to maintain perfusion, but once cardiac function deteriorates beyond a point, they hasten its decline (**Figure 8.4**).

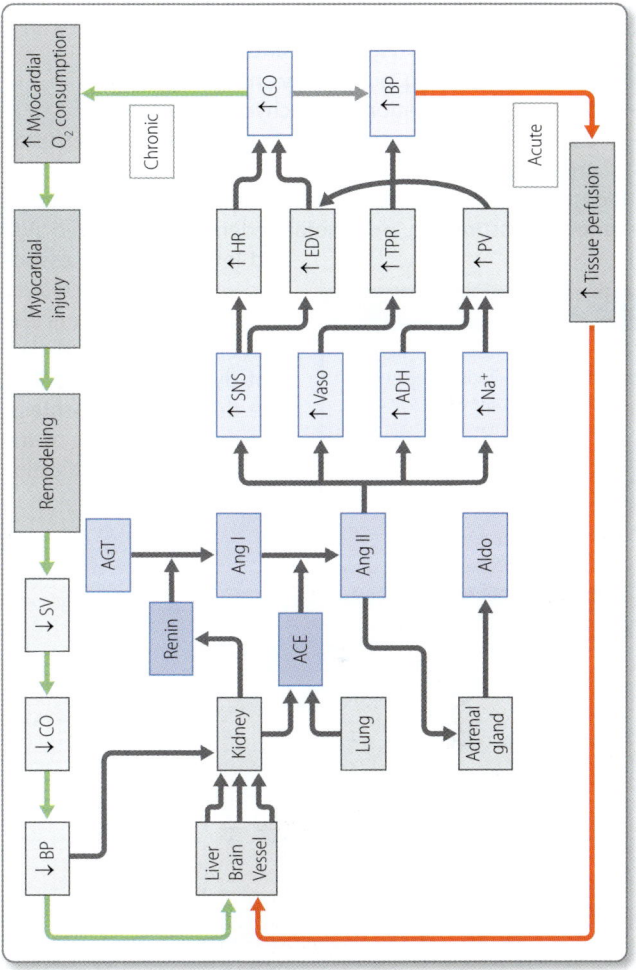

Figure 8.4 The pathophysiology of heart failure. ACE, angiotensin-converting enzyme; ADH, antidiuretic hormone; AGT, angiotensinogen; Aldo, aldosterone; Ang I, angiotensin I; Ang II, angiotensin II; BP, blood pressure; CO, cardiac output; EDV, end-diastolic volume; HR, heart rate; PV, plasma volume; SNS, sympathetic nervous system; SV, stroke volume; TPR, total peripheral resistance; Vaso, vasoconstriction.

Clinical features

Patients present with (**Figure 8.5** and **Table 8.5**):
- Fluid retention, e.g. pulmonary and ankle oedema
- Signs of compensation, e.g. tachycardia
- Cachexia due to a catabolic state, reduced tissue perfusion and inflammation

Right-sided HF is associated with features of raised systemic venous pressure (e.g. peripheral oedema and elevated JVP) and left-sided HF is associated with increased left atrial and pulmonary pressure (e.g. pulmonary oedema and resultant dyspnoea) (**Table 8.6**). The degree of breathlessness is a key aspect of the NYHA functional classification (**Table 8.2**).

> **Clinical insight**
>
> *Non-cardiogenic pulmonary oedema* is caused by, high altitude, decreased plasma oncotic pressure as a result of low albumin and increased alveolar capillary permeability in acute respiratory distress syndrome.

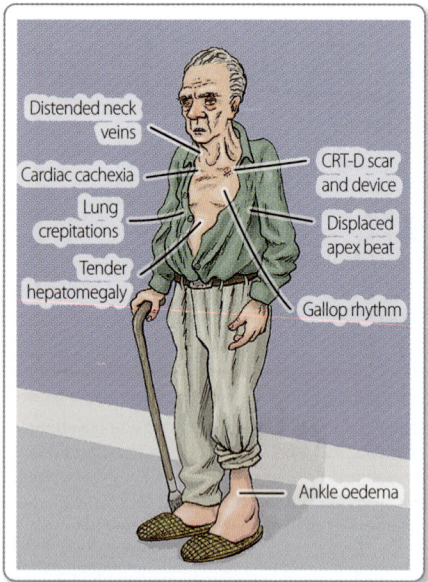

Figure 8.5 Common signs of heart failure.

Clinical features	Sensitivity (%)	Specificity (%)
Symptom		
Orthopnoea	21	81
Oedema	23	80
Paroxysmal nocturnal dyspnoea	33	76
Dyspnoea	66	52
Signs		
Tachycardia	7	99
Raised jugular venous pressure	10	97
Third heart sound	31	95
Peripheral oedema	10	93

Table 8.5 Clinical features of heart failure and their sensitivity and specificity.

Symptom or sign	Right-sided heart failure	Left-sided heart failure
Peripheral oedema	Prominent	Not prominent
Oedema	Systemic	Pulmonary
Organomegaly	Liver	Cardiac
Raised jugular venous pressure	Prominent	Not prominent
Dyspnoea	Not prominent	Prominent
Gastrointestinal	Prominent	Not prominent

Table 8.6 Clinical features of right-sided and left-sided heart failure.

Investigations

All patients require blood tests, ECG, chest X-ray and echocardiography. Exercise tests are also commonly performed to inform management and prognosis.

Coronary angiography may also be done to assess for CHD, the most common cause of HFrEF.

Blood tests: Blood tests are performed to rule out other causes of breathlessness, e.g. anaemia, and assess severity – brain natriuretic peptide (BNP) is a marker of disease severity (**Table 8.7**).

Electrocardiography: Common abnormalities seen on ECG include:
- **Coronary heart disease:** Q waves, T wave inversion, prolonged QRS [i.e. bundle branch block (BBB)]
- Left ventricular hypertrophy, especially in HFpEF
- Prolonged QRS duration (i.e. BBB) - a marker of severity
- **Arrhythmias:** Atrial fibrillation and paroxysmal ventricular arrhythmias

Chest X-ray: Chest X-ray may show (**Figures 8.1** and **8.6**):
- Pleural effusions of fluid accumulating between the layers of pleura
- Kerley B lines from fluid accumulating between the interlobular septa
- Bilateral perihilar markings (classically batwing-shaped) from the collection of alveolar fluid
- Upper zone venous vessel enlargement from pulmonary venous hypertension
- **Cardiomegaly:** Increased cardiothoracic ratio (>50%)

Blood test	Assessing for
Full blood count	Anaemia or infection
Urea and electrolytes	Renal failure
Liver function tests	Liver failure
Thyroid function tests	Thyroid disease
Lipid profile	Hypercholesterolaemia
Glucose	Diabetes mellitus
Natriuretic peptides	Disease severity

Table 8.7 Blood tests in patients with suspected heart failure.

Chronic heart failure

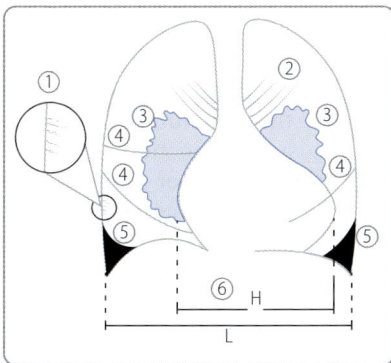

Figure 8.6 Chest X-ray features of heart failure: (1) Kerley B lines (2) upper lobe venous diversion (3) ill-defined peri-hilar (batwing) shadowing (4) fluid in the oblique and horizontal fissures (5) pleural effusions, and (6) increased cardiothoracic ratio, where the width of the heart shadow (H) is >50% of the width of the lung (L) fields.

Echocardiography: Echocardiography is performed on diagnosis to:
- Measure the ejection fraction and distinguish HFrEF and HFpEF
- Assess valves
- Measure chambers
- Identify LVH. An echocardiogram showing normal systolic function does not exclude HF. There may still be:
  – Valve disease
  – Diastolic dysfunction
  – Pericardial disease
  – High-output HF

> **Clinical insight**
>
> Patients can be shocked by a diagnosis of heart failure, particularly by the term 'failure'. Conversely, if their symptoms are mild, some may not comprehend the seriousness of the diagnosis.

Magnetic resonance imaging: Cardiac magnetic resonance imaging (MRI) can provide high-resolution structural and functional assessment of:
- Ventricular volumes
- Wall thickness
- Chamber dimensions
- Ventricular systolic functions
- Myocardial ischaemia

- Myocardial scarring
- Infiltrative disease.

> **Clinical insight**
>
> An increased concentration of brain natriuretic protein (>400 pg/mL) strongly suggests heart failure. BNP is released by myocardium in response to stretch. It increases renal natriuresis and causes vasodilation, thereby decreasing blood pressure.

Exercise tests: These include the 6-minute walk test to assess functional capacity and monitor progress, and cardiopulmonary exercise testing to assess exercise capacity, inform prognosis and assess the need for heart transplantation.

Management

Lifestyle modification, medication and device therapy aim to:
- Treat the cause
- Reduce symptoms
- Reduce aggravating factors
- Improve prognosis and quality of life

Key evidence-based therapy recommendations of the 2013 ACCF/AHA guidelines are shown in **Table 8.8**.

Stage	Recommended therapy
A	Control HTN and dyslipidaemia in accordance with HTN guidelines to lower HF risk
	Control other risk factors: Obesity, diabetes, and smoking
B	ACEI (ARB or Entresto - ARNI if ACEI not tolerated) + β-blocker + SGLT-2 inhibitors (empagliflozin or dapagliflozin) + mineralocorticoid antagonists (spironolactone or eplerenone) for patients with: • Reduced EF + previous ACS or MI (↓ HF symptoms, ↓ mortality) • Reduced EF without previous MI (↓ HF symptoms)
	Statins for patients with: • ACS history (↓ HF symptoms, ↓ CV events)

Table 8.8 Key treatment recommendations for heart failure stages A to D: treatments with class I evidence in the 2013 American College of Cardiology Foundation/American Heart Association (ACCF/AHA) heart failure guidelines. *Continues overleaf*

Stage		Recommended therapy
		BP control in accordance with HTN guidelines for patients with: • Structural heart changes and no ACS history (↓ HF symptoms)
C		Specific patient education to self-manage HF care
		Exercise training is safe to improve functional status
		Long-term anticoagulant therapy in patients with AF and another cardioembolic risk factor (HTN, diabetes, CVA history, and ≥75 years). Choice of agent depends on patient's clinical profile
	HFrEF	Pharmacological measures as listed for A and B (4 morbidity and 4 mortality), i.e. ACEI (or ARB) + β-blocker + SGLT-2 inhibitors (empagliflozin or dapagliflozin) + mineralocorticoid antagonists (spironolactone or eplerenone) if needed: • Loop diuretic if volume overloaded in NYHA class II–IV • Hydralazine + nitrate if still symptomatic African-American and NYHA class III–IV IV iron therapy – if ferritin is <100 ng/mL or if ferritin is between 100 and 299 along with a transferrin saturation < 20%. For symptomatic benefit.
		ICD therapy (4 mortality from sudden cardiac death) in patients with HREF at >40 days after MI and: • Non-ischaemic dilated cardiomyopathy or CHD, with both LVEF ≤ 35% and NYHA class II or III symptoms • LVEF ≤ 30% and NYHA class I
		Cardiac resynchronisation therapy for patients with LVEF ≤ 35%, LBBB with QRS ≥ 150 ms and NYHA class II, III or ambulatory IV symptoms
	HFpEF	Systolic and diastolic BP control
		• SGLT-2 inhibitors: Empagliflozin and dapagliflozin • Diuretics to relieve volume overload symptoms
D		Treat cardiogenic shock with IV inotropic support until definitive treatment
		Cardiac transplantation

ACEI, angiotensin-converting enzyme inhibitor; ACS, acute coronary syndrome; AF, atrial fibrillation; ARB, angiotensin II receptor blocker; CHD, coronary heart disease; CKD, chronic kidney disease; CVA, cerebrovascular accident; EF, ejection fraction; HFpEF, heart failure with preserved ejection fraction; HFrEF, heart failure with reduced ejection fraction; HTN, hypertension; ICD, implantable cardioverter-defibrillator; LBBB, left bundle branch block; LVEF, left ventricular ejection fraction; MI, myocardial infarction; NYHA, New York Heart Association; SGLT-2, sodium-glucose cotransporter-2.

Table 8.8 Continued

Lifestyle modification

All patients should be encouraged to:
- **Exercise:** A tailored rehabilitation program of structured aerobic exercise is safe in stable patients, improves functional capacity, quality of life and reduces morbidity
- Moderate alcohol intake; abstain in alcohol cardiomyopathy
- Quit smoking
- Restrict fluid (to <1.5 L/day) and salt (to <6 g/day) intake to minimise fluid retention symptoms. Advise patients to monitor their weight and seek medical advice if it increases >2 kg in 2 days
- **Receive vaccinations:** Influenza (yearly) and pneumococcus (once)

Patients should be made aware of driving restrictions.

> **Clinical insight**
>
> Heart failure is a syndrome not a diagnosis. The underlying cause must be investigated and treated.

Medication

Medications can improve symptoms, prognosis and target underlying cause.

Heart failure with reduced ejection fraction: First-line treatment for all patients is a β-blocker, an angiotensin-converting enzyme (ACE) inhibitor, SGLT-2 inhibitors (empagliflozin or dapagliflozin) + Mineralocorticoid antagonists (spironolactone or eplerenone). Patients are started on low doses and titrated until stable. Long-term monitoring is performed in primary care.

A diuretic is prescribed in proportion to symptoms to relieve fluid retention and congestion. Patients should be monitored for renal function and electrolyte derangement when dosages are started or changed.

Digoxin is used to control heart rate in patients with atrial fibrillation or advanced HF.

Heart failure with preserved ejection fraction: SGLT-2 inhibitors – empagliflozin and dapagliflozin. Treatment, therefore, involves aggressive management of underlying hypertension, diabetes, weight control and lipid control.

Diuretics reduce symptoms of fluid retention and β-blockers reduce heart rate and increase diastole.

Devices

Cardiac resynchronisation therapy and implantable cardioverter defibrillators improve prognosis for HFrEF patients whose heart chambers contract dyssynchronously or who are prone to life-threatening ventricular arrhythmias.

> **Clinical insight**
>
> Depression is common in patients with heart failure and generally correlates with disease severity. Physicians need to directly ascertain if patients are depressed, as outcomes are worse in patients with untreated depression.

Surgical management

Primary valve disease indicates valve repair or replacement, and CABG is indicated in those with severe CHD. Patients with severe symptoms despite medical therapy (i.e. NYHA class 3 or 4) may be considered for:
- Mitral valve repair for mitral regurgitation – surgical or mitral valve clip
- Left ventricular restoration
- Insertion of a left ventricular assist device (**Figure 8.7**)
- Heart transplantation - the only curative option

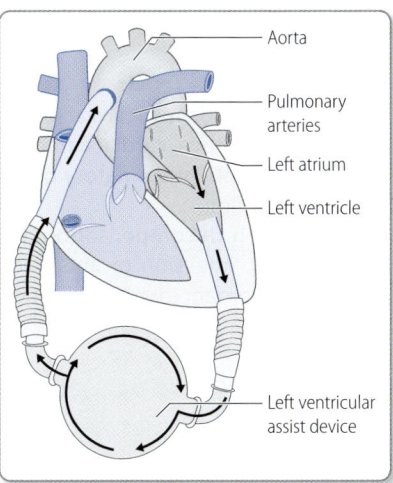

Figure 8.7 A left ventricular assist device in situ.

Heart transplantation is contraindicated in the elderly, renal failure, irreversible pulmonary arterial hypertension and other severe non-cardiac disease.

Prognosis

The prognosis for chronic HF is worse than the prognosis for many cancers. Around 35% of patients with a new diagnosis will die within 12 months, and approximately 50% in 5 years.

Severely symptomatic (NYHA class 4 or ACCF/AHA stage D) patients with a poor prognosis likely require palliative care.

8.3 Acute heart failure

Chronic HF symptoms appear slowly over time and worsen gradually. In acute HF, symptoms develop suddenly and are initially severe.

65% have acute-on-chronic HF, 30% have new (de novo) disease, and 5% are nearing the end of their life.

Epidemiology

Patients are typically in their mid-70s. Half of cases have HFrEF, and half have HFpEF. Two-thirds of patients are known to have CHD, and one-third have diabetes, chronic kidney disease, COPD or atrial fibrillation.

Aetiology

Common causes of de novo failure include myocardial infarction, acute valvular dysfunction, arrhythmia, cardiac tamponade, medications [e.g. non-steroidal anti-inflammatory drugs (NSAIDs)], IV fluids or thyroid dysfunction.

Acute-on-chronic HF occurs with decompensation, for example, due to severe illness (e.g. infection or anaemia), negatively inotropic drugs, non-concordance with medication or thyroid dysfunction.

Prevention

Prevention measures include:
- Adequate monitoring

- Ensuring medication concordance
- Detecting and treating arrhythmia early
- Managing intercurrent illnesses (e.g. pneumonia) or comorbidities aggressively

Clinical features

Patients present with fatigue, oedema, cough, breathlessness and severe orthopnoea.

Signs include tachycardia, tachypnoea, hypertension (**Table 8.9**) and a third heart sound. Signs of fluid status and tissue perfusion are used to guide treatment (**Table 8.10**). An elevated JVP and peripheral oedema are commonly seen and reflect right-sided decompensation.

Severe presentations are usually a result of left-sided failure causing severe pulmonary oedema, evident as reduced oxygen saturations and inspiratory crepitations.

Blood pressure	Prevalence (% of cases)	Presentation
High (>150 mmHg)	50	Symptoms with abrupt onset (hours or days)
Normal (120–149 mmHg)	40	Symptoms with gradual onset (days or weeks)
Low (91–119 mmHg)	9	Hypoperfusion
Very low (<90 mmHg)	1	Cardiogenic shock

Table 8.9 Blood pressure in patients with acute and severe de novo heart failure.

Haemodynamic state	Treatment
Wet and cold	Vasodilators and additional diuretics
Wet and warm	Diuretics and additional vasodilators
Cold and dry	Inotropes and intra-aortic balloon pump
Warm and dry	The aim for all patients with heart failure

Table 8.10 Treatment of patients with acute heart failure in various haemodynamic and clinical states.

Investigations

All acutely ill patients are assessed using resuscitation guidelines (e.g. the ABCDE approach) to prioritise treatment.

Investigations are the same as for suspected chronic HF, but with an emphasis on urgent echocardiography (where available) if the diagnosis is unknown.

ECG changes are usually non-specific, but chest X-ray will demonstrate pulmonary oedema (**Figure 8.1**).

> **Clinical insight**
>
> In cardiogenic shock the heart is unable to pump enough blood for the body's basic needs. It is defined as SBP < 90 mmHg in the presence of low urine output, poor peripheral perfusion, confusion or lactate > 2.0 mmol/L.

> **Clinical insight**
>
> Breathless patients with normal oxygen saturation (94–98%) are not given oxygen as there is no evidence of benefit.

Management

Management is determined by haemodynamic state and clinical stage (**Table 8.10**). Once stable, therapy for chronic HF is started.

Medication: Initial management, ideally in a coronary care unit or high-dependency unit, includes: Wet, signs of fluid overload; dry, absence of these; cold, signs of reduced tissue perfusion; warm, absence of these.

- Intravenous loop diuretic to remove excess fluid
- Intravenous morphine to reduce stress and to venodilate
- Intravenous glyceryl trinitrate to vasodilate and accommodate excess fluid
- Cessation of administration of inappropriate drugs (e.g. NSAIDs)
- Inotropes to augment cardiac output where a reversible cause of cardiogenic shock is identified

Non-pharmacological management: Initial management also includes:

- Sitting patient up
- Stop IV fluids (except in acute right ventricular failure)
- Oxygen if hypoxic (saturations < 94%)

- Continuous positive airway pressure (CPAP) ventilation in patients with pulmonary oedema and significant dyspnoea and hypoxia
- **Monitoring of fluid balance:** Urea, electrolytes, urine output and body weight
- Fluid intake restricted to <1.5 L/day
- Invasive ventilation if respiratory failure occurs

Prevention of cardiovascular disease

chapter 9

Despite decreasing mortality attributable to cardiovascular disease (CVD) in the developed world, the global incidence is increasing. This is due to both increasing incidence in the developing world and ageing populations. Coronary heart disease (CHD) is the most preventable form of CVD and has become the primary cause of global morbidity and mortality. CVD encompasses a wide variety of congenital and acquired conditions, including peripheral artery disease, diseases of aorta, cerebrovascular disease, and heart disease. Atherosclerotic CVD is a subset of CVD caused by atherosclerosis, including CHD, atherosclerotic cerebrovascular, aortic and peripheral artery disease.

Primary prevention is intervention before atherosclerotic disease is clinically evident. This focusses on diet, lifestyle education, management plans and medical interventions to lower cardiovascular risk factors. Atherosclerosis can be slowed and even reversed by changes in diet and lifestyle. However, recent evidence suggests health promotion via counselling and education produces only mild reductions in risk factors, with marginal impact on CHD morbidity and mortality. The main benefit is seen in high-risk hypertensive and diabetic patients.

Secondary prevention is aimed at the early detection and treatment of all atherosclerotic disease. Peripheral vascular disease is under-recognised as a forerunner and comorbidity of CHD.

9.1 Preventive measures

Calculating cardiovascular risk

Primary prevention hinges on an assessment of cardiovascular risk. Risk factors are categorised as non-modifiable, modifiable and emerging (lipid and inflammatory markers) (**Table 9.1**). Most are atherogenic, i.e. they increase the amount or rate of atherosclerosis in arteries. The three major modifiable

Class	Risk factors
Modifiable	Smoking, physical inactivity, atherogenic diet, BMI ≥ 25 kg/m^2, hypertension (e.g. BP > 140/90 mmHg), hyperlipidaemia (e.g. total cholesterol < 5 mmol/L/190 mg/dL) and stress
Non-modifiable	Age, sex and family history/genetic
Emerging	C-reactive protein, fibrinogen, homocysteine, arterial calcification and lipoprotein(a)

BMI, body mass index; BP, blood pressure.

Table 9.1 Cardiovascular risk factors.

> **Clinical insight**
>
> C-reactive protein (CRP) is an acute phase protein produced by the liver and correlates with levels of systemic inflammation. Atherosclerosis is a systemic inflammatory and metabolic disease.

factors are smoking, hyperlipidaemia and hypertension. Modifiable risk factors account for approximately 50–70% of CVD events and deaths worldwide. They may also account for up to 90% of the population attributable risk of first acute myocardial infarction (MI) and stroke.

Risk score calculators (e.g. www.qrisk.org) use data from large population studies to predict the risk of a future cardiovascular event. Most report a person's 10-year risk; 20% or over is usually considered high risk and indicates primary prevention strategies should be adopted.

Risk calculations are used to guide treatment intensity and monitor progress. As many interventions are behavioural, it is essential to promote patient understanding and involvement in setting and making risk calculation targets.

Patients who are already high-risk, and therefore unsuitable for many risk calculators, include those over 75 years or with proven:
- Atherosclerosis
- Hypertension
- Type 1 or 2 diabetes mellitus

- Renal dysfunction
- Inherited dyslipidaemia

Risk factor reduction

Interventions aim to reduce modifiable risk factors:
- Smoking cessation
- Physical activity – at least 30 minutes, five times a week
- Healthy eating
- Maintain a healthy body weight (BMI < 25 kg/m^2)
- Blood pressure < 140/90 mmHg
- Total cholesterol < 5 mmol/L (190 mg/dL)
- Normal glucose metabolism
- Avoidance of stress
- Antiplatelet medication (e.g. aspirin)

Primary interventions should begin with diet and weight decrease, an increase in physical activity and smoking cessation.

Behavioural change

Shared decision-making interventions and motivational interviewing can help to guide and prioritise cardiovascular risk reduction strategies. There are three levels to encouraging behavioural change in patients:

1. *Brief advice:* Opportunistic conversation raising patient's awareness and assessing their desire to change
2. *Brief interventions:* Structured advice providing more formal help, e.g. arranging targets and follow-up
3. Motivational interviewing to examine their motivation and help them to act. This involves listening and patient-centred counselling skills that support patients to explore their ambivalence about changing their health-related behaviours (**Figure 9.1**).

Smoking

Smoking is decreasing in much of the developed world, but still increasing in the developing world. It is the leading preventable cause of CVD. Smoking causes nearly 20,000 deaths from CVD in the UK every year. The risk of heart attack is up to four times greater and the risk of stroke up to two times

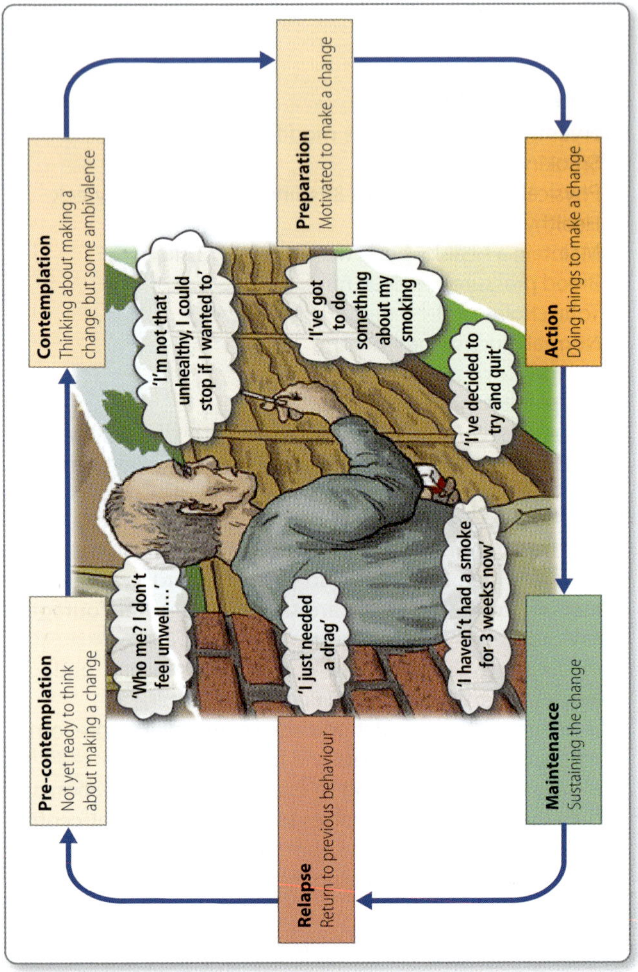

Figure 9.1 Motivational interviewing as informed by Prochaska and DiClemente's model of behavioural change. This example concerns smoking cessation, but the theory is applicable to any behaviour.

greater for smokers. Smoking even a few cigarettes daily is associated with an increased risk of stroke and MI.

Smoking is atherogenic as it causes endothelial cell dysfunction, an increase in platelet and macrophage adherence to the endothelium, is prothrombotic and proinflammatory, and it induces tissue remodelling.

Smoking cessation is proven to be beneficial in established atherosclerosis as stopping smoking can lead to a reduction in the atherosclerotic burden. After 1 year of not smoking, the excess risk of CHD falls to 50% of that of current smokers. After 15 years, the risks of heart failure, CHD, and stroke resemble those of a non-smoker. Over 8% of all smoking-related deaths are due to second-hand smoke exposure. Smoking cessation is also effective in secondary prevention, with significant reduction in 5-year mortality post-MI or in patients with known CHD.

Physical activity

A sedentary lifestyle is associated with urbanisation and a western lifestyle. It increases coagulopathy, decreases cardiovascular fitness, and is associated with depression, obesity, type 2 diabetes mellitus, and metabolic syndrome. More than 5 million deaths worldwide are attributed to physical inactivity. In the UK alone, it causes one in 10 premature deaths from CHD, and one in six deaths overall. More than 20 million adults in the UK are failing to meet Government guidelines for physical activity, and that women are 36% more likely to be considered physically inactive than men.

A common goal is 30–60 minutes of exercise of sufficient intensity to cause shortness of breath, 3–5 times a week. Secondary prevention often requires detailed programmes and medical supervision for high-risk patients.

Adequate sleep

Inadequate sleep is an independent risk factor for CVD events. All individuals should aim for a habitual sleep duration of 7–8 hours nightly. Inadequate sleep duration has been associated with an increased risk of MI and increased incidence of CVD risk factors and subclinical non-coronary atherosclerotic plaque burden, although limited evidence exists to confirm that improving sleep duration or quality reduces CVD events.

Diet

An unhealthy diet is atherogenic due to high fat and salt intake and is associated with being overweight or obese, and with type 2 diabetes mellitus and metabolic syndrome. A healthy diet is therefore the cornerstone of CVD prevention.

Specific diet education and plans may be needed (**Table 9.2**), though exact recommendations vary. A healthy cardiovascular diet includes daily whole grains, nuts, unsaturated fats, fruit and vegetables, fish and moderate (1–2 units) alcohol intake.

Component	ESC recommendation	AHA/ACC recommendation
Saturated fatty acids	<10% calories	5–6% calories
Trans-unsaturated fatty acids	As little as possible	Reduce
Salt	<5 g/day	Reduce (e.g. <2.4 g/day if hypertensive)
Fibre	30–45 g/day	Diet emphasises intake of vegetables, fruits, and whole grains; includes low-fat dairy products, poultry, fish, legumes, non-tropical vegetable oils, and nuts; with limited intake of sweets, sugar-sweetened beverages, and red meat
Fruit	200 g/day (2–3 servings)	
Vegetables	200 g/day (2–3 servings)	
Fish	Twice a week (≥1 oily)	
Alcohol	♀ ≤1 glass (20 g)/day ♂ ≤2 glasses (20 g)/day	Average of: ♀ ≤1 glass (20 g)/day ♂ ≤2 glasses (20 g)/day

Table 9.2 Guidelines for diet proportions to prevent cardiovascular disease. Based on the European Society of Cardiology (ESC) 2012 guidelines and the American Heart Association/American College of Cardiology (AHA/ACC) 2014 guidelines.

Adherence to Mediterranean-style or plant-based diets offer optimal cardiovascular benefit.

Weight

Obesity is approaching global epidemic proportions. It is associated with CVD, hypertension, type 2 diabetes mellitus, metabolic syndrome, dyslipidaemia, raised inflammatory markers, certain cancers, Alzheimer's disease and sleep apnoea. Although commonly measured in BMI, central obesity, i.e. an increased waist-to-hip circumference or waist-to-weight ratio, is a stronger risk factor for CHD (**Table 9.3**).

Blood pressure

Hypertension is the most common risk factor for CVD and should be screened for whenever possible. The increased stress on arterial walls increases arterial damage, inflammation and atherogenesis. A reduction in diastolic blood pressure by 6 mmHg leads to a 15% decrease in CHD

> **Clinical insight**
>
> Garlic slightly lowers cholesterol, inhibits platelet aggregation and may lower blood pressure.

Weight	BMI (kg/m^2)	CHD risk	
		Waist circumference ≤ 102 cm/≤88 cm	Waist circumference > 102 cm/>88 cm
Underweight	<18.5	...	...
Normal	18.5–24.9	...	...
Overweight	25.0–29.9	↑	↑↑
Obesity, class I	30.0–34.9	↑↑	↑↑↑
Class II	35.0–39.9	↑↑↑	↑↑↑
Class III	≥40	↑↑↑↑	↑↑↑↑
BMI, body mass index.			

Table 9.3 The increased risk of coronary heart disease (CHD) in overweight and obese people.

> **Clinical insight**
>
> The metabolic syndrome includes any three of:
> 1. Abdominal obesity
> 2. Low high-density lipoprotein (HDL)
> 3. Hypertension
> 4. Fasting hyperglycaemia
> 5. Hypertriglyceridaemia
>
> Its prevalence in the US is >20% of persons ≥20 years old and >40% of those >40 years.

risk, and a 42% decrease in cerebrovascular accident risk. Isolated systolic hypertension is also a major risk factor for IHD.

Recommended targets are <140/90 mmHg or <130/80 mmHg in chronic kidney disease.

Self-monitoring and management of hypertension is important in primary and secondary prevention of CHD. Central to this is clear communication with patients and support from medical professionals.

Therapy targets the patient's cardiovascular risk score, blood pressure and evidence of end-organ damage guide management.

Salt reduction initiatives: Population-wide programmes to reduce salt intake are considered one of the simplest and most cost-effective ways to reduce blood pressure and improve global public health. They involve food industry regulations and package labelling. Most countries with salt reduction programmes have maximum intake targets of 5–8 g/day. The average intake in the UK, e.g. in 2011 was 8.1 g/day. It is estimated by the Consensus Action on Salt and Health (CASH) in the UK that a reduction to 6 g/day would decrease the average risk of MI by 16% and cerebrovascular accident risk by 22%.

Lipids

High levels of low-density lipoprotein (LDL) cholesterol are atherogenic. Elevated triglycerides also increase risk. Screening or investigation of CHD involves a full fasting lipid profile. A key risk indicator appears to be the ratio of total or LDL cholesterol to high-density lipoprotein (HDL).

Familial hypercholesterolaemia: Familial hypercholesterolaemia should be excluded if the patient has a strong family history of premature CHD. It is an autosomal dominant inherited disorder of cholesterol metabolism. It is undiagnosed in as many as 90% of patients because cholesterol is often not checked in people under 40 years of age.

Early identification with a simple fasting lipid blood test is important to allow prompt treatment. All patients with definite, possible or suspected familial hyperlipidaemia are referred to a specialist centre for diagnosis and management.

Therapy targets: Therapy aims to decrease LDL cholesterol and increase HDL cholesterol. This is achieved by medication (statins in the first instance), a healthy diet and increase in physical activity. Most recent guidelines do not recommend specific treatment targets for primary prevention, but recommend assessing the individual patient's clinical findings, lipid profile and family history. The European Society of Cardiology 2011 targets are already given, (Chapter 5, Hyperlipidaemia, Table 5.5).

The UK's National Institute for Health and Care Excellence (NICE) recommends a target LDL of <1.4 mmol/L (<~100 mg/dL) in secondary prevention.

Statins: Statins exert their effects in the liver and are very effective at lowering LDL cholesterol. They are uniformly prescribed to patients with CHD, regardless of starting cholesterol level, because they reduce cardiac events and total mortality. If a single agent does not control lipid levels, combination therapy is required.

> **Clinical insight**
>
> Statin side effects include myositis (i.e. muscle aches), rhabdomyolysis, and moderate or severe liver dysfunction.

Diabetes

Uncontrolled diabetes is a pro-inflammatory and pro-infective state. A person with diabetes has a two-fold greater absolute risk of CVD than a non-diabetic.

It is atherogenic due to glucose disruption of structural proteins, largely via the formation of advanced glycation end-products: permanent bonding to and disruption of proteins [e.g. haemoglobin A1c (HbA1c)]. This includes structural proteins of small vessels (i.e. microvascular disease) and the walls of larger arteries, which promotes atherosclerosis–macrovascular diabetic disease.

Coronary heart disease prevention in diabetic patients requires aggressive management of diabetes mellitus and of all cardiovascular risk factors: weight management, physical activity, blood pressure and cholesterol. Targets are often lower than for non-diabetics.

Stress

Although there is mixed evidence on the link between stress and CHD, there is a strong association with depression, social isolation and poor social support.

Chronic neurohormonal activation increases heart rate and blood pressure: life events, work stress, anxiety, type A personality traits. Consistently raised cortisol inhibits immune housekeeping function, which can promote arterial wall damage. In western cultures, stress is also associated with poor diet, low socioeconomic status, smoking, increased alcohol intake and lack of physical activity.

Acute stress and anxiety can promote arrhythmias, a pro-thrombotic state and an CHD event in established disease.

Aspirin

Aspirin decreases the risk of a first MI by a quarter to a third. Primary prevention in those with a 10% 10-year risk involves low dose (e.g. 75 mg) aspirin. It is also beneficial in secondary prevention of MI and ischaemic stroke.

The increased risk of gastrointestinal or cerebrovascular bleeding must be considered.

9.2 Secondary prevention/cardiac rehabilitation

Secondary intervention includes regular blood pressure checks, monitoring of fasting lipids, and diet and lifestyle advice, as well as medications including aspirin, statins, angiotensin-converting enzyme (ACE) inhibitors, and β-blockers.

Cardiac rehabilitation provides continued information and support to achieve the many lifestyle modifications required after a heart attack. Patients can meet in groups over a period of several weeks and are given a supervised exercise programme. This allows them to meet other people who have been through the same experience and to regain confidence in getting back to a full and active lifestyle. Use of expert patient or patient forum services can also be a valuable source of information and support.

Management of stable angina

Stable angina represents stable CHD. All patients with new onset of chest pain with a possible ischaemic cause are referred for further investigation. In the interim, patients should be immediately started on aspirin 75 mg once daily, and should undergo the following investigations:
- ECG to look for evidence of ischaemia
- Fasting lipid profile
- Haemoglobin A1c

Secondary prevention is started as soon as possible. Many patients require a lipid-lowering agent, preferably a statin (these drugs are thought to have pleiotropic effects). If a patient has angina attacks more than twice a week, regular anti-anginal medication is started and the patient is referred to a cardiologist for further assessment.

Index

Note: Page numbers in **bold** or *italic* refer to tables or figures respectively.

A

Abdomen 120
Abdominal aorta *21*, 104
    branches of **21**
Abdominal bruit 201
Abdominal examination 287
Abdominal ultrasound 138
Abnormal dilations 166
Accelerated idioventricular rhythm 244
Acetyl carrier protein 73
Acetyl coenzyme A 75
    carboxylase activity, regulation of *75*
    synthesis 72
Acidosis 257
Acute coronary syndrome 233, 235, 236, 301
    diagnosis of **237**
    types 235
Acute kidney injury 202
Acute limb ischaemia, symptoms of 170
Adductor longus *121*
Adenosine 156
Adenosine
    diphosphate 65, *66*, 71, *75*, 126, *153*
    monophosphate *71*, *75*
        cyclic 50
    triphosphate *38*, 50, *71*, 75, *75*, *78*, 126
Adequate sleep 313
Adrenal glands *21*
Adrenal steroids 211
Adrenal vessels 21
Adrenocorticotropic hormone 200
Aerobic exercise, regular 181
Alcohol 147
    unit of 147
Aldosterone 63, *295*
Aldosterone-blocking diuretic 197

Aldosterone–renin ratio 201
Allergy history 100
Alpha-blocker 159
    doxazosin 197
Amiloride 197
Amiodarone 156, 259, 277, 283
Amphetamines 101
Amyloid disease 252
Amyloidosis 262
Analgesics 242, 243
Angina 90, *91*, 92, 94, 207, 227, 230, **234,** 237
    managing 241
Angiotensin 160, *295*
    receptor blockers 161, *161*, *196*, 233, 301
Angiotensin-converting enzyme *196*, 233, *295*
    inhibitors 159, 196, 197, 242, 243, 301, 302, 319
        mechanism of action of *161*
Angiotensinogen *295*
Ankle
    oedema 104
        causes of **98**
    swelling 95
Ankle-brachial pressure index 136
Anterior tibial
    artery *121*
    tendon *121*
Anti-anginal medication **163**
Anti-arrhythmic medication **155**
Anticoagulant 151, **152**
    novel oral 153, 283
Anticoagulation 282
    systems 67
Antidiuretic hormone 61, *157*, *295*
Antidote 152
Anti-inflammatory medications 248

Index

Antiplatelet
    and antithrombotic therapy 242
    drugs 153
        mechanism of action of *153*
    medication 154
    therapy 243
Antithrombins 68
Anxiety 318
Aorta *139, 143, 293*
    arch of *3*
    ascending *139*
    descending *3, 139*
Aortic annulus *139*
Aortic arches 27
Aortic coarctation 200
Aortic dissection 91, 202
Aortic regurgitation 116, 118
Aortic root 8
Aortic stenosis 116, 118
Aortic valve *6, 8, 115, 139, 143*
Aortography 144
Apex beat 114
    abnormalities of 116
Apolipoprotein 80-82, *84, 85,* 86
    B 212
    functions of 81
Arachidonate 74
Arrhythmia 96, 237, 244, 249, 255, **255,** 256, *257,* 298, 304
    detect 136
    electrical evidence of 238
    mechanism of 252, 276
    pathophysiological mechanisms of *257*
    temporary 166
Arterial bypass 164
Arterial coronary artery bypass grafts **165**
Arterial development 26
Arterial dominance 12
Arterial graft 165
Arterial pulse 103, 107
Arterial repair 166
Arterial supply 9
Arterial tree, first vessels in *57*
Arterial ulcers *120*
Arterioles 16, *17*
Artery
    arcuate *121*
    circumflex *10*
    diagonal *10*
    elastic 16, *57*
    facial *19*
    left anterior descending *10,* 11
    lingual *19*
    maxillary *19*
    obtuse marginal *10*
    occipital *19*
    popliteal 120, *121*
    suprascapular *19*
    vertebral *19*
Ascites 104
Aspirin 234, 243, 318, 319
Assessment tools 146
Asthma 94
Asystole 246
Atenolol 156
Atherogenesis 174
    initiation of 176
    level of 210
Atheroma
    debris deposits of 173
    degree of 172
Atherosclerosis 21, 101, 169, 171, 177, 179, 181, 206, **214,** 310
    complications of *177*
    progression of *173*
    risk factors for **179**
    signs of 221
    site of **178**
Atherosclerotic plaque, accumulation of 89
Athletic training 259
Atrial and ventricular ectopic beats 108
Atrial arrhythmias 135, **135**
Atrial fibrillation 108, 113, 155, 256, 259, 260, 270, *272,* 278, **279,** *281,* **282, 283,** 301
    ablation 284
    clinical features of 280
    management of acute 282
    permanent 284

pre-excited 270
prevalence 278
types 278
Atrial flutter 155, 256, 269, *270*, 273
Atrial natriuretic peptide 62
Atrial septal defect 117
Atrial septation 24
Atrial stress 279
Atrial systole 42
Atrial tachycardia 259, 260, 270
Atrioventricular nodal re-entry tachycardia 96, 267
Atrioventricular node *12*
Atrioventricular reciprocating tachycardia 268
Atrioventricular re-entry tachycardia 96
Atrioventricular septation 24
Atrioventricular valves
 close 43
 open 44
Atypical angina 229
Augmented vector
 foot *130, 226, 251*
 left *130*
 right *130*
Auscultation 114, 122
Autonomic nervous system activity 51

B

Bachmann's bundle *12*
Bainbridge's reflex 47
Baroreceptor 58
 activation 48
Benzodiazepine 155
Beta-blockers 196, 242, 243, 259, 277, 283, 302, 319
 cardioselective 234
Beta-oxidation **75**
Bicuspid valve *115*
Bile acid sequestrants 150, 219
Bill's blood test results **207**
Bill's chest pain 206
Bisoprolol 156
Blood
 composition 64
 constituents **64**

flow 44
flow, non-laminar 177
lipid measurements, non-fasting 214
supply and drainage 9
test 125, 192, 207, 238, 298, **298**
urea nitrogen 207
volume, control of *61*
Blood pressure 28, *42*, 56, 57, 122, 188, *189*, 250, *272, 295*, 305, **305,** 310, 315
 checks, regular 318
 control of 58
  short-term mechanisms of *59*
 determinants of 57
 diastolic *57*, 186
 mean arterial *57*
 measurement of 190
  opportunistic 183
 monitoring, ambulatory 136, 184, 185, *189*, 190
 regulation, long-term *61*
 symmetry 123
 systolic *57*, 186
 targets
  for reducing **194**
  monitoring 198
 transmit *57*
Blood vessels
 flow through *56*
 walls of *14*
Body mass index 184, 194, 201, 233, 310
Brachiocephalic trunk *3*
Brachiocephalic vein
 left *3*
 right *3*
Bradyarrhythmia 258
 non-cardiac causes of 259
 symptomatic 263
Bradycardia 258, 262
 asymptomatic 263
 episodes of 260
 non-cardiac causes of **259**
 treatment for symptomatic 263
Brain
 natriuretic peptide 126
 regions, influence of higher 60

Breath, shortness of 270
Breathing pattern 103
Broad pulse pressure 123
Bronchus
    left main *3*
    right main *3*
Brugada's syndrome 100
Brush border lipase inhibitors 150
Bundle branch block 267, **275**
Bundle of His *12*, 13

C

Cachexia 296
Caffeine 101
Calcium 65, 201
    deranged 259
Calcium-channel
    antagonists 234
    blockers 33, 96, 156, 162, 196, *196*, 259
Calf tenderness 120
Capacitance vessels *17*
Capillary refill time 107
Capillary wedge pressure 145
Carboxylic acid **69**
Cardiac action potential *32*
Cardiac arrest 245
Cardiac axis 131, *132*
    deviation 132
Cardiac biomarkers 125, *126*, **126**
Cardiac catheterisation 143
Cardiac causes 102, 105
Cardiac conduction pathway 12
Cardiac cycle 28, 41, *42*
Cardiac disease **102**
Cardiac imaging 137
Cardiac ischaemia, acute 90
Cardiac magnetic resonance scan *143*
Cardiac muscle *28*
Cardiac nuclear medicine 142
Cardiac output 45, 54, *295*
    increasing 294
Cardiac pain 91
Cardiac pauses 265
    causes of 265
Cardiac preload 45

Cardiac rehabilitation 318, 319
Cardiac resynchronisation therapy 303
Cardiac rhythms, causes of **108**
Cardiac subtypes 126
Cardiac surface 5
Cardiac syncope 95
Cardiac tamponade 304
Cardiac tumours, benign 105
Cardiomegaly 298
Cardiomyocyte 28, *28*, 34
    contraction 36
    depolarisation 32
    ion channel, types of 31
    membrane *30*
    potassium channels 156
Cardiopulmonary exercise testing 137, **137**
Cardiopulmonary resuscitation 245, 246
Cardiovascular anatomy 2
Cardiovascular centre of medulla *40*
Cardiovascular disease 309, **314**
    prevention of 309
    risk factor for 101
Cardiovascular examination 103, **103**, 184, 206
Cardiovascular physiology 27
Cardiovascular risk
    assessment of 145, 309
    calculating 309
    factors 310
Cardiovascular surgery 164
    surgical scars of *114*
Cardiovascular symptoms 90
Cardiovascular system *1*
    development of 22
Cardioverter defibrillators 277
Carnitine shuttle 70
Carotid artery 18
    common *19*
    external 19
    internal 18, *19*
    left common *3*
    main branches of external 20
    right common *3*
Carotid bifurcation *19*
Carotid Doppler ultrasound 138
Carotid pulse 108, *112*

Carotid sinus 19, 20
Carvedilol 156
Catecholamines 201, *257*
Catheter *11*
    ablation 273
    access 143
Caudal segments 24
Cell membrane 36
Cerebrovascular accident 301
Cerebrovascular bleeding 318
Cerebrovascular disease 183
Chambers and valves 5
Characterising pain, SOCRATES
  mnemonic for **92**
Chemoreceptor 60
    stimulation 48
Chest 113
    discomfort 248
    leads 128
    radiography 137
    X-ray 238
Chest pain 90, 205, 227, 230
    aspect of 92
    causes of 90, **90, 224**
    differentiating **92**
    exertional central 237
    type of 229
Chlorthalidone 197
Cholesterol 77, 80, *84, 85*, 86, *87*, 222
    absorption 79
    bad 125
    biosynthesis of *78*
    effect on 149
    ester 80
    esterification 79
    good 127
    lowering medications **149**
    metabolism 28, 76
    raised total 192
    synthesis 77
        regulation of 79
    very high total 207
Cholesteryl ester *84, 85, 87*
    transfer protein *84, 85, 87*, 88
Chronic airways disease 99
Chronic fatigue syndrome 97
Chronic heart failure 289

Chronic kidney disease 199, 233, 301
Chronic obstructive pulmonary disease
  94, 286, 287
Chronotropic incompetence 259, 262
Chylomicron 80, 82, 83
Chylomicronaemia 208
    syndrome 214
Chylomicrons 83, *84, 85*, 87
Citrate shuttle 72
Clopidogrel 243
Clotting cascade *151*
Clubbing
    digital 105
    stages of 105
Coagulation cascade 66
Coagulation system, enzyme of 65
Coenzyme A 75
Cold right foot 169
Collapsing pulse 107
Common fibular nerve *121*
Compensation, signs of 296
Computed tomography 141
    coronary angiography 142
Condensing unit 73
Conducting tissue, circuit of 254
Conduction block 252
Conduction pathway 35
Conduction tissue 26
Conservative management 146
Constrictive pericarditis 113
Continuous positive airway pressure
  ventilation 307
Contractility 46
Corneal arcus 214
Coronary angiography 144, 241
Coronary artery 26, 165
    blood flow 89
    bypass grafting 114
        triple *165*
    calcium score 141
    disease 89, 223, 256
    haematoxylin and eosin staining
        of *174*
    lumen inhibiting blood flow 230
Coronary blood flow 52, *53*
Coronary catheter *10*
Coronary flow reserve 52

Coronary heart disease 10, 89, 146, 154, 155, 160, 163, 183, 205, 214, 217, 223, **229**, 230, 249, *257*, 279, 285, 286, 298, 301, 309
    arrhythmogenesis 254
    development of 228
    increase risk of 60, 315
    prevention 318
    risk 315
        factors, signs of 230
Coronary vessel
    blockage 228
    vasospasm 230
Cortisol 201
Cranial nerve 40
Cranial segments 24
C-reactive protein 310
Creatine kinase 126
Crepitations 119
Culprit vessel 227
Cushing's syndrome 200
Cutaneous tissues *17*
Cyanosis, peripheral 106, *107*
Cyanotic congenital heart disease 105
Cyclic guanosine monophosphate 50
Cyclo-oxygenase *153*

D

Dan's chest pain 223
Dapagliflozin 302
De novo
    failure, causes of 304
    vessel formation 22
Deep fibular nerve, medial branch of *121*
Deep vein thrombosis 94, 95, 98
Depression 303
Diabetes 229, 317
    control of 174
    mellitus
        type 1 310
        type 2 287, 310
    uncontrolled 317
Diabetic retinopathy 123
    stages of 124
Diet 148, 314
    and exercise 218
    unhealthy 314

Digoxin 282, 302
Dihydropyridine 162, 259
Diltiazem 33, 249
Direct current cardioversion 283
Disease progression stages 290
Disopyramide 273
Distal convoluted tubule 63
Diuretic 157, **158**
    amiloride 197
    type of 158
Door-to-balloon time 244
Doppler echocardiography 140
Dorsal aortae 27
Dorsalis pedis artery 120, *121*
Dronedarone 283
Drug 154, 160
    anti-anginal 162
    anti-arrhythmic 154
    anticoagulant *151*
    antihypertensive 159, 160, 196
    anti-platelet 153
    class 155
    diuretic *157*
    group 149, 154, 234
    history 100
    lipid-lowering 149, 150
Dysbetalipoproteinaemia 208
Dyslipidaemia 209
    management of 213
Dyspnoea 93, 214, 237, 297
    causes of 94
    symptoms of 95, 95

E

Early after-depolarisations 254
Echocardiography 138, *139*
    signs 135
Ectopic beats 252
Einthoven's triangle *130*
Ejection fraction 301
    preserved 292
Electrical activity 267
Electrocardiogram 237, *272*
    analysis of 131
Electrocardiography *42*, 127, 184, 185, 192, 231, 238, 298
    12-lead *128*

elements 133
    intervals of *131*
Electrochemistry 257
Electrolyte disturbance 262
Electrophysiological investigations 277
Electrophysiology 28, 276
Element 133, 134
Elevated cyclic adenosine
  monophosphate 257
Emergency treatment 264
Empagliflozin 302
Encephalopathy 202
End-diastolic volume *295*
Endocardial tubes 22
Endogenous lipoprotein pathway *85*
Endogenous pathway 84
Endothelial injury 174
Enzyme 73
Eplerenone 302
Essential hypertension 185, 187
  modifiable risk factors for 187
  non-modifiable risk factors for 187
  pharmacological treatment of *196*
Esterification 79
Estimated glomerular filtration rate 184, 185, 192, 201
Excessive caffeine consumption 101
Excessive vagal tone 262
Exercise 147, 218, 222, 302
  testing 136, 300
  tolerance test 136
Exogenous lipoprotein pathway *84*
Exogenous pathway 83
Extensor hallucis longus tendon *121*
Extensor retinaculum, inferior *121*
Extracardiac relation 5
Extracellular changes 257
Extracellular concentration 29
Ezetimibe 150

F

Familial hypercholesterolaemia 219, 317
  diagnosis of 222
Family medical history 100
Fatty acid 127
  co-linkage to coenzyme A 70
  metabolism 74
    regulation of 74
  oxidation 70
  synthase 71, 72, **75**
    complex, domains of **73**
  unsaturation of 74
Femoral artery 120
  and vein *121*
Femoral nerve *121*
Femoral tibial arteries *121*
Fetal heart circulation *25*
Fibrates 150, 219
Fibrillation 279
Fibroannular rings *12*
Fibrosis causes electrical conduction 258
Finger clubbing 105, *105*
Fish oil supplements 219
Flavin adenine dinucleotide 75
Flecainide 273, 283
Flexor digitorum longus *121*
Flexor hallucis longus *121*
Flexor retinaculum *121*
Fluid balance, monitoring of 307
Foam cell
  formation *176*
    and accumulation 175
  proliferate 175
Fondaparinux 242
Four cardiac surfaces, structures and
  borders of **5**
Frank-Starling
  curve *46*
  law 45, 47, *294*
Fredrickson classification **210**
Free fatty acids *84*, *85*, *87*
Free radical damage 174

G

Gallop rhythm 116
Gastro-oesophageal reflux disease 92
Gated ion channels 31
Gaucher disease 212
Gender 229
Global blood pressure control **59**
Glomerular filtration rate 200
Glomerulonephritis 202

Index

Glycated haemoglobin 216
Glycerol 71
    esters of 127
Glyceryl trinitrate 92, 163, 237
Glycoprotein 66
Glycosuria 230
Guanosine triphosphate 50

H

Haemodynamic 53, 173
    state 305
Haemoglobin, glycated 179
Haemorrhage
    cerebral 202
    intra-plaque 177
    small splinter *106*
    splinter 105
Haemostasis 28, 63
Hair, skin, eyes and mouth, signs of **111**
Hands 104
Head and neck 109
Heart *2*
    and great vessels, surface anatomy of *3*
    autonomic control of 27, 39
    beats 1
    block 135, 260
        complete 250, *251*, 252
        types of **260**
    catheterization
        left 144
        right 144
    conduction pathway *12*
    development of 22
    function 184
    inferior surface of *11*
    rhythm 246
    surgery 262
    transplantation 166, 303, 304
Heart disease 96
    atherosclerotic 89
Heart failure 94, 100, 163, 233, 285, 292, *294*, **298**, *299*
    acute 237, 304, 305
    biventricular 110
    cause of 291, 291, 292
    classification of progression of 291
    clinical features of 297
    functional classification of 290
    left-sided 297, 297
    pathophysiology of *293, 295*
    right-sided 110, 297, 297
    signs of *296*
    treatment of 276
    with preserved ejection fraction 289, 292-294, 301
Heart murmurs 117
    detection of 118
Heart rate 47, 107, 132, *295*
    causes of
        fast **108**
        slow **108**
    intrinsic 36
Heart sound *42*, 43, *112*, 114, **116**
    abnormal *118*
    normal *118*
    physiological basis of 43
    reflect 115
    third 297
Heart tube *23*
    looping, precision of 24
Heart valves *115*
    anatomy of *6*
Heaves 114
Heparin 68, 152
Hepatic apolipoprotein E and B-48 receptors 84
Hepatic disease 212
Hepatic triglyceride lipase *87*
Hepatitis 212
Heterozygous familial hypercholesterolaemia 220, 221
High-density lipoprotein 80, 82, 83, *84, 85, 87*, 127, 149, 185, 207, 217, 233
Holter electrocardiography monitoring 266
Home blood pressure monitoring 190
Homozygous familial hypercholesterolaemia 220, 221
Hormone 60, 61
    influencing blood pressure 61
Hydralazine 162

Hydroxy-3-methylglutaryl coenzyme A
  78, 86, 149
Hyperaldosteronism, primary 200
Hyperbilirubinaemia 288
Hypercholesterolaemia 149, 208, 229, 230
Hyperglycaemia 174
Hyperhomocystinaemia 174
Hyperkalaemia 262
Hyperlipidaemia 205, 208, **214**
  causes of secondary 211
  evidence of 206
  management, secondary 217
  type of 205, 208
    primary 218
Hyperlipoproteinaemia
  combined 208
  mixed 208
  primary 210
Hypertension 116, 135, 183, 186, *189*,
  301, 310, 315
  complications of 191
  control of 174
  end-organ damage in 192
  global burden of *188*
  investigations for secondary 201
  isolated stage 1 193
  management of *189*
  secondary 198
  self-monitoring and management
    of 316
  stages of 186, 193, 194
Hypertensive emergencies 202
Hypertensive retinopathy 123, *124*
  grading of signs of 125
Hypertriglyceridaemia 208
Hypertrophic cardiomyopathy 116
Hypoalbuminaemia 288
Hypothermia 259
Hypothyroidism 259, 262

I

Immune dysregulation 177
Implantable cardioverter defibrillators
  277, 301, 303
Infarct, site of 227
Infarcted pathology 178

Infective endocarditis 105
  signs of 105, *106*
Infiltrative disease 252
Inflammatory cell 173
Influences conduction velocity 254
Influenza 302
Inherited cardiac conditions **100**
Inherited dyslipidaemia 311
Inorganic phosphate *75*
Inotropes
  negative 47, 47
  positive 47, 47
Inotropism 39
Interim treatment 264
Intracellular cholesterol transport 85, *86*
Intracellular concentration 29
Intracranial pressure, increased 259
Ion channels, different gating
  mechanisms of **31**
Irreversible pulmonary arterial
  hypertension 304
Irritable bowel syndrome 97
Ischaemia 247, 257
  causes 257
  precipitate signs of 231
Ischaemic heart disease 89, 194, 223
Ischaemic pain 179
Ischaemic pathology 178
Ischaemic symptoms 238
Ivabradine 163

J

Janet's results **185**
Janeway lesion 106, *106*
Joint hypersensitivity syndrome 97
Jugular vein
  drains, internal 112
  left internal *3*
  right internal *3*
Jugular venous pressure 250
  raised 297
Jugular venous pulse 103, 109, *111,
  112*
  waveform 112
  waves of 113
Juxtaglomerular apparatus *161*

K

Kidneys, arteries and veins of *21*

L

Labetalol 156
Lecithin cholesterol acyl transferase 87, *87*
Left atrium 5, *7*, 116, *139*, *293*
Left bundle branch block 117, 238, 301
Left coronary artery 9, 10, *10*, *139*
    flow 52
    left-sided angiogram of *10*
Left subclavian
    artery *3*, *139*
    vein *3*
Left ventricle 6, *7*, 116, *139*, *143*, *293*
    3D echocardiogram of *141*
Left ventricular
    diastolic dysfunction 294
    ejection fraction 233, 301
    failure, back pressure from 290
    hypertrophy 116, 279
    restoration 303
    systolic dysfunction 116, 256
    thrombus 247
Left ventricular assist device
    in situ *303*
    insertion of 303
Lesion, treatment of 232
Levine's sign *91*
Lifestyle
    changes 181
    modification 218, 302
Limb leads 129
Lipase activity, regulation of *71*
Lipid 28, 316
    absorption 80
    functions 69
    levels 219
    metabolism 68
    profile 125, 211, 212
        fasting 319
        full 216
    rich 173
    transport, functions in 83
Lipid-lowering agent 319
Lipogenesis 71, 74
Lipolysis 69
    regulation of 70
Lipoprotein 80
    carrier 81, 82
    chemical composition of 80
    esterification 80
    intermediate-density 80, 82, *84*, *85*, *87*
    metabolism 83
    properties of 82
    structure *81*
Liver *143*
    disease 214
    function tests 216
Loop diuretics 157
Loop of Henle *157*
Low-density lipoprotein 80, 82, *85*, 86, 125, 149, *176*, 192, 207, 212, 217, 222, 233
    cholesterol, high levels of 316
    levels 207
    optimal 217
Lower limb 119
    pulses of *121*
Low-molecular weight heparins 153
Lung *143*
    disease, chronic 116
Lysosomal acid lipase 86

M

Macrophage calcification 177
Magnesium
    correction of 276
    deranged 259
Major vessels, structure and function of **15**
Malonyl
    coenzyme A synthesis 72
    transferase, formation of 72
Masseter muscle *19*
Massive pulmonary embolism 91
Mediterranean-style diet 181
Membrane
    depolarisation 48
    ion transport 41

Metabolic adaptation 51
Metallic heart valves 152
Metanephrines 201
Metformin 249
Metoprolol antagonise β1-adrenoreceptors 156
Mevalonate, formation of 77
Microsomal enzymes 74
Mineralocorticoid antagonists 302
    receptor 159
Minimally invasive repair 166
Mitral regurgitation 118, 291, 303
Mitral stenosis 116, 118
Mitral valve 5, *6, 7, 115, 139*
    prolapse 100
    repair 303
Mr Bayliss' electrocardiograph *226*
Mr. Goldman's electrocardiogram *251*
Mr. Marks' presenting features **286**
Multifocal atrial tachycardia 108
Murmur 118
Muscle receptors 60
Muscular arteries 16, *57*
Myocardial anaerobic respiration 230
Myocardial cell death 236
Myocardial contraction, mechanism of *38*
Myocardial infarction 126, 154, 163, 166, 225, 233, 236, 244, **255**, 256, 258, 262, 279, 301, 304
    complications of 244
    recurrent 247
Myocardial ischaemia 202, 228, 258
    acute 254
Myocardial metabolic 230
Myocardial necrosis 246
Myocardial perfusion *142*
Myocardial relaxation 40
    abnormality of 294
Myocardial repair and support 167, **167**
Myocardial sarcomeres *37*
Myocardial structures, rupture of 246
Myocardium 9
Myofibril 36
    contraction 36
Myogenic autoregulation *51*

Myogenic response 51
Myoglobin 126
Myosin light chain kinase 50
Myosin-head binding, cycles of 38

N

Nail abnormalities 103
National Institute for Health and Care Excellence Guidelines 214
Natriuretic peptides 126
Neck and face, arteries of *19*
Neovascularisation 177
Neurohormonal activation, chronic 318
Niacin 219
Nicorandil 163
Nicotinamide adenine dinucleotide 75
    phosphate 75, *78*
Nicotinic acid 151
Nitrates 162, 234
Nitric oxide 50, 234
    donor 163
Nodular lesions 205
Non-cardiogenic pulmonary oedema 296
Non-pacemaker cardiomyocyte *35*
Non-ST-elevation myocardial infarction 223, 235, 237, 242
Non-steroidal anti-inflammatory drugs 92, 200, 304
Non-sustained ventricular tachycardia, paroxysms of 244
Noradrenaline **41**
Norepinephrine **41**
N-terminal pro-brain natriuretic peptide 126
Nuclear medicine 140

O

Obesity 147, 315
Obstructive liver disease 212
Obstructive sleep apnoea 200, 259
Oedema 297
    non-pitting 99
    peripheral 297
    pitting 99
Omega-3 fatty acids 219

Optic disc oedema *124*
Organ system 191
Organomegaly 297
Orthodromic atrioventricular reciprocating tachycardia *269*
Orthopnoea 93, 287, 297
Orthostatic hypotension 250
Osler nodes 105
Outflow tract septation 25
Oxidation 75
Oxygen saturation *272*

P

Pacemaker 263, *264*
- action potentials of *35*
- hierarchy of 35, 36
- potentials 35
- site 36

Palmar erythema 106
Palmitate release unit 73
Palpation 114, 120, 122
Palpitations 94
- causes of 96
- duration of 96, *96*

Parasympathetic activation 59
Parasympathetic nervous system 40
- inhibition of *59*

Parathyroid hormone 201
Paroxysmal atrial fibrillation, management of 283
Paroxysmal nocturnal dyspnoea 93, 287, 297
Percutaneous coronary intervention 164, *164*
- and surgery 242-244

Pericardial rub 117
Pericarditis 92, 248
Pericardium 13
Peripheral arterial disease 171
Peripheral resistance 294
Peripheral vascular disease 154, 179, 183, 214, 217
Permanent pacemaker 96, *264*
- insertion, complications of 263

Peroxisome proliferator-activated receptor 149

Phenylalkylamine 155
Pheochromocytoma 199, 202
Phosphate 75
Physical activity 313
Physical inactivity 310
Pigtail catheter 144
Pill-in-the-pocket 284
Plaque
- cells die 178
- erosion 177
- rupture 175

Plasma volume *295*
Plateau 33
Platelet *66*
- activation 65
- aggregation 65

Pneumococcus 302
Pneumonia 92, 94
Pneumothorax 91, 263
Poiseuille's equation 54
Polycystic kidney disease 199
Popliteal tibial arteries *121*
Popliteal vein *121*
Posterior tibial
- arteries 120, *121*
- tendon *121*

Potassium 201
- channel blockers 234
- deficiency 276
- deranged 259
- sparing diuretics 159

Prasugrel 243
Precapillary sphincters 18
Primitive heart tube, segments of **23**
Proliferative diabetic retinopathy *124*
Propafenone 273, 283
Propranolol 156
Prostaglandin 74
- biosynthesis *76*

Protein 73
- C system 68

Pubic tubercle *121*
Pulmonary artery *143*, 145
- left 3, *112*
- main *112*
- right *112*

Pulmonary capillary wedge pressure 144, 145
Pulmonary disease 291
Pulmonary embolism 90, 92, 94
Pulmonary embolus 291
Pulmonary trunk *3*
Pulmonary valve *6*, 9, *115*
Pulse 120
- character 108, *109*
- irregularly irregular 280
- peripheral 104
- pressure *109*, 122
  - narrow 123
- rhythm 107
- volume 109

Pulseless electrical activity 246
Purkinje fibres *12*

Q
QRS duration 267

R
Radial pulse 107, 250
Radiation 91, 118
Rating pain 93
Reduction unit 73
Refractory hypertension 198
Regulatory troponin complex 38
Remnant particles 83
Renal artery stenosis 199, *199*
Renal dysfunction 311
Renal failure 304
Renal juxtaglomerular apparatus 62
Renal ultrasound 201
Renin–angiotensin–aldosterone
- cascade *63*
- system 62, 188, 294

Respiration 109
Respiratory rate 103
- and breathing pattern, signs of 110

Resting membrane potential 29
Reverse cholesterol transport 86
- lipoprotein pathway *87*

Rheumatoid arthritis 262
Rheumatoid conditions 262
Rhythm 108, 135
- disturbance 291

Right atrium 8, *112*, 113, 117, *139*
Right coronary
- artery 11, *11*, *53*, *165*
  - flow 52
- ostium *11*

Right ventricle 9, *112*, 113, *139*

S
Salicylic acid 154
Salt and health, consensus action on 316
Sarcoidosis 262
Sarcolemma 36
Sarcomere *37*
Sartorius *121*
Septum
- interatrial *139*
- interventricular *139*

Severe de novo heart failure **305**
Shock
- cardiogenic 170, 237
- septic 170

Simon Broome criteria **222**
Single-photon emission computed tomography 231
Sinoatrial node *12*
Sinus
- arrest 265
- arrhythmia 108
- bradycardia 259
- node
  - disease 259
  - dysfunction 259
- pauses 259
- rhythm 108, 112, *269*, 276
  - normal *266*
- tachycardia 259, 288

Six-minute walk test 136
Skin lesions 205
Smoking 229, 311
- cessation 147, 313

Sodium, deranged 259
Sodium-glucose cotransporter-2 301
- inhibitors 302

Index

Sotalol 156
Spironolactone 197, 302
Squalene epoxide, formation of 78
Stable angina 90, 227, 230
    management of 319
Staging heart failure disease progression 290
Statins 77, 150, 234, 242, 243, 317, 319
ST-elevation myocardial infarction 223, 235-237, 243
Stimulus 31
Stony dullness 119
Stress 318
    acute 318
    chronic 60
    echocardiography 140, 231
    testing 180
Stroke 280
    volume 45, *295*
Subclavian artery *19*
    right *3*
Subclavian vein, right *3*
Sudden cardiac death 100
Supraventricular tachycardia 96, 244, 270, 271, **271,** *272,* 275
    cause of 254
Surgical management 164
Sympathetic activation 59, 258
Sympathetic nervous system 39, *59,* 61, *295*
Syncope 250
    causes of 97
Systemic lupus erythematosus 212, 262

T

Tachyarrhythmias 266
    broad complex 267
    narrow complex 266, 267
Tachy-brady syndromes 260
Tachycardia 266, 273, 296, 297
    management of *272*
Tachycardiomyopathy 270
Tar-stained fingers 230
Temporal artery, superficial *19*
Thiazide 211
    diuretic 159
        long-acting 197

Thienopyridines 154
Thoracic artery, internal *19*
Three-dimensional echocardiography 140
Thrombin 65
Thromboembolic disease 20
    risk of 282
Thromboembolism 166
    risk of 284
Thrombolysis 67, 243
    mechanism of *68*
Thromboxane *66*
Thyrocervical trunk *19*
Thyroid
    artery, superior *19*
    cartilage *19*
    function tests 271
Thyroid-stimulating hormone 201, 207
    level 216
Tibial nerve *121*
Ticagrelor 243
Tilt table test 136
Tissue plasminogen activator *68*
Torsade de pointes 254, *274*
Total cholesterol 127, 222
Toxins 174
Trabeculated right atrial appendage 8
Trachea *3*
Trans fats 222
Transient partial repolarisation 33
Trans-oesophageal echocardiography 140
Transthoracic echocardiogram *7, 8*
Transthoracic echocardiography 138
Transvenous pacing 265
Transverse cervical artery *19*
Tricuspid regurgitation 113
Tricuspid stenosis 113
Tricuspid valve 6, 9, *112,* 113, *115, 139*
    base of *139*
Triglyceride 80, 82, *84, 85, 87,* 127, 149, 212, 233
    chronic raised blood concentration of 205
Triglyceridehydrolysis 70
Troponin 126
    concentration 237

Tunica
    externa 15
    intima 14
    media 15

U

Ulcers 120
Ultrasound 138
Underlying cause 291, 292
Unipolar leads 129
Unstable angina 223, 227, 235, 236, 242
Urea and electrolytes 125, 216, 271, 298
Urinalysis 192

V

Vagal manoeuvres 271
Vagal stimulation 271
Vagus nerves
    left 40
    right 40
Valve repair 166
Valvular dysfunction 291
    acute 304
Valvular heart disease 279
Vascular dysfunction 291
Vascular endothelial cells 175
Vascular inflammation 175
Vascular smooth muscle 48
Vascular tone 49
Vasculogenesis 22
Vasoactive chemicals 49
Vasoactive compounds, mechanisms of **49**
Vaughn–Williams classification **155**
Veins 18
Vena cava
    inferior *3, 21,* 55
    superior *3,* 55
Venous duplex ultrasound 138
Venous graft 165, **165**
Venous return 12
Ventricles contract 43

Ventricular diastole 44
Ventricular ectopic beats 244
Ventricular ejection 44
Ventricular fibrillation 246, 277, *278*
    survivors 278
Ventricular pressure increases 43
Ventricular rate 266
Ventricular relaxation 44
Ventricular septal defect 117, 246
Ventricular septation 24
Ventricular systole 43
Ventricular tachycardia 246, 254, 256, *272, 273, 275*
    complex *274*
    types *274*
Ventriculography 144
Venules 18
Verapamil 33
Very-low-density lipoprotein 80, 82, *84, 85, 87,* 212
Vessels, development of 26
Virtual electrocardiography leads **130**
Von Gierke disease 212
von Willebrand factor *66*

W

Waveforms *131*
Weight loss 218, 222
Wolff–Parkinson–White syndrome 268, *269,* 273

X

Xanthelasma 103, 119, *213,* 230
Xanthoma 206, 214
    around eyelids, small *119*
    intimal 175
    planum 213
    tendinosum 221, 222
    tuberosum 213
Xanthomata 104
    lipid deposits *119,* 205